D0882407

JUN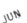

Listen to Your Body

A Gynecologist Answers Women's Most Intimate Questions

COMPLETELY REVISED AND UPDATED

Niels Lauersen, M.D., Ph.D.,
and Eileen Stukane

A Fireside Book
Published by Simon & Schuster
New York   London   Toronto   Sydney   Singapore

FIRESIDE
Rockefeller Center
1230 Avenue of the Americas
New York, NY 10020

FIRESIDE and colophon are registered trademarks
of Simon & Schuster, Inc.

Designed by William P. Ruoto

Manufactured in the United States of America

10   9   8   7   6   5   4   3   2   1

Library of Congress Cataloging-in-publication Data

Lauersen, Niels H.
    Listen to your body : a gynecologist answers women's most intimate
questions / Niels Lauersen and Eileen Stukane.—Completely rev. and updated.
        p. cm.
    Includes index.
    1. Gynecology—Popular works. I. Stukane, Eileen. II. Title.

RG121.L353 2000
618.1—dc21   00-058844

ISBN 0-684-85411-2

Acknowledgments

This new, updated *Listen to Your Body* owes its existence to our friends and patients. To each and every person involved in the realization of the first edition of *Listen to Your Body,* we extend our deepest gratitude.

The research material was gathered by Lori Leeds, Zoë Graves, Maryellen Kurkulos, and Kathleen H. Wilson, who also helped us refine the completed manuscript. Our appreciation goes to each of them.

The manuscript was transcribed and typed by Yvonne Brenner, who gave us insightful comments.

The original artwork was done by Lauren Purinton Rand, Pauline Thomas, Ellen Felten, Lynne Cooper, and Judith Lief. We also thank Tom Saltarelli, Joan L. Wacks, and Alexander Marshall for photographic work.

Special acknowledgment goes to our agents, Diana Price, Joyce Frommer, and Ellen Levine, for their acumen and enthusiasm.

We also extend our gratitude to our legal adviser, Richard Allen, for his interest and advice on this project.

Many others helped us in so many ways that we can do no more than list them by way of saying thank you: Ellen Black, Mary Parvin, Dana Dolan, Lynn Ramsey, Catherine Houck, Marlene Baragano, Patricia Honig, Adrian Rothenberg, Anne Jackson, Tom Ripa, Dr. Victor Reyniak, Dr. Howard Hochberg.

Questions asked directly by patients or written in letters from women who live in the United States and Canada have been used as the basis of our effort to arm women with information about their bodies. We deeply appreciate the questions and comments from these women. They have often suffered unnecessarily because they were unable to find the proper medical help, but perhaps their suffering has not been needless. It is hoped that their experiences, as portrayed in this book, will help other women to recognize their problems in order that they may obtain proper treatment.

We finally wish to extend our gratitude to Angela Miller, Jack Artenstein, and the staff of Simon & Schuster who helped us make *Listen to Your Body* a reality.

We also give our thanks to the staff at Berkley Books for keeping *Listen to Your Body* alive and available to our readers (in paperback for almost twenty years)—you made us a bestseller!

To our shining lights at Simon & Schuster, our editors: Betsy Radin Herman, who started us off; Patricia Dalton Medved, who moved us along; and Marcela Landres, who was there at the end with her contagious enthusiasm and bright intelligence. We also owe a debt of gratitude to assistant editor Anne Bartholomew who has added her sparkle to this new edition and heroically managed to keep us organized.

And finally, we thank our readers, who never let us forget that *Listen to Your Body* was their bible. Your interest guaranteed this update, and in the world of health care, we are always ready to be your guides.

Niels H. Lauersen, M.D., Ph.D.
Eileen Stukane
New York City
2000

To the improved health care of women throughout the world.

Contents

Editor's Note

In an effort to clarify the writing, when the authors refer to a woman's doctor, they use the male gender pronouns—*he, his, him*. The authors have given the book's hypothetical gynecologist a masculine identity to distinguish the doctor from the patient, who is always a woman and thus is referred to with female gender pronouns—*she, hers, her*. This doctor/patient gender identification must not be viewed as political or chauvinistic labeling; the distinction is made only to avoid confusion. The fact remains, however, that the overwhelming majority of OB/GYN specialists are men, a situation that, for the benefit of both patients and doctors, the authors hope will soon change. Many women are now entering OB/GYN training programs, and today a woman often has the opportunity to select a female or male doctor of her choice.

Preface

It is the year 2000, the beginning of our journey into the twenty-first century, an historic year in many ways—especially for *Listen to Your Body*. For the first time since its publication almost twenty years ago, *Listen to Your Body* has been updated. What you hold in your hands is a volume of answers to the health questions of today's twenty-first-century women.

The *Listen to Your Body* of 1982 emerged as a book of answers to the thousands of letters I had received after the publication of my first book, *It's Your Body*. Women were still in the early years of the health movement that would transform the doctor/patient relationship forever. The godlike figure of the doctor with the unquestioning patient before him would soon fade into memory. Health partnerships evolved as the best doctors focused on becoming more responsive to their patients' needs and questions, and self-empowered women became more assertive and inquisitive.

Listen to Your Body was on the front lines helping to forge those partnerships between women and their doctors. Many women have told me how this book reflected their own situations, and how they relied on the advice within its covers. Over and over, I have heard women refer to *Listen to Your Body* as their "bible." In the first edition I wanted to provide women with medical information and insights that were not easily available. For example, I explored the mind/body link in medicine, a connection that had few advocates back then, but today is taken for granted. In this new *Listen to Your Body* my goal is, again, to contribute to the empowerment of women in their health partnerships with their doctors by arming them with the latest medical findings.

This new *Listen to Your Body* provides a forum for recent letters from contemporary women. Since letter-writers openly revealed intimate details of their personal lives, the original correspondences have been altered to protect identities. In addition, initials and cities have been changed to prevent recognition of the writers. In this latest edition, I delve into issues such as the latest attitudes toward PMS, the current treatments for endometriosis, and the complexities of hormone replacement therapy. The new *Listen to Your Body* also offers an understanding of the range of sexually transmitted diseases women may be exposed to today, and it simplifies the world of infertility and assisted reproductive technology.

With this new twenty-first-century edition of *Listen to Your Body*, my co-author and I continue our commitment to taking the mystery out of medicine and improving the health partnerships of all women and their doctors. I also invite women who have questions and concerns to contact me personally. I will do my best to answer your questions, as I have responded to the women in this book.

Sincerely,
Niels H. Lauersen, M.D., Ph.D.
The New York Medical Center for Reproductive Medicine
784 Park Avenue
New York, NY 10021
212-744-4222
E-mail: NLauersen@aol.com
Web site: www.DrLauersen.com

1.

Becoming a Partner in Your Own Health Care

A DOCTOR IS NOT A GOD

The doctor's phone was ringing, patients were flowing in and out of the waiting room, and the doorbell was being pressed once more. It was an afternoon filled with activity, charged by movement everywhere but within the doctor's inner office. There the bustle evaporated into quiet. Sunlight warmed the mahogany desk where the doctor, sitting with his patient, leaned forward to hear her words.

She was an articulate woman with self-assured eyes and an easy smile. Ten years before, when she was in her twenties, she had undergone an operation that she later learned was unnecessary. After that, she haunted the local library and voraciously read books about her body. She wanted to know what questions to ask whenever she had a quirk or an ailment, and she shopped for a doctor who, during a visit, would set aside time to listen and talk to her.

This resourceful woman became the rarest and best type of patient. No longer did she view the doctor as a god. Now she saw him as a partner, an educated mortal who would help her stay healthy. Calmly, she asked her doctor/partner the things she wanted to know about herself. As she spoke, she glanced toward her lap and a sheet of paper with her handwritten questions. She had learned to be relaxed, to use this mahogany desk as a bridge toward more

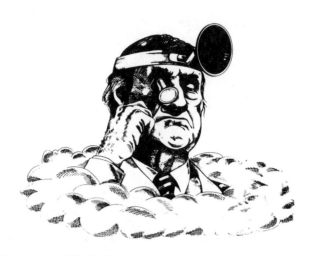

1-1   **"The Doctor Is Not God."** *Reproduced by permission from Marcia Stamer Dugan/*The Miami Herald.

information. And the doctor responded. His forward gesture diminished the distance between them and placed them in the throes of a new movement.

The beginning of a real partnership in health care is at hand. He is one of many competent doctors and leading physicians who are beginning to change, who are trying to talk to, and not at, their patients and listen to their complaints. She is among the growing number of women who are becoming extremely health conscious and well-informed, very sensitive to the signs from their bodies, and genuinely more expressive. The old doctor/patient relationship can be overthrown and replaced by the give-and-take understanding of people such as these who are committed to better health care for women. But the message must be allowed to spread through women's networks to every feeling person.

The thousands of letters I've received after my lectures and seminars on women's health care have shown me that when women dismissed what their intuitions told them about their own bodies and the treatments they were receiving, they were often left physically and mentally scarred. Discovering the despair that this lack of proper medical attention has caused has been heartbreaking. If women had been more informed about and more in tune with their bodies, many lives would have been free from anguish and changed for the good.

Until all doctors decide to descend from Olympus, women can receive the health care they deserve only by learning about the intricacies of their bodies, by beginning to trust their intuitions, and by becoming active partners in their own health care. When I heard Karen's story, a truly shocking event, I thought that no one incident could more clearly illustrate what happens when a partnership doesn't exist and a woman succumbs to fear, rejects her instinctive feelings, and becomes a victim of medical incompetency. If only she had listened to herself.

Karen's Story

Karen was half undressed. She had started to peel off her navy blue leotard when she glanced in the locker room mirror. Now, with the top of her leotard dangling around her waist, she stared at her familiar, naked breasts. Her nipples practically touched the glass as she leaned toward her reflection. She wasn't imagining the lump. There it sat, high on her left breast, parallel to her armpit and directly below her collarbone. She pressed it with the index and middle fingers of her right hand. It wasn't mushy, like some of the lumps she had felt before her period. It was hard, round, and small, like a medium-size cultured pearl.

Usually, after teaching two exercise classes, Karen's face flushed to a radiant crimson. Immobilized in front of the mirror, she watched that rosiness fade to the color of a blanched almond. *My God,* she thought, but before her nervousness over the lump could escalate, she was distracted by Emily's sliding grip on her leg. Karen bent down and collected the four-year-old into her arms.

Has it really been four years since I left the dance troupe? Karen wondered to herself. She had intended to return, but when Emily was born with Down's syndrome, Karen, who was only twenty-six at the

time, decided to stay home with the child. The experts had said that
Emily was educable, and Karen wanted to give her the time and
attention she needed for learning. Emily was so good-natured and
cuddly that Karen and her husband, Don, eventually nicknamed her
Precious. She captivated everyone, including the owners of the
health club where Karen had started to work. They even allowed
Karen to bring her to exercise and yoga classes. Karen considered
herself lucky. She kissed her daughter on the cheek and tickled her
behind the ear.

After she lowered Emily to the floor, Karen yanked a sweater over
her head and finished dressing. She tried not to think about the
lump. She would make an appointment with her gynecologist, ask
him to examine her. She pressed the lump again. She was sure she
had never felt anything like it before.

Karen is a pseudonym for a real, concerned woman. Since Emily was
born she has been especially careful about her health because she
feels particularly protective toward her daughter. If anything happens to her, Karen feels, Emily would suffer her loss severely.

The essence of her story, which I have momentarily interrupted,
is well known by women. Gynecologists have heard many patients
describe medical problems which they had thought were either
"nothing" or "trouble" at first. Then something happened. Women
listened to their bodies, but after they visited doctors, they listened
to their doctors and those early body signals were forgotten. The
medical checks-and-balances system tilted. Karen's destiny would
have been different had she held her locker room feelings, disturbing
though they were, in her mind.

Karen sat at the edge of the table, raised her arms over her head, and
watched her gynecologist frown as he felt the lump from every
angle. She was a young woman with no history of breast cancer in
her family, but she knew those facts wouldn't save her from the disease. She also knew that the nugget in her breast matched descrip-

tions of breast cancer symptoms that she had already read about in magazines. She wasn't surprised when her gynecologist sent her to a surgeon named Fielding for an opinion.

Dr. Fielding told her to take off her blouse and lie on the table. He could be positively sure that the lump was a benign cyst if he could aspirate it, draw out liquid from it with a syringe. Karen felt that she must have reached the outer limits of her courage if she could remain motionless on a table while a man injected a needle into her breast. Nothing happened. No liquid surged up through the needle. "It's cancer, isn't it," she said to Dr. Fielding, whose face, from her vantage point on the table, looked like a Mount Rushmore carving. "No, now don't jump to conclusions," he said. He appeared to have enormous girth, and his voice seemed to resonate with a commanding timbre. *Of course he's right. I'm jumping to conclusions,* she thought to herself.

"Well, we'll have to watch it, but I don't think you have anything to worry about," Dr. Fielding told Karen as she, now fully dressed, sat in his office. She watched him pull out a sketch of a breast from his desk drawer, pencil in a circle where her lump was located, and put the paper into her file folder. He asked her to come back in a year, and at that moment Karen decided to bury her sense of foreboding.

She continued to teach her classes. She was a former dancer and a health culturist who knew her body so well she could predict the arrival of her period practically down to the hour. She was aware of the lump's presence. *Still there? Yep, still there,* she would say to herself. Once in a while, when Emily grabbed her breast in play, she would shiver a little. Then she would remind herself of Dr. Fielding's words. Nothing to worry about. For Emily's sake, there should be nothing to worry about. When she and Don made love and he caressed her breast and felt the lump, she would joke about it. "I'm providing a new diversion," she'd tell him, but he wouldn't laugh. He wanted her to see another doctor.

Twelve months after her final visit, she returned to Dr. Fielding. This time he didn't aspirate the lump. He just felt it, said it hadn't grown, and told her he'd see her in another year. So Karen never paused in her activities. When she wasn't doing leg lifts or demonstrating yoga breathing, she was singing *Sesame Street* songs to Emily.

During the holidays, Karen feasted a bit too heartily and gained five pounds, but she amazed herself by dieting and losing more than she had anticipated. Ten pounds disappeared in four weeks. She hadn't been so slim since her dancing days. She felt lithe and sexy. One night she and Don made love in that indescribable way only two people who know each other very well can share. But afterward he looked troubled. With his head on the pillow and his gaze toward the ceiling he said, "There's another lump. Lower this time." Karen's right hand went to her left breast and she felt it. Her weight loss had made the second lump obvious.

Dr. Fielding reassured her that the second lump was probably nothing to worry about either, but he might as well take it out. He performed a biopsy on Karen in the office. While he was operating he kept saying that the lumps looked like nothing more than "little fibrocystic tumors." "I'm only sending this to the lab for procedure's sake," he mumbled.

When Karen returned to have her stitches removed, Dr. Fielding was as even-tempered as ever. The last suture out, he told her the incision had healed beautifully. Then he walked to the sink behind her to wash his hands. As she was midway through buttoning her blouse, she realized that Dr. Fielding was talking to her. She could hardly hear him over the sound of running water. And he was facing the wall to boot. He was telling the wall something about "bad cells." He was soaping his hands and garbling the word *masectomy*.

"*What?*" she cried out.

And finally he turned off the faucets, pivoted around, and repeated himself. "The lab found some bad cells. I'm afraid that we'll have to schedule you for an operation to remove the rest of them. You'll have to have a masectomy," he said, and walked into his adjoining office.

Karen lay back on the table and cried. He hadn't even said *cancer.* Didn't he think she knew what she had? For almost two years she had been walking around with a fatal disease. Letting it spread. She could have died. Maybe she would die right now. Who would watch over Emily? What would Don do? Why hadn't she taken care of this sooner? Seen another doctor? Why had she believed this Dr. Fielding? That day in the locker room she'd known it was bad. She'd known, but she'd let a cloud of fear cover her perceptions.

Karen underwent a modified masectomy, including the removal of two positive lymph nodes. If she had received the right treatment sooner, there might not have been any lymph node involvement at all. But these days, two years after chemotherapy and radiation treatments, she's still a star instructor at the health club, a loving mother, and she's becoming an optimist again. She says she won't feel really super, though, until she passes the five-year mark. (Then, her survival rate will officially change, because the odds are good that cancer won't return after five disease-free years.)

At the time of her relationship with Dr. Fielding, Karen had been fearful of her body's basic warning: a visible, touchable lump. She chose to transform Dr. Fielding's words into sacred scripture, when her instincts had told her that this lump was definitely something to worry about. Right from the start, she had intuited bad news.

Karen's success as a dancer and as an exercise instructor depended upon her body's fitness. And like a broker evaluating the Dow Jones Index, she could gauge the importance of every little and big change in her body. She recognized when she should slow down and when she should push herself harder. She really hadn't needed a doctor to tell her that the lump was an ominous sign; she had seen a portent of illness in the locker room mirror.

On her first visit to Dr. Fielding, however, this remarkably aware woman suspended her awareness. After the aspiration episode, she suppressed the throbbing knowledge in her brain and clung to the words of an incompetent physician—a man who knew less about her body than she did. She was understandably scared, but she allowed her fear to override her intelligence. In a moment that was crucial to her well-being, Karen relinquished her role as a partner in her own health care. She listened to and abided by one man's judgment. And by permitting Dr. Fielding to become a god of sorts, Karen set up that old-fashioned kind of doctor/patient relationship that continually blocks better health care. The meeting of a woman and her doctor should be a time for sharing.

Doctors aren't gods and women aren't really mystified by their bodies. Even the women who were relegated to menstrual huts once a month by horrified tribesmen, even they surely knew they were healthy. If Karen had relied on her instincts, she would have thought *I need a second opinion* when she heard Dr. Fielding tell her that she had nothing to worry about and that he didn't want to see her for a year. She would have sought the right kind of care and avoided two years of harboring dangerous cancer cells and unrelenting emotional strain.

Whenever Emily touched her breast, Karen had shivered not so much from pain as from fright. She was afraid that she would have to face what she knew was true. She didn't want her husband to talk about seeing another doctor. Yet if she had consulted a different physician, she might have stopped the disease at a less worrisome stage. Early on, another breast specialist could probably have performed a lumpectomy to remove the lump, and then a plastic surgeon could have corrected any disfigurement with reconstructive techniques. The cancer might have been halted without the need for a mastectomy and chemotherapy, and Karen might not be anxiously awaiting the fifth anniversary of her surgery.

It's tragic, but Karen suffered the all-too-common double misfortune of not heeding her body's messages and of encountering a man who didn't do his job. There were clear mistakes made by Dr. Fielding. Even if he thought the lump was benign, he should have explained fibrocystic breast disease to Karen and told her to monitor the lump at home. A fibrocystic breast lump would have been slightly painful to her touch, and after her next menstrual period it would have changed shape and become less sore. In fact, it might have diminished in size and completely disappeared due to the hormonal changes brought on by menstruation. If Karen had kept a close check on the lump and if it had remained the same after her period, had *not* become smaller, and if Dr. Fielding were acting responsibly, he would have asked her to come back to the office for another examination. He never should have allowed her to go for more than two months without reexamining her breasts. Dr. Fielding had already aspirated the mass and discovered the lack of fluid. The solidity of the lump should have caused thoughts of cancer to spring into his mind at the start.

As was particularly clear in Karen's case, many doctors cannot face cancer, so a woman has to be courageous enough to accept what her body is telling her. During the two years that Karen was under Dr. Fielding's care, he never discussed the possibility of cancer with her. A capable physician, feeling the hardness and the contour of Karen's lump, would have been highly suspicious. If a doctor cannot absolutely rule out the disease, and especially if he thinks cancer is likely, he sends a woman for a mammogram and a possible proper biopsy. Yet even when Karen's biopsy finally made cancer impossible to hide from any longer, Dr. Fielding still tried to avoid it. He turned his body away from hers, faced a wall, ran water into a sink, and mumbled her need for surgery into the air.

Now, it's possible that if Karen had visited the doctor with a companion who would have been her patient advocate, the facts might have come out sooner. An advocate can take a more objective position and ask questions a patient may forget. Dr. Fielding might have responded differently to an advocate than to his patient. So while a woman is learning to trust her body awareness and to become more assertive in the way she gets information from her doctor, she might ask her partner or a friend to come along when a health concern is at the forefront.

Every woman who confronts a Dr. Fielding who does not discuss her condition with her should find another doctor.

A WOMAN AND HER DOCTOR,
THE NEW PARTNERSHIP

Women can be their own health protectors without suffering
through life-threatening scares like the one Karen survived, but with
knowledge. It's time to remove the blinders from both sides of this
partnership. Women are no longer Victorian maidens and doctors
don't have to examine them under covers anymore. It isn't necessary
for gynecologists to be as remote as historian Carl N. Degler, author
of *At Odds*, tells us they were in the 1800s: "Most physicians,
throughout the nineteenth century, in order to avoid any charges of
impropriety, bent over backwards not to appear too familiar. As a
result, lights were dim during the examination, and the examination
and delivery were by touch only; if instruments were used they had
to be manipulated under covers! One male writer even pointed out
proudly in justification of modesty, that one of the greatest male
obstetricians had been blind!"[1] Dr. Fielding, with his impaired mental vision, acted like a man of the last century.

You probably won't find any blind obstetricians in delivery rooms
today, but you might run into a lack of communication between a
woman and her doctor, and that in itself is a kind of blindness that
leading physicians are trying to cure. The best doctors are now realizing that they can give women the most complete medical care only
if women are well-informed. A smart doctor won't automatically
prescribe the pill to a woman if she wants birth control; instead, he'll
explain all the different forms of contraception, and together they'll
decide what suits her needs. An informed woman will want to feel in
control of her body, will take time to listen to the latest findings, and
will become one half of a better health collaboration.

Of course, the idea of a woman's having a command of herself did
not evolve easily in America. When a woman talked about taking
"control of her body" in the nineteenth century, she meant that she
said no to her husband once in a while when he wanted sexual intimacy and she didn't. In older, European societies, women were
bolder sooner. They were more conscious of their sexual options, the

intricacies of their bodies, and their health. Openness between a woman and her doctor happened many years ago. In fact, not just women but men *and* women were encouraged to learn more about medicine from their European doctors. During the first half of the twentieth century, birth control champion Margaret Sanger let people know that sexual pleasure and procreation could be separated, and American men and women began to grasp their physical choices. The women's liberation movement, which began in the late sixties, spawned important books like *Our Bodies, Ourselves*[2] in the early seventies, and women began to understand their right to be heard. They also enjoyed a deeper comprehension of their bodies and their power. But equality in the doctor's office still hadn't happened.

LETTERS OF FEAR, FIGHT, AND FRUSTRATION

Although contemporary women have influenced the medical establishment and many physicians have been happy to regard their practices as doctor/patient partnerships, there's still a great dilemma at hand. A doctor must always ask himself, "What is the right treatment?" and a woman must seriously consider, "Am I getting the right treatment?" Like the creaking of a time-worn building, the question "What is right" is constant. For every woman the answer comes with an understanding—of her body and herself.

My hope was that the publication of my first book, *It's Your Body: A Woman's Guide to Gynecology*,[3] would foster that understanding and would arm women with enough information to find the most impeccable care for themselves. However, the thousands of letters I received as a consequence of that book have shown me that many women are full of questions no one has ever answered, and that the lack of proper medical care is frightening, much worse than I had ever imagined. Some of the letters describe medical ignorance and malpractice so severe they have altered the course of lives. I cannot help but be deeply touched by so many moving stories and searching questions.

> . . . *My doctor really neglected me. After the cesarean section that brought me my daughter, I was semiconscious in my hospital bed . . . pneumonia following the operation. For the first week my doctor never came to my room. I only saw him on the eighth day, when he took out my stitches from the cesarean. In ten days I left the hospital . . . I never had regular periods anymore and I began to hurt all the time. My doctor said nothing was wrong. After two years of pain I went to another doctor who said that the incision from my cesarean had not healed. My uterus and ovaries were infected . . . I was twenty-five years old and I had to have a hysterectomy. Now I can't ever have any more children . . . Why wouldn't a doctor notice that a patient hasn't healed? I know my husband would really like to have a son. Why, why, would a doctor do something like this?*
>
> —B.L., Phoenix, Arizona

> . . . *After five years of taking birth control pills, I became infertile. There were D & Cs, tests, hormonal medications, laparotomy and laparoscopy, and finally my doctor told me I had a tipped uterus. He repositioned it surgically, but according to my present doctor, this operation was not only unnecessary but the source of my continued infertility and abdominal pain. Due to poor postoperative procedures there is much scar tissue on my ovaries and surrounding areas. Intercourse always hurts. . . . What do I do? I'm thirty-three and this new doctor says I should undergo a hysterectomy at thirty-five if I do not become pregnant. He says that hysterectomy will be the only real end to my pain. I am confused and worried about my future and my life. . . . My husband and I are in the process of adopting a child, so pregnancy is not so important, but I am living in great distress.*
>
> —G.D., Columbus, Ohio

I am twenty-three years old and working toward my master's in business administration, but sometimes, during my ovulation and period, I am in so much pain I cannot study. The tears run from my eyes uncontrollably. . . . When my ordeal began two years ago I went to a gynecologist who told me that he didn't know what was going on, said it was all in my mind. I finally sought out a gynecologist here in Boston and he diagnosed endometriosis and put me on contraceptive pills and painkillers. Still, the pain during ovulation and menstruation is almost too sharp to bear. I sometimes find I'm clutching myself around the stomach in the middle of a class. . . . Now my doctor says that pregnancy might end the endometriosis, and perhaps I should consider having a baby. I have aimed my life toward a career and I am not even married. Isn't this suggestion extreme? If I have the child maybe I should ask the doctor to raise it!

—R.V., Boston, Massachusetts

I am an enlisted female soldier, and in all my eight years of service I have yet to find a good, efficient, reliable, military doctor. . . . So many females are ruined for life because of these quacks. . . . Several female soldiers have had miscarriages because they were given medication to start their periods when they had tubal pregnancies. The doctors had told them they weren't pregnant. . . . Instruments used during examinations have caused miscarriages. . . . Many women have had infections after operations because instruments have not been properly sterilized. . . . Either these doctors are not trained as efficiently as civilians or they just don't care.

—P.Y., Miami, Florida

I am thirty-three years old and I am suffering with endometriosis. I've never been able to conceive a child, though I have tried for years, especially after my doctor did major surgery and scraped everything out. That was six years ago. Three years ago he suggested a hysterectomy. I don't want to have surgery but I need to find some relief. I am in a lot of pain during ovulation and for one week with each period. Is there a drug that might help me? Is there anything that might help me?

—C.K., Little Rock, Arkansas

I am eighteen years old and just married. I have had herpes type I ever since I was a little girl. Nobody ever told me that it was a type of STD. I read about it in school and really freaked out. My doctor just tells me not to worry. Will I still be able to have a child? Is it contagious? Why won't someone give me a straight answer?

—S.T., Des Moines, Iowa

I'm twenty-one years old and I've been on painkillers for three years. I've had surgery six times, had a total of six bleeding cysts removed, had a tubal infection, and I still have scar tissue and adhesions on my tubes, ovaries, and large intestine. My doctor wants to remove my female organs because I am always in so much pain, and intercourse is almost unbearable. He's afraid I'm going to become addicted to the painkillers, too. I've had three or four opinions and they're all the same—my organs must go. Is there anything I can do? I have one child but I always thought I'd have more than one. Please help me.

—E.N., Albany, New York

I've been married almost two years and I'm twenty-four years old. Before I was married I only had sex with one man other than my husband, but that other man really got around. Now that I am a married woman you can imagine my embarrassment to have blisters around my vaginal area. My husband has never had sex with anybody else, and I think I may be giving him herpes. I think the blisters that come and go are herpes blisters, but my doctor can't give me a definite answer. What can I do? Did I get herpes before I got married? Why are they coming out now?

—A.H., Milwaukee, Wisconsin

The suffering of these women brings me sorrow, but the thoughtlessness of their doctors causes rage. There are never enough questions a woman can ask about her body, and she deserves a doctor who is willing to answer every query. By talking to, not at, each other, women and their doctors are involved in an ongoing movement toward better health care.

Women and men have the right to know the subtleties of their bodies. With these letters as my forum, personal questions, secret questions—and I hope, your questions—will be answered. And everyone's goal will be the same—excellent health through shared information.

2.

How to Find a Competent Physician You Can Trust

"Love all, trust a few. . . ."
—Shakespeare, *All's Well That Ends Well*

When you choose the person who will be your doctor you're entering into a health partnership. A woman and her doctor, when they really learn to trust one another, can share a lifetime of experiences from her first hesitant questions about contraception, through the births of her children if she has any, through every case of the willies, to the crest of her maturity. Trust will hold their partnership together as long as they're nourishing it with honesty and good communication. But as in any relationship where trust, which is always specially given, is not handled with care, there can be a change of heart.

A woman who loses confidence in her doctor loses trust in him, too, and repairing damaged trust is about as easy as building snow castles in spring. So whether a woman is looking for a doctor because she is young and just beginning to want gynecological care, or because she has moved to a new town and needs a checkup, it's just as likely that lost trust is sending her on a search. Sometimes there is no way to make a shattered partnership whole again, even though a woman might have trusted her doctor at first.

WHEN TRUST IS LOST

In one situation of lost trust, a woman I'll call Laura gave up the doctor who had helped her to become pregnant after four frustrating years of infertility. Everything was splendid until one night near the eighth month of her pregnancy when Laura's water broke at home. Her husband rushed her to the hospital.

Fearful that a premature son or daughter would die, the expectant father was drenched in perspiration and visibly trembling by the time Laura's doctor joined them in the labor room. They had waited two hours for him.

"Don't worry. Everything will be fine," the doctor assured them as he examined Laura. "The baby is in the correct position. Its heart rate is normal. You will have an easy and natural vaginal delivery," he announced. "Just relax and remember your Lamaze."

Laura breathed deeply.

The obstetrician patted her on the arm, looked at his watch, and excused himself.

Hours passed and Laura was still in labor. She wondered why the doctor hadn't come back to reassure her. She hadn't seen him since he had checked the time and left. Her husband was there, of course, but she couldn't shake the feeling of having been abandoned by the person who had cared for her for months, the person she had come to trust and depend upon for guidance and moral support. No one in the hospital seemed concerned about her or her baby, no one but an intern who stopped by on his rounds and perfunctorily examined her. She was delighted to see a medical man enter the room, but her pleasure changed to anxiety when she noticed his look of consternation.

"It's a breech . . . you know that, don't you?" he asked with an assuming nod.

"A breech? That's ridiculous," argued Laura. Her voice was quivering. "My doctor said everything was perfect. You must be making a mistake. Where is my doctor?" she pleaded in a close-to-hysterical cry.

"Yes, where is he? Please get the doctor," pressured Laura's husband, who had never fully calmed himself.

"Well, I don't know, but we'll have to find him, because this is definitely a breech," said the intern.

Laura's husband and the intern had the doctor paged—no response. They called his office—no response. Frantic, they left a desperate message on his service. "We're trying to find your doctor," the intern told Laura as he held her hand. Tears of despair were spilling onto her cheeks when the obstetrician finally arrived in his cashmere coat, white silk scarf, and black dinner jacket. He had left not only the premises but the neighborhood as well. While Laura's state of alarm had grown impossible for her to contain, he had been miles away, shaking hands at a friend's testimonial dinner.

Laura tried to figure out why he had gone so far from her. Even she knew that a premature birth could be very difficult and risky. She quickly questioned him, but he wasn't cooperating. Without any explanation, she was wheeled into the operating room for a cesarean section. Her world was in rapid motion. She didn't understand how circumstances could change so fast. Why hadn't her own doctor diagnosed the breech right away? Why couldn't she still give birth naturally? He was the same obstetrician who had told her months ago that even in the event of a breech, she would still be able to deliver vaginally. Yet near the moment of birth, the time that every pregnant woman imagines for months, he was hurrying her into surgery. Her doctor didn't acknowledge any of her attempts to get information. She felt ignored, shocked, and eventually, hurt.

Laura's new daughter was a well and happy baby after a few days of intensive care, but Laura herself never recovered emotionally. She felt permanently robbed of her rights as a mother. She and her husband had prepared themselves for natural childbirth and parent bonding, and she saw no reason why they hadn't been allowed to follow through. Even the day after the cesarean, her doctor had avoided any conversation about the breech. It wasn't surprising that before she left the hospital, Laura had decided to shop for another physician, someone who wouldn't break his promises and manipulate her. "I don't trust him anymore," she admitted to her husband.

Through friends, Laura found a new doctor who reviewed her records and told her and her husband how absolutely right her doctor had been in doing the cesarean. Statistics show that the powerful force of natural childbirth is sometimes too much for a premature breech baby to survive unharmed. There's a very high risk that this fragile newborn would have had brain damage if permitted to come into the world naturally. A premature breech has a much better chance of escaping damage if he or she arrives by cesarean section.

Laura's confidence in her doctor had diminished when he had misdiagnosed the breech, but she couldn't forgive him, strongly mistrusted him, for failing to explain the reason for the cesarean. He might have done the right thing for her baby, but he had made her feel pushed around and used. If he had been more sensitive and communicative, she probably would have remained a loyal patient, but he lost her. Laura looked for a different physician, as many women in her situation would have.

Working Out a Health Partnership

There is always a doctor with whom you can create a fresh partnership. However, sometimes a woman might not want an instant and permanent separation from her doctor, as Laura did. Another woman might feel that her doctor is basically competent, and even though he might have done something to antagonize her, she might decide to try to stay with him. Usually there is a point just before trust is completely destroyed, when, if a woman cares to, she can awaken her doctor to his shortcomings and strengthen their relationship.

One woman had believed in her doctor during his early days of practice, when he had spent a lot of time consulting with her and explaining everything that he was doing. She had trusted him and praised his manner and skill. After he had cured an infection in her tubes, she had wanted contraception and, like true equals, she and he, together, had decided on an IUD for her.

Years passed. One day she read that IUDs might damage a woman's tubes and she was anxious to talk to him. She was considering the possibility of becoming pregnant and she wanted his advice about her prospects Were her tubes all right? She arrived for her appointment, but now his practice was flourishing and she felt like a numbered part on an assembly line. She was whisked into a gown, into the examining room, into his office, and he barely gave her time to think about her questions.

If she hadn't known him very well she would probably have lost faith in him and looked for another doctor, but given the positive experiences she'd had with him in the past, she was reluctant to change doctors. She made an effort to bring back the communication they once had by doing something that many of us do not take the time to do: write a letter. In the letter, she told him that she knew he had a thriving practice now and she didn't mind if she had to wait to see him, but when they were face-to-face, she wasn't getting the care she deserved. She reminisced about the way he used to talk to her and supply so many facts about her health that she used to feel like she was the doctor by the end of their visits. She explained that his empathy wasn't the same anymore, maybe because he was overworked and frazzled. "Perhaps it's time to reduce your patient load?" she wrote. "You may notice that I used to send my friends to you, but I don't anymore."

Her doctor trusted her integrity and responded to the letter. She had exercised her half of their partnership. She had made her needs known, as every woman who cares about her health should. The doctor telephoned, apologized, and softened his approach with all his patients. Trust was reestablished and the "marriage" weathered the crisis.

It's often difficult to speak your feelings in person. You might love your doctor or be dismayed by him, but either way, you should, since you're his partner, tell him in a letter. The quiet art of writing letters—which tangibly place friendship and remembrance in one's hands—is all but gone. If your doctor has proved he is competent, it's not only fair, it's warm and gracious of you to be honest with him and show that you are concerned about your health care. Writing a letter to your doctor is more than appropriate—it's impressive.

Of course, if he has lost your trust, as Laura's doctor did, then you must not let your shared history prevent you from finding an easier partnership. With or without the mail, a doctor who loses his patients gets the message that he needs a new style.

Instinct will tell you if your doctor is taking your trust for granted and giving you less-than-thoughtful advice. Then you're faced with holding on or finding someone new. Each woman's body ultimately offers the final solutions. If the signs say "Go" and not "Stay," there are certain essential measures of a new doctor's know-how to look for and find. Without these qualities there can be no trust. Now, if you desire an obstetrician, ask your partner to join you in figuring out a doctor's competency quotient. A husband and wife should, together, pick the person who will help them have their son or daughter. That's really where the partnership that characterizes natural childbirth begins.

HOW TO JUDGE A DOCTOR'S COMPETENCE

The usual way a woman finds a new doctor is by asking her friends whom they recommend and gathering names. Everyone has special preferences. Some women are only interested in women doctors, some want doctors who are older and more fatherly, others like physicians who mingle with the jet set on weekends in Monte Carlo. A woman and her doctor must be emotionally compatible so that their communication is open and their partnership is solid, but the foundation of their relationship should be his ability to understand and treat her unique medical needs.

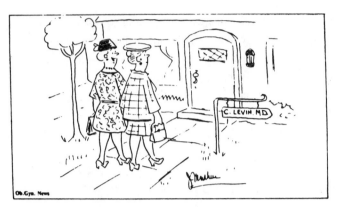

"*I've already diagnosed my ailment, but I
thought I'd get a doctor's opinion anyway.*"

2-1   *Reproduced by permission of the artist, Jeffrey J. Monahan, and* Ob. Gyn. News, *Rockville,
Maryland.*

A woman should always have choice on her side by evaluating the qualifications of several doctors before she narrows the field to one. She can make a list of candidates by talking to women who have similar lifestyles. A twenty-seven-year-old single working woman might ask other women who are young, single, and professional whom they consult for their health problems. A married woman with three children is likely to have a doctor more in tune with the concerns of married women. By confiding in women who are like you, you're in a much better position to find a doctor on your wavelength.

If you've just moved to a new community, call the doctor you've left behind and ask him to suggest the outstanding physicians in the area. Co-workers and neighbors will probably be happy to tell you whom they've discovered, and after you've exhausted your personal contacts, the state or county medical society can provide you with the names of local gynecologists and obstetricians. If you're interested in putting yourself in the care of a woman doctor specifically, the American Medical Women's Association in your area can give you their references. Women's health collectives have sprung up in many areas of the country, and your local chapter of the National Organization for Women (NOW) should be able to give you the phone number of any collective you would like to locate. A women's health group will have names of women doctors readily available.

Once you have your list of physicians, it's time to be a detective. The *Directory of Medical Specialists,* which you can find in the reference section of your local library, at a medical library, at most county medical societies, or in many doctors' offices, gives a physician's birth date, specialty, the medical school where he was educated, the hospital where he was trained, membership in professional organizations, and current hospital affiliation. The best hospitals are connected to universities, associated with medical schools, or part of large medical centers. So it's important to note where a doctor trained and where he works today.

If a doctor completed his residency at a highly reputed hospital complex and he's still working at such a center, he is probably one of the best in his field. Good hospitals have good doctors, because the members of a hospital community keep tabs on one another. The interns and residents are always judging the staff doctors and vice versa, so a staff doctor is actually working in front of an audience. In fact, nurses and interns often know who the best doctors are, and they are always willing to tell you. When you find out the hospital affiliation of a doctor in whom you're interested, you might try to get in touch with a nurse or an intern at the hospital. Then you'll have inside information on the doctor's competence. But it isn't likely that a doctor will be at a well-known hospital unless he is quite able. These centers are wrapped in red tape—there are ethical committees, supervisory boards, review boards, all kinds of overseers—to scrutinize and screen doctors constantly.

Does Board Certification Really Matter?

At smaller, less-restrictive hospitals, doctors are sometimes not as up-to-date in their fields and it's possible that not all of them are board-certified. The *Directory of Medical Specialists* tells you whether a doctor is certified by the American Board of Obstetrics and Gynecology. A board-certified doctor—today about 30 percent are women, and their ranks are growing—has completed three to five years of residency, has passed a required number of board examinations, and holds the official title of "diplomate" of the American Board of Obstetrics and Gynecology.

There are many doctors who call themselves gynecologists without being board-certified diplomates. They might be physicians of good judgment, but they are practicing outside the guidelines of the board and they are not bound to live up to its standards. Also, an uncertified doctor is not receiving the board's regular mailings, which provide news of current breakthroughs in obstetrical and gynecological research and treatments. He might be ignorant of the latest developments in his field.

When a doctor is not certified by the board, he doesn't risk being expelled from it and having his career ruined. Certified doctors, however, rather proudly carry out their duties within the rules and regulations of the board. Board-certified doctors are known to provide quality medical care at respected institutions.

A Doctor Is Only As Good As His Hospital

The hospital where a doctor has received an appointment is important not only because it's a measure of his professional competence, but also because it's the place where you will be treated. A doctor who operates out of a small, architect's dream of a hospital with a kitchen supervised by a Cordon Bleu chef and rooms shaded by damask drapes might not be able to perform the latest tests. This type of hospital doesn't usually have any modern facilities—except, maybe, in the kitchen.

Large medical centers are not pretty places with delectable cuisines, but they generally have the best equipment for the most advanced treatments. If you're planning to have a baby, you'll want to know that your obstetrician works at a hospital with an intensive care nursery for premature deliveries. If you think surgery is in store for you, you'll surely feel safer knowing that the hospital in which you'll be operated on has a skillful staff of anesthesiologists. Death or the quality of your future life can depend upon the technology available. If a woman knows a competent, caring doctor with access to the latest scientific equipment, even if he's miles away, she should make every effort to consult with him. What seems like a hassle at first might turn out to be the least complicated course.

When a woman's health is at stake, miles should not matter. For example, having a first child at over thirty-five is a high-risk situation, and it's worth covering a little distance to find a perinatologist, an obstetrician who specializes in high-risk pregnancy, to care for you and your baby in well-equipped surroundings. For infertility, an emotional condition as well as a physical problem, a woman needs the insights of a doctor who has unshakable knowledge about all the modern tests and evaluations. (It's significant to realize that there are only a few experts at large medical centers who are completely familiar with infertility. Many, many gynecologists have been known to bill themselves as experts though they have actually impeded conceptions.) If there is some question of cancer, it's absolutely a must to seek a cancer specialist associated with either a large cancer hospital or a hospital that's part of a cancer research center for a first or second opinion. (For the leading cancer care center nearest you, call 1-800-4CANCER, the National Cancer Institute's cancer information line. All information at the NCI, including new treatments and clinical trials, is accessible through this number.)

Travel should not deter a woman who wants better health and/or a baby. The best doctors are at the best hospitals. Remember, though, they might not be next door to your home.

Do the Best Doctors Charge More?

Sometimes a doctor's fees are based on his high-overhead office. Don't be dazzled by his prices. You should be paying your physician for his competence, not his fancy address. It's quite appropriate to call his office to inquire about the fee for a visit before you decide to make an appointment.

If strawberries from the same harvest are selling for a dollar a quart at the supermarket and three dollars a quart at the gourmet shop, where are you going to make your purchase? The "comparative" principle is the same in shopping for doctors. After you learn qualifications, affiliations, and get some idea of a doctor's competence from his patients and hospital sources, you should have a sense of his abilities. Background and know-how being equal, choose a doctor who is charging you for his skill, not for his collection of French impressionist paintings.

If you visit a second-opinion doctor and he says you need surgery, get an estimate of the cost from several qualified surgeons, and call your insurance company to find out what will be covered. When it comes to your health, money, naturally, should not be an object, but remember that the fees might vary from one competent physician to another as much as the prices at Sears and Tiffany's.

WHY IS IT SO DIFFICULT TO FIND A HIGH-CALIBER DOCTOR?

When two people get together, the relationship that develops is not always an easy one, and the doctor/patient partnership is no exception. Many women have left doctors' offices, never to return, and they don't want to experience similar physicians again. Had some women heeded their own mind-and-body signals immediately they would have admitted that trust had disappeared and switched doctors sooner than they did.

Sometimes the relationship could have been a bit better if a husband or lover had shared in a woman's quest for better care; after all, her birth control or pregnancy changes his lifestyle, too. When a woman's mate decides to become involved in her relationship with her doctor, the three-way communication—mate, woman, and doctor—can frequently alter the partnership for the benefit of all. But as positive as it would be for a woman's loved one to join in her pursuit of a doctor, for the most part women still do the job alone. Therefore, it's important to know that improved health care begins with you and your knowledge of your rights.

The letters I've received have focused for me the dilemma that women throughout the world are facing. They're looking for doctors they can consider their own for their lifetimes. But they're mystified by the strange situations and wrongheaded information they encounter in their searches.

I have included some of these letters here so that perhaps your hunt for a high-caliber doctor will be easier. As these real-life episodes illustrate, the perfect doctor/patient partnership won't exist until women are able to feel confident in their right to be inquisitive consumers of medical services. I hope these stories, with their personal probing questions, and the answers that follow will bolster the confidence that every woman needs.

What Do You Do When You Have to Leave the Doctor You Love?

Shortly after I moved to a new town I became pregnant for the fifth time. My neighbors told me that the local doctor was good so I went to him. I hated him. Everything inside me told me to leave him, but my husband just said I was spoiled because I had adored the doctor where we used to live. I told myself that he was probably right and I tried to adjust to this new guy, but the pregnancy was different from all my others.

I couldn't hold my water and I had to keep several changes of underwear at work. The doctor never checked anything, he just said it was normal for me not to be able to control my bladder. My blood pressure skyrocketed and I began to retain fluid, but no matter how much I begged he wouldn't give me water pills. I knew something was wrong with the child I was carrying. It didn't kick and move the way the others had, and I told the doctor. He had a lot of trouble finding a heartbeat, but he told me everything was fine.

Two days after my appointment with the doctor, I gave birth to a dehydrated, dead baby boy.

I am finally getting over the depression I suffered after the stillbirth. I now travel back to my original doctor for care, because, needless to say, I am afraid to trust anyone in the medical profession but this one doctor I have known for years.

—B.E., (name of town withheld)

This is a horror story, clearly an example of how a doctor should not be. He didn't pay attention to anything she was saying, and he failed to treat her with modern medication. Her instincts were immediately correct. Her husband disagreed with her judgment and stopped her from finding another physician, but apparently he never went to the doctor's office with her.

I strongly advise that, at least a few times during the pregnancy, a husband should visit the obstetrician with his wife. A father-to-be is a member of a natural childbirth partnership and he should keep himself informed all along the nine-month way. What kind of delivery does the obstetrician foresee? How long will his wife be able to work? Does he like the obstetrician's attitude? When a husband participates, he can judge the doctor with firsthand information, and his wife won't be alone in her ruminations. And when it comes time to hear the baby's heartbeat, a husband and wife can listen to it together. Of course, this doctor didn't even let the woman hear the heartbeat by herself.

Many women change obstetricians during the course of their pregnancies. There are so few times a woman is pregnant in her life; she owes it to herself to find someone in whom she has confidence, a doctor who is backed up by a reputable hospital with all the latest equipment. Even if she has to travel to find a terrific obstetrician, she should.

Now, this woman, considering her high blood pressure, might have done better with a perinatologist, a doctor who specializes in high-risk pregnancies. She should have been told to stop work and she might have been advised to enter the hospital for tests supervised by a specialist in cardiovascular diseases. She didn't even know that she was running the risk of early labor, and a small hospital might not have had the facilities for monitoring her circulatory condition or taking care of her premature baby.

Since she trusted her former doctor, she should have asked him to recommend a physician in her new neighborhood when she began to have doubts about her doctor's judgments. She also could have called the nearest medical center, asked for the head of the obstetrical department, and requested recommendations from his office. Once she received the names of a few physicians, she could have done her detective work, as described earlier in the chapter, to determine the doctor with the greatest competency.

What Happens When a Doctor Becomes Outraged?

I live in a town of under 10,000 people and everyone uses the same doctor, a man whose word is trusted in the community. I've known him for years and I have always gone to him for my yearly checkups. I'm forty-five and the last time he examined me he said I had fibroid tumors and I should have them removed surgically. I've read enough to know that fibroid tumors might disappear after menopause and I mentioned that to my doctor. I have no discomfort or pain, so I thought I'd rather not have surgery and see if, in time, the tumors go away. My doctor became very angry with me; he even raised his voice and told me that if I didn't trust him I should go find another doctor. I decided that was just what I would do.

Since he is the only gynecologist in town, I traveled to another community and sought a second opinion. The second doctor agreed that we should wait and observe the fibroids. I'm very happy with him and I've decided to make him my doctor. But my first doctor is still mad. This is a small town and everybody knows everybody. We all go to the same church, have children in the same school, and talk gets around. He has started to make insulting comments about me

*and my family, to tell false, unflattering stories about us, and I'm
afraid people are starting to wonder what the facts really are. I've
felt so uneasy lately that I've tried to talk my husband into moving.*
                                    —L.V., (name of town withheld)

Here a doctor's personal pride has come into account. He has
always been viewed as the god in town. No one challenged him. No
one competed with him. It's important in small towns, where
women have few choices, that they band together to share information and form active community groups. A strong women's organization might be able to work with a nearby hospital administration
to attract a new physician to the area. There should always be selection for you and competition for doctors.

This woman was definitely right to seek a second opinion. The
worst thing a person can do is to submit to treatment that time
proves totally unnecessary and deeply upsetting. Thank goodness
she didn't think that an additional doctor's visit and travel were too
much of a rigmarole. It's always extremely important to avoid
unneeded surgery, no matter how inconvenient a trip to a faraway
doctor might be.

I hope this woman has friends to whom she can impart her story.
I'm sure she is a respectable citizen in the town and she should voice
her opinions about the local doctor. Maybe she'll find that others
agree with her. As people begin to recognize her predicament, perhaps the doctor will be the one who thinks about moving.

Can a Woman Switch Obstetricians in the Middle of Her Pregnancy?

*I was in my fifth month when I found out my mother had breast
cancer and had to have a mastectomy. I became worried and
nervous and totally preoccupied with her operation and recovery.
In the middle of everything I went for my regular doctor's visit
and my obstetrician suddenly couldn't find the baby's heartbeat.
He said that my uterus was smaller than it should be and perhaps*

the baby had died. He told me to return in two weeks for more testing.

The stress in my life was so severe I didn't know what to do. Someone at my husband's office gave us the name of the doctor who had delivered his son and in a panic I made an appointment with the new doctor. He used an ultrasound technique to show me that the baby was fine and I remained with him until the birth of my healthy little girl.

I just want to say that I don't think I would have worried about my original doctor if he had not been so offhanded about my baby's life. I wouldn't have thought it a good idea to change obstetricians during a pregnancy, but I'm very glad I did.

       —N.K., Scranton, Pennsylvania

This woman could have continued to trust her doctor if he had only explained the newer methods for determining whether or not a baby is alive. She didn't have to wait two or three weeks to find out. Amniocentesis or ultrasonography could have told her almost immediately.

Amniocentesis is the withdrawal and analysis of a sample of the amniotic fluid around the fetus. Ultrasonography is a high-frequency acoustical way of getting X ray–type pictures of what's going on inside the uterus with no harmful effects on a mother or her child. High-frequency sound is projected into the body and the sound waves return, like an echo in the Grand Canyon, to produce a reflection of the fetus on a television-like screen. A woman can glance at the screen and see the fetus moving, just like on live TV.

If for some reason the baby had been dead, this woman would not have had to carry it to term. A doctor can induce early labor with a new type of prostaglandin suppository. So the emotional stress of living with a lifeless unborn can be removed right away. There was no reason for the doctor to send her home to suffer—unless, of course, he *wanted* her to switch obstetricians.

Whenever a pregnant woman starts to mistrust her obstetrician, she should reflect on her feelings and discuss them with her family.

Does she want to see another doctor? If she honestly feels she does, she must not hesitate.

"You're Just Nervous, Honey"

In the past few years I've been to three doctors and they've all told me the same thing. I have unusually high blood pressure. However, one at a time they dismissed this finding. The first doctor put his hand on my shoulder and said, "You're just nervous, honey." The two other doctors told me, "Learn to take life a little easier."

Meanwhile, I also suffer from menstrual cramps and these doctors suggested that I take birth control pills to alleviate the pain. Since I had read the pros and cons of the pill I decided against it.

I made an appointment with a fourth doctor, and finally I think I have found someone who stands out from the crowd. He said that even compensating for the fact that I might be nervous in a doctor's office, my blood pressure was very high. He gave me an EKG which showed no abnormalities, but he emphasized the importance of blood pressure pills. I began taking them and now my pressure is normal.

This doctor told me that if I had taken the birth control pills, with my high blood pressure, I "wouldn't be here today." I'm so happy I trusted myself instead of those thoughtless doctors.

—F.M., Point Pleasant, New Jersey

This very alert and informed woman was saved by her own intuition and because she was listening to her body. Her experiences show the importance of reading as much as you can and feeling, inside, what's right for you.

Today, many women consult only one doctor, a gynecologist, for all their problems. A gynecologist has become a primary physician to such a great extent that medical students are being encouraged to learn more general medicine when they're training in gynecology. That doesn't mean that a gynecologist should treat heart problems, but he should check your blood pressure on every visit and send you to a cardiovascular specialist if there are any signs of trouble.

A woman should get full value from every meeting with her doctor. If he forgets to take your blood pressure, remind him. Ask him what it is and write it down so you can make a comparison the next time.

It's indisputable malpractice to put someone with high blood pressure on birth control pills. If this courageous woman hadn't listened to herself, as her current doctor told her, she might have been dead. Fortunately, today she's a living example for everyone to follow.

Hold On to Your Organs

I am fifty, well into menopause, and on my fifth doctor in fifteen years. I don't take hormones, am a firm believer in vitamins, and I've held on to my organs, but it has been a fight. Every doctor wants me to part with all or part of my reproductive system. They say that if my organs are removed I won't have to worry about them becoming a source of cancer. This seems like outright malpractice. The doctors might as well have suggested that I cut off my finger so I won't break a nail.

My latest Pap test was fine as usual. I don't know why these doctors think that just because a woman has reached menopause she wants to lose part of her body! I feel great.

         —D.W., Chicago, Illinois

For years, this woman has been trying to find a doctor she can trust. One certainly has to doubt the need for surgery since it's now fifteen years since the first suggestion was made and she's still fine. Judging from the letter, there appears to be no pathology and only her intuition saved her from a knife-happy surgeon.

Many doctors like to suggest that women who reach menopause have hysterectomies just to avoid the possibility of getting cancer in the uterus and ovaries. There's absolutely no reason for this surgery. Yes, doctors should do everything possible to reduce the risk of cancer, but no organs should be considered optional. We don't remove lungs to eliminate lung cancer, so it should follow that we don't take out a woman's uterus to prevent uterine cancer.

Fortunately, when it comes to cancer of the uterus, there are ways to detect the disease at an early stage. The Pap smear for cervical cancer, abnormal bleeding after change of life for uterine cancer—both offer warnings. There are few sure methods to determine the presence of ovarian cancer, but we do know that almost 7,500 healthy ovaries would have to be removed in order to prevent one death! With this ratio, ovarian surgery should hardly be encouraged. In the overall view, only 3.8 of the 14,500 yearly deaths from ovarian cancer would be prevented, but how many physical and emotional problems would the removed ovaries cause? There are no figures to answer that question.

Ms. W.'s story shows that women must keep searching for several opinions until they find someone they can trust. Hopefully, this fifth doctor will be the one to make the difference for her. If women never stop being active partners in their own health care, always take on positive attitudes, and keep themselves fit with exercise, diet, and vitamins, the level of unnecessary surgery could be greatly reduced.

IT'S NOT ALL BAD

So far I've presented letters from women who have had difficulties finding physicians they can trust. Their plights are real, but there are good doctors out there for them. Many excellent physicians are treating women who write letters of appreciation and notes of praise, thanks, and love.

Recently a woman wrote these touching words to the doctor who had performed her myomectomy, an operation to remove her fibroid tumors:

> *The experience of being operated on and of slowly recovering has taught me my body's limits as well as its strengths. There is no memory that I need to suppress or push aside.*

I'm not sure which contributed more to my feelings of comfort and security: my complete confidence in your knowledge and skill, or my pleasure in your cheerful, reassuring manner. I shall never forget how I felt as I was wheeled into the operating room—as if I were surrounded by people who cared about me and knew exactly what they were doing. I could face this trial with utter serenity. And I can't tell you how nice it was to know that after a day of pain and discouragement, your smiling face would appear in my room—weekends and all—to comfort and cheer me.

Finally, it was obvious even to an amateur like me that both your abilities and your niceness had earned you the respect of the people most qualified to judge—the nurses and doctors you work with.

"For where there is love of man, there is also love of the art. For some patients, though conscious that their condition is perilous, recover their health simply through their contentment with the goodness of the physician."

—HIPPOCRATES

When Should a Woman Look for Her First Gynecologist?

I am only fifteen years old. I have never had a pelvic examination but I have always wondered what the doctor does. I have never taken my clothes off in front of a man before. I don't know if I could do it, even for a doctor. I don't like it in gym when I have to undress with my classmates.

The problem is my mother. She wants me to see a doctor for a vaginal examination. She says that since I've had my period for three years, it's time. Is she right? I've never had any problems and I've never had sexual intercourse.

I don't think I could live through it. I embarrass easily and I would die if a doctor saw me naked.

—S.R., Corpus Christi, Texas

With today's good nutrition, it's not uncommon for a woman to reach menarche (the onset of menstruation) at age ten. Girls find themselves living with monthly cramps and worrying about contraception before they've even started to wear panty hose.

When a woman's periods become regular—one or two years after her first signs of spotting—it might be time for her first gynecological checkup. A young woman might have monthly pain, heavy bleeding, or frequent bleeding. There might be any number of unforeseen conditions that could easily be treated with a visit to a gynecologist. A young woman might want to talk first with her mother or a favorite teacher about what she is going through, but a doctor is probably going to be the best person to help her.

Of course, a menstrual problem is not the only reason a young woman might want to embark on her first visit to a gynecologist. The high rate of teenage pregnancies shows that today's young women are making decisions about sexual relations very soon after their menstrual cycles begin. If a teenage girl is thinking about having sex with her boyfriend, her thoughts alone should send her to a gynecologist. She should try to talk to a doctor about birth control and the consequences of intimacy before she becomes physically involved. No young woman should become her boyfriend's lover if she feels he is pushing her into sex before she's ready. But if you're a sensible woman who has established a deep friendship with one young man who you feel is special and important, a doctor's visit might be the wisest move you could make.

A mother who suggests that her daughter visit a doctor during her mid-teens, while she is still a virgin, is understandably concerned and protective. With so many teenagers becoming pregnant, being exposed to sexually transmitted diseases (discussed in greater detail in *You're in Charge: A Teenage Girl's Guide to Sex and Her Body*, by Niels H. Lauersen M.D., Ph.D., and Eileen Stukane, a Fawcett/Columbine book), she wants her daughter to have the proper counseling and an early examination as part of her health education. Armed with information, a young woman will be able to avoid an unwanted pregnancy and plan an unburdened life.

Mother's Gynecologist?

If a young woman has a close, give-and-take relationship with her mother, she might be happy to go to her mother's gynecologist. Some young women might be embarrassed to tell their mothers that they're thinking about sex, and they would rather visit a Planned Parenthood office or a high school—or college—clinic, where they can find or be referred to doctors. Certain teenage girls might request women doctors.

The doctor a girl visits for the first time should not reveal any of her secrets. Even if he is her mother's doctor, he should be ethical. He should not break the understood vow of silence the two of them share. If you don't trust him, don't go to him. Your doctor must be compatible, understanding, and responsive to your needs.

Your mother should not be in the examining or consultation rooms if you don't want her there. However, if you're nervous and want your mother in the examining room, the doctor should permit her presence. Afterward, she should not be included in your private consultation unless you'll feel more comfortable with her sitting in the chair next to you.

What to Expect During an Examination

A woman's first gynecological experience can be an excellent introduction to a lifetime of learning about, and understanding, her reproductive health. If a doctor does not follow the procedure as it's described below, you could ask him for a more complete examination. If he is reluctant to comply, you might feel more comfortable with another doctor. Here's what to expect:

Either in his office or in the examining room when you're fully gowned, the doctor will ask you for your personal history. If you have never had sexual relations, don't be too shy to tell him. Whether you're in the office or the examining room, you'll both be sitting and having a face-to-face conversation.

After your chat, you'll be asked to urinate so that your bladder is empty and the doctor can have a better chance to examine your organs. Also, you're providing urine to be tested for sugar and protein content that might indicate upcoming diabetes and kidney problems. You'll change into a gown and wait in an examining room where a nurse will probably take your blood pressure before the doctor enters. You'll be wearing an open gown, but you should never be completely nude.

The first thing the doctor will do is to feel your neck to be sure that there are no abnormal lymph nodes and the thyroid gland is not enlarged. Then he will check your breasts one at a time for lumps and examine your abdomen. If he notices any excessive hair growth, he should explain the possibility of excessive male hormones to you. The doctor should communicate with you throughout the examination so that you can monitor your body when you're by yourself. Then it's time for the internal.

You will be lying on your back on the examining table with your knees bent and your legs apart. The doctor will sit on a chair facing your legs. He will shine a light on your genital area and examine your outer vulva. Then, using an instrument called a speculum, he will look inside the vagina and check the cervix, the mouth of the womb. The speculum comes in various sizes, and the doctor should choose the size that's right for you. A woman who knows she has a narrow vaginal opening might suggest that he use a small speculum. If a woman is a virgin, he might entirely disregard the instrument and examine her with a swab. If a doctor does use a speculum, it should be warm, and there's nothing wrong with a woman asking her doctor to take the chill off the instrument with a heating pad or hot water.

During the speculum examination a doctor can see only a woman's vagina and cervix; he cannot peer into her uterus and study her ovaries. A physician can outline the size and the shape of the uterus and the ovaries, however, by gently pressing on the organs with both hands. The finger of one hand is placed inside the vagina to steady the organs. The other hand is rested outside the abdomen,

PELVIC EXAMINATION

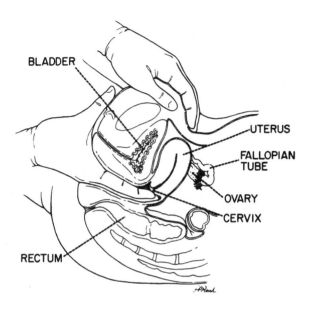

BLADDER

UTERUS

FALLOPIAN TUBE

OVARY

CERVIX

RECTUM

2-2   **The Internal Examination.** A doctor examines a woman's internal organs through a bimanual examination while the woman is lying on her back on the examining table with her legs in the stirrups. As pictured, during this examination the doctor inserts the index and middle fingers of one hand into the vagina until he reaches the posterior fornix (the space behind the cervix). His thumb remains on the outside of the vulva, but he should carefully avoid touching the clitoral area. The other hand is resting on the woman's abdomen, and if she relaxes her abdominal muscles the doctor should be able to palpate the uterus to define its shape and size. He can also determine if the uterus is anteverted, located in the front next to the bladder, as shown in the illustration. If the uterus is retroverted (tilted), it will be pointed downward toward the rectum, which, in the illustration, is located beneath the doctor's internally positioned fingers. The doctor can also palpate the ovaries and tubes (the grayed organs to the right of the uterus) by moving his hands to the side of the uterus.

and by moving the hand in a circular motion the doctor can tell if there are any abnormalities. All this should be done with great sensitivity and at no time should a woman feel any severe pain, although there might be some discomfort.

The entire internal should be done slowly and gently, without embarrassment to the doctor or to the woman. (Remember, you are gowned, and not totally naked.) A woman should feel free to ask her doctor to explain what he is doing as he is doing it. There should be no mystery for you to ponder after you leave a gynecologist's office.

Can a Woman Under Eighteen Have a Gynecological Examination Without Her Parents' Consent?

According to the Alan Guttmacher Institute, in recent years the laws governing minors' access to confidential reproductive health care have remained largely unchanged. No state explicitly requires parental involvement for contraception, prenatal care, STD (sexually transmitted disease) diagnosis and treatment, or drug and/or alcohol abuse. In these areas, states either have no laws or they have enacted laws favoring the rights of minors. In twenty-three states and the District of Columbia, a minor has the explicit right to seek contraceptive services from a gynecologist by law. In twenty-seven states and the District of Columbia, laws authorize a pregnant minor to obtain prenatal care and delivery services without parental consent, and in forty-nine states and the District of Columbia, laws give women under eighteen the right to visit a gynecologist on their own for diagnosis and treatment of sexually transmitted diseases. (State laws become more restrictive when the health issue is an abortion. The number of states with laws requiring parental involvement rose from eighteen to thirty between 1991 and 1997.)

3.

Menstrual Cramps Are Real

A SLAP IN THE FACE

As soon as Judy saw the faint brown stains on her panties she brought the undergarment to her mother. All her friends had their periods and she had been dying to get hers, too. "Well, this is the beginning of your womanhood, Judy. You're finally growing up," said her mother as she looked at the soiled white cotton. Then, for no apparent reason, Judy's mother gently slapped her on the side of her face. Judy wondered if she had done something wrong, but no, then her mother hugged her and brought her up to the master bedroom, where a box of Kotex was being saved for this moment.

It took years, but by the time she told the story to her doctor, Judy had learned that the slap was a time-honored custom. Her mother had simply been carrying out a tradition, but neither she nor her mother had known what the slap was supposed to mean. It was Judy's grandmother, the matriarch of the family, who finally explained that the slap was intended to bring good health. For generations, menstruation must have been regarded as a sickness.

Today, with all our increased knowledge about women's bodies, most people know that menstruation is a natural process and not a disease, but it still continues to be shrouded in mystery. One can understand how menstruation might have *originally* been considered a weird or magical event. Imagine primitive man watching primitive

woman bleed for five days without dying. He must have been totally
awed and frightened.

Civilization progressed, but the facts about menstruation
remained elusive. Take the word *menstruation*, for instance. It comes
from the Latin word *mens*, meaning "month," but *month* is a deriva-
tion of *moon*—in Greek *moon* is *mene*. The ancients were still identifying the monthly cycle as something cosmically controlled, like the
phases of the moon. Thus, the interpretations of menstruation are
mind-boggling.

A number of religions that remain with us today viewed—and
sometimes still view—this very healthy and natural occurrence as
repugnant. When Muslim women are menstruating, they are not
allowed to enter mosques. Women of the Greek Orthodox faith,
early in the twentieth century, were forbidden communion during
their menstrual periods. At one time in the Catholic Church's
history, intercourse during menstruation was a sin. Even though
menstruation gives a woman a wondrous internal cleansing, in the
orthodox Jewish faith a woman's "clean" days are *after* her period,
when she is immersed in a purifying bath. Women's bodies have
been featured in an enormous number of myths and misconceptions.

And Freud, with his ridiculous "penis envy" theory, furthered
misunderstanding. Paula Weideger, in her book *Menstruation &
Menopause*, explains that according to Freud, menstruation, like loss
of virginity, childbirth, and menopause, is a time when a woman
becomes furious because she doesn't have a man's penis. "Freud,
then, believed that banishing a woman from sight, forbidding her to
touch utensils shared with a man, or prohibiting sexual relations
between man and menstruating woman are rational actions that
men must take to protect themselves. The menstrual taboo spares
man from witnessing the rage of woman's castration anxiety, and
from being reminded of his own castration anxiety, which would be
elicited by the sight of genital bleeding."[1]

Menstruating women have been blamed or credited for everything from blight to harvests of plenty, from causing death to curing
illness. Through it all, women have remained silent. In *My Mother/*

My Self, Nancy Friday describes the day she started menstruating and the way her mother skidded around the subject. "She caught me off guard with a new voice: 'Well, how does it feel to be a woman?' . . . I leaned far out the car window, my pigtails flying behind. My answer was appropriately lost in the wind. They were the last words my mother was to utter on the subject. . . . I am still working on her question about how it feels to be a woman. But I never have understood the secrecy about menstruation."[2]

MENSTRUATION IS NO MYSTERY

The letters I have received have shown me that many women, through no fault of their own, don't understand the physical and emotional changes they go through every month. Even many doctors don't comprehend the hormonal fluctuations and the impact they can have on a woman's body. A menstrual period is actually the end result of a delicately balanced interplay of nervous signals and hormonal responses. The famous kidnapping of Patty Hearst in 1974 offers an example. Her menstrual period was said to have stopped for a long time during her days of captivity. When she was retrieved from the underground and tried as a bank robber, she was reported to have menstruated almost continuously for more than a year. Once a woman learns how her menstrual cycle works, she can understand why a female who is under severe stress might either lose her period or bleed without pause.

During the menstrual cycle, which is the time from one period to another, complex but wonderfully designed hormonal fluctuations occur in a woman's body. If a woman could visualize what is happening, she could understand not only menstruation but conception, contraception, premenstrual tension, menstrual cramps, and menopause. So much can be revealed through the menstrual cycle. Very personal questions about menstruation are in this chapter's letters from concerned women, but it's best to remove the menstrual mystique before these questions are answered.

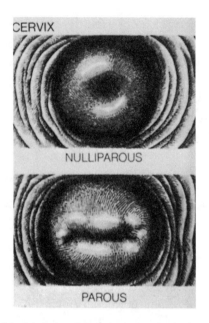

3-1 **The Cervix.** The cervix is viewed through a vagina that has been opened with the aid of a speculum. The pleated area surrounding the cervix is the vaginal wall. The opening in the center of the cervix, the external cervical os (the mouth of the womb), leads into the cervical canal, which connects the vagina to the uterine cavity. By inserting a finger into her vagina, a woman will be able to identify the cervix, a hard protrusion similar to the tip of her nose. Note that the cervix differs in the nulliparous, a woman who has not borne children, and the parous, a woman who has had a natural birth. A woman must examine her own cervix to identify the mucus in order to determine her fertility.

The Ebb and Flow of the Feminine Cycle

A few days after menstruation, as the blood starts to diminish, the hypothalamus of the brain, which controls the menstrual cycle, sends a hormonal message—the Releasing Factor—to the pituitary gland. The message doesn't have to travel far because the pituitary is located just below the hypothalamus.

When the pituitary receives the message, it releases the Follicle Stimulating Hormone (FSH), which travels through the blood to the ovaries, and then the action begins. The ovaries start to work and all the little follicles, the potential egg cells in the ovaries, begin to

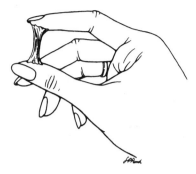

3-2   **Spinnbarkeit.** At the time of ovulation, if a woman is fertile, the mucus from the cervix can be threaded for several inches between two fingers. The mucus has a clear, thin consistency similar to raw egg white. This ability to thread the mucus is called "spinnbarkeit." The presence of abundant, stretchable cervical mucus usually indicates a high estrogen level and shows that a woman's fertility is at its peak.

grow and to produce the female hormone estrogen. A woman's skin might start to feel smoother as her estrogen builds. The estrogen will also effect the cervical mucus:

- The First Mucus Check (Before Ovulation): The mucus secreted by the cervix, the mouth of the womb, is tactile, visible evidence of the events happening inside a woman's body.
- Right after menstruation the mucus is usually not noticeable, but toward the middle of a woman's cycle the mucus makes an appearance. A woman can thread out the mucus from her vagina with two fingers and if it has the clear, thin consistency of a raw egg white, that's her sign that estrogen is increasing. This phenomenal ability to thread the mucus is called "spinnbarkeit," meaning stretchability.

As the estrogen increases, it sends a "slow down" message back to the pituitary. At about this time a woman's breasts are becoming a little bigger and one of the ovarian follicles, for some unknown reason, is beginning to surpass the other egg cells in its development. That one egg cell, called the Graafian follicle, or the follicle (egg)-of-the-month, bubbles out on the outside of the ovary. This bubble contains the egg that's destined for a trip to the womb.

• The Second Mucus Check (During Ovulation): The mucus in the cervix, when the egg is about ready to be released, is in abundance and a woman should be able to feel the wetness in her vagina and to thread the mucus for several inches. (The consistency of the mucus varies from woman to woman. One woman describes it as "rubber cement" and another as "gloppy glue.") Also, the cervix, which had been closed and facing backward, begins turning forward and opening, thereby making it easier for the sperm to move into the uterus (see figure 3-2). If a woman wants to become pregnant, she could insert a finger into her vagina and if her cervix is open and her wetness is at a peak, she has arrived at the best time for conception.

About thirteen or fourteen days into the cycle, the pituitary responds to the increased estrogen by sending out the Luteinizing Hormone (LH) and stopping the FSH. The LH makes the Graafian follicle burst and eject a mature egg cell—this release of the egg is *ovulation*. The egg then strikes out on a five-to-seven-day journey inside the Fallopian tube to the womb.

The scar tissue that's left behind after the egg pops out becomes the corpus luteum, the producer of progesterone, the pregnancy hormone. Progesterone causes the lining of the uterus to change into a soft, spongy nest rich in blood vessels and glandular tissue that is the perfect bed for the egg coming down the tube. The hormone also relaxes the uterus to give the egg a better chance to implant itself into the endometrium, the transformed uterine lining. Also, progesterone alters the cervical mucus.

• The Third Mucus Check (After Ovulation): Once progesterone enters into the cycle, the mucus decreases in amount and rather than being clear and stretchy, it becomes cloudy and thick. It loses its stretchability. It is almost as if the cervical mucus changes to

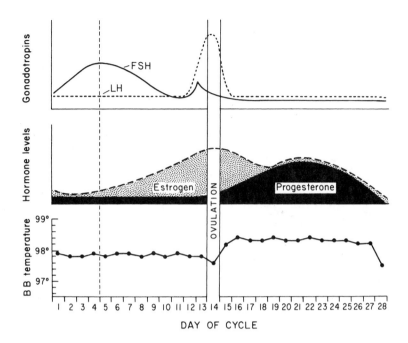

3-3 **The Menstrual Cycle.** The top curves illustrate the fluctuations in the gonadotropins, the brain hormones, during the menstrual cycle. The middle curves indicate the fluctuations of the female hormones—estrogen and progesterone—during the twenty-eight-day cycle. The bottom curve indicates the Basal Body Temperature (BBT) fluctuation. Day One marks the first day of menstrual bleeding. The FSH will stimulate estrogen production from the ovaries. The estrogen, in turn, will prime the cervix and increase the cervical mucus in preparation for ovulation. When the estrogen reaches a peak, it will trigger LH release. The LH will then stimulate ovulation. After ovulation, the estrogen and progesterone will increase and cause the body temperature to rise, a sign that ovulation has taken place.

create a natural diaphragm that prevents vaginal bacteria and germs from entering a clean, protected uterus. The egg is being given the best environment for growth.

Estrogen and progesterone increase together after ovulation, as the LH drops off (see figure 3-3). There are a number of side effects that come from the surge of estrogen and progesterone during this last half of the menstrual cycle. They are specifically covered in chapter 4 and chapter 5.

Meanwhile, as the menstrual cycle nears an end, if the egg is fertilized and pregnancy occurs, estrogen and progesterone levels stay high. But if there is no fertilization, the brain doesn't get the stimulus it needs to maintain the corpus luteum. The corpus luteum disintegrates, progesterone and estrogen levels drop rapidly, and menstruation is triggered. The endometrium—the enriched spongy lining of the uterus—which is useless without a pregnancy, leaves the body as menstrual blood. On this first day of a woman's period, one cycle has just ended and another is beginning. A woman has arrived at Day One of a brand-new cycle.

HOW YOUR MOOD HAMPERS YOUR HORMONES

The brain's pituitary is a sensitive gland that responds to every rise and dip in a woman's emotional makeup. Since the pituitary starts and stops the hormones that regulate menstruation, if the pituitary is thrown off, so are your hormones and so is menstruation. It's the domino principle applied to biology. One thing sets off another, that sets off another, that alters menstruation. And no one can say what that first trigger might be—a mood that overtakes you, a stressful situation, even a flight in an airplane can make the difference.

It's not at all extraordinary for college students living away from families and pressured by exams to experience amenorrhea—the loss of their periods—sometimes for a whole semester. A counselor at a college freshman dormitory used to tell her female charges, "Don't worry, when you go home for Christmas vacation, your period will come." As soon as they left their tense campus lives and returned to the relaxed atmospheres of their homes, these young women sent tranquil messages to their pituitaries, and the pituitaries responded by orchestrating normal hormonal flows.

The pituitary reacts with a woman. In extreme cases, women have been known to be in such intense emotional states that they have not only arrested their periods, they have created false pregnancies.

As a resident I was called in to evaluate a woman who had entered labor. She had never been seen in our hospital before. She said that she had been without her period for nine months and she was swollen, as if she were with child, but I could not hear the heartbeat of the baby. I was afraid the unborn might be dead so I sent her for an X ray of the abdomen. There was no sign of a fetus. The woman had never conceived. The expectant father, who was waiting outside the labor room with brand-new baby clothes, refused to believe the news. The "mother" screamed, cried, breathed in gasps, and began to menstruate—which shows how a drastic mood change can start as well as stop a period.

Women who haven't menstruated and are worried that they're pregnant often begin to bleed the second they hear that their pregnancy tests are negative. In an unusual instance of menstrual breakthrough, a bride's maid of honor began bleeding between the wedding and the reception, because during the service she had fallen down the altar steps, ripped her red silk dress, and damaged her shoes. The embarrassment of losing her balance and dignity in front of three hundred wide-eyed viewers had overturned her inner equilibrium, too. Clearly, the feminine cycle reflects feelings.

MENSTRUAL CRAMPS ARE REAL

Doctors are like explorers discovering new continents when they hit upon something never before known in medicine. In 1957, Dr. V. R. Pickles and his colleagues at the University of Sheffield in England must have felt a rush of excitement when they were able to isolate a "menstrual stimulant" in menstrual fluid. That first bit of news is now common knowledge about the cramp-causing hormonelike substances called prostaglandins, which are produced in many tissues of the body, but most significantly in the lining of the uterus.

Six years after Pickles and his group discovered their "menstrual stimulant," they were able to identify it as prostaglandins, and therein they made a tremendous breakthrough for women. They found that females who had excruciating menstrual cramps had more prostaglandins than women who were less bothered. We still don't know why some women have more prostaglandins than others. Maybe it's genetic. But women who produce a lot of prostaglandins have monthly menstrual packages that often include cramps, nausea, vomiting, diarrhea, headache, fatigue, and nervousness.

Women don't experience these symptoms until their periods are about to begin because during most of the monthly cycle prostaglandins are held in check by progesterone. Just before menstruation, progesterone drops and prostaglandins rise. The mouth of the womb, from which the blood usually flows, tightens. The prostaglandins in the menstrual blood trapped within the womb are absorbed by the uterine muscles, released, reabsorbed, and released again in a circular fashion. It's a vicious cycle. As the prostaglandins follow their circuit, the uterus contracts and cramps with ever more intensity, and until the menstrual blood flows from the vagina, taking with it the prostaglandins, women feel terrible. They are suffering very real pain, which is clinically called primary dysmenorrhea (secondary dysmenorrhea involves pain brought on by a pelvic disorder—such as infection, endometriosis, fibroid tumors pressing on nerves, or a poorly placed IUD).

As prostaglandins are released, the uterus contracts and cramps, resulting in what might be called a charley horse of the womb. Sometimes the uterine contractions can be more pronounced than they are during childbirth. And if the blood is not allowed to escape through the vagina it could back up, first into the Fallopian tubes and then into the abdominal cavity, making already unbearable cramps even more blindingly painful. This could lead to endometriosis, and a woman should ask her doctor to check for the condition (see chapter 7).

In the past, when women bore children at earlier ages, doctors heard fewer complaints about menstrual cramps. Today, when childbirth is often postponed, more women are suffering dysmenorrhea.

Biology doesn't evolve as fast as society. It's frightening to know that menstrual cramps are the single greatest cause of lost working hours and schooldays among young women. Studies have estimated that over 140 million working hours are lost annually as a result of menstrual pain. More than half of the menstruating women in this country have cramps! The pain is real and expensive.

TREATMENT OF MENSTRUAL PAIN

Men, women, doctors—everyone—must be made to understand that menstrual cramps are not merely "in women's heads." The painkillers and tranquilizers that have been prescribed by doctors for menstrual cramps are treatments for symptoms, not causes. If plentiful prostaglandins make menstrual pain, it logically follows that the way to alleviate cramps, and possibly other unwanted effects of menstruation, is going to involve medication that inhibits prostaglandins. Women started to use this medication—nonsteroidal anti-inflammatory drugs, or NSAIDS—in the 1980s for menstrual pain.

The frustration and despair felt by women who knew that every month of their menstruating lives was going to be riddled with pain was eliminated. The key to cure comes from *treating causes, not symptoms.* Women educated themselves, listened to their bodies, and finally educated their doctors. The latest menstrual cramp relievers might not be known to many physicians. For the health movement to continue, women must ask questions and get answers, and keep the doctor/patient partnership in a constant state of evolution.

Is There Any Relief?

What can I do when one or two days out of every month I have cramps so severe that I vomit four or five times a day? The cramps start at the beginning of my period and sometimes I'm lucky because they go away overnight—I'm only in bed for a day. When they last two days my complexion almost looks green and even if I could, I

*wouldn't want to leave the house. I've tried taking aspirin but
with the vomiting and all, it doesn't stay down. I become exhausted
from all the retching and pain.*

*Next month I'm supposed to be a bridesmaid, but I'm afraid the
wedding will happen at the time of my period. Is there anything I
can do? I'm only twenty years old. Am I going to go through twenty
more years of living like this?*

— J.B., Mobile, Alabama

*I've tried everything—aspirin, heating pads, birth control pills,
codeine, even childbirth (I have a six-month-old daughter), but
nothing has lessened the severity of my menstrual problems. My
doctor is very sympathetic and he wants to try the birth control
pills again, but I just don't want to take them. I am also leery of
drugs that make me drowsy because I have a new baby to care for.
Yet once a month I break out in a cold sweat, and I must live
through a couple of days of cramps, vomiting, and diarrhea. It's not
right to have to suffer so much.*

— N.T., New York, New York

*I've watched my daughter writhe between the sheets of her bed,
her head on a sweaty pillow, the tears rolling down her cheeks. She
is in such pain from her periods that I feel like crying for her. She
puts heating pads on her stomach, takes Tylenol, even drinks an
occasional glass of wine, which someone told her might help. Often
the cramps make her vomit and she becomes ashen, like a corpse. The
doctors say she'll outgrow the pain, but how can she live like this?
She's only fifteen and she has already lost the joyfulness of youth.*

— L.L., Hartford, Connecticut

All the symptoms of dysmenorrhea—cramps, vomiting, nausea,
paleness, and sweating—which are mentioned by the women who
wrote the above letters are due to high prostaglandin levels. We have
learned to respect the powerful prostaglandin hormone, which is
produced all over the body, in men as well as in women. If a man or

a woman is given prostaglandins in any form, he or she will show exactly the same symptoms as described in the letters, and sometimes there will be fever and fainting, too. The effects of prostaglandins can be so overpowering that they will debilitate the nerves and a person will weaken and pass out.

Every woman who is suffering menstrual cramps or any of the accompanying symptoms should see her doctor to make sure that her abdominal pain is not being caused by infection or tumors or one of several different types of pelvic diseases. If a doctor can rule out serious pelvic problems, then prostaglandins are probably the cause and a woman can be treated.

Since aspirinlike medication prevents the body from releasing prostaglandins, a woman who has not tried aspirin before might take two aspirins four times a day for two days *before* her period starts, and during the first days of her flow. Prostaglandins are more efficiently blocked when the aspirin, or any other antiprostaglandin drug, is taken *before menstruation*.

The NSAIDs, Over-the-Counter Antiprostaglandins. It's clear from the letters that many women cannot tolerate aspirin, or that aspirin does not bring relief. These women might try Midol, the time-honored, over-the-counter, aspirinlike drug, or one of the nonsteroidal anti-inflammatory drugs/NSAIDs.

Besides curbing cramps, Midol and the most popular NSAIDs—generically known as ibuprofen and naproxen sodium—will also reduce menstrual flow. Since they can irritate the stomach, however, these drugs should be taken with some food, a cracker or a glass of milk.

One or two tablets of Midol Maximum Strength Cramp Formula four times a day, one day *before* and during the first few days of menstruation, have been known to provide positive changes.

The same dosage of one or two tablets, four times a day, one day *before* and during the first few days of menstruation, also works for Advil, Nuprin, and Motrin tablets. Each of these brand-name NSAIDs contains 200 milligrams (mg) of ibuprofen, a drug traditionally used to fight arthritis but now FDA-approved for relief of menstrual cramps. Another NSAID, Aleve, contains 200 mg of naproxen and 20 mg of sodium.

Most women, even those who have irregular periods, usually know their bodies well enough to guess when their periods are about to arrive. You have a much better chance for relief if you start an NSAID *prior to menstruation,* whenever you have that first sign that your period is coming. I've noticed that many women try each of these drugs but eventually settle on the one they feel is right for them.

Prescription Antiprostaglandins. You might wonder why you would want a prescription for an antiprostaglandin medication, since so many of these drugs are available over-the-counter. The reason I recommend prescription NSAIDs to my patients is that individual tablets are available in higher doses by prescription, and I feel that the release of the drug is improved. Also, although many NSAIDs are sold over-the-counter, a wider variety of these FDA-approved drugs for treating dysmenorrhea is available by prescription. Among them are Anaprox (naproxen sodium), Cataflam (diclofenac potassium), Naprosyn (naproxen), Motrin (ibuprofen), Orudis (ketaprofen), Ponstel (mefenamic acid), and Voltaren (diclofenac sodium).

I Feel Better When I Begin to Flow

I've had horrible menstrual cramps ever since I was twelve years old. The pain starts twenty-four hours before my period and it grows and grows until I have to go to bed. Finally, the flow starts and everything is fine again. But those twenty-four hours are a nightmare. I asked my family doctor to give me something for the cramps. I begged him for years, but he said that I was just imagining them. After I reached my twenties and married, I went to another doctor who gave me Ponstel. This drug helps me a little bit, but I still have to lie down until the flow starts. Is there anything else I can do?

—C.G., Winston-Salem, North Carolina

The cramps this woman is enduring are clearly due to a high level of prostaglandins. She feels better when she starts to flow because the menstrual blood, which contains the prostaglandins, is being released from her body, and as prostaglandins diminish, so does cramping. I would suggest a higher dosage of Ponstel (mefenamic acid) for Ms. G. If an increased amount of the drug still is ineffective, Motrin, Anaprox, or one of the other prescription NSAIDs might be better for her. Although all NSAIDs inhibit prostaglandin production, a woman often has to find the one that is "right" for her.

While trying to find relief, this woman—and every woman— must remember that menstrual cramps are real. A doctor who says you're imagining them is old-fashioned and misinformed. Such an uneducated response to the pain of menstrual cramps sends a message that you need to find another doctor.

The Far-Reaching Effects of Menstruation

I'm thirty-two years old, have two preschool children, and I am at my wits' end. I have extreme cramping a week before my period and for the first three days of my very heavy flow. My mood swings are irrational. I also have pain in my lower back. I've been to many doctors. Some physicians have prescribed birth control and hormone pills but I cannot stand the side effects. It is taking all my energy to control myself, especially with a one-year-old and a three-year-old in the house. I've recently turned to prayer. My present doctor suggested a vaginal hysterectomy to remove my uterus, and the idea of no periods and no pain does seem appealing. However, I thought I should seek a second opinion but when I did, the doctor I consulted said, "Women complain too much about their periods." Where do I go from here?

—B.A., Lancaster, Pennsylvania

Although there are medical meetings, professional seminars, and published studies to provide information about the treatment of menstrual cramps, many doctors still don't know what is going on inside a woman's body. Many physicians do not want to spend the money to go to meetings where they can learn the latest developments. Hormonal surges during the menstrual cycle can bring on an array of biological and psychological changes. Unfortunately, some doctors still do not recognize the complexity of these symptoms.

No woman should agree to a hysterectomy before she has tried all other avenues of treatment. Nowhere does this woman say she was given either an over-the-counter or prescription NSAID (see pages 69 to 70), and one of these drugs might help her. Recently a woman with severe menstrual cramps had to be pushed into my office in a wheelchair. After two months of menstruation with Motrin, she has no more symptoms and she now walks very jauntily into the building. Her pain came from high prostaglandins, and Ms. A's might too.

The Caring Father

I am the father of five daughters and my oldest daughter has been stricken with crippling pain ever since she began her periods at age twelve. I have felt drained and tortured all the times I have seen her become incapacitated for two or three days before her period. I have watched her go through these heartbreaking spells and I can only say they are agony to witness. Even though my daughter is in her twenties and married now, I cannot give up on my efforts to try to help her. Is there a drug she can take or a doctor she should see? There must be a way I can end my child's suffering.
                                        —W.K., Minneapolis, Minnesota

It is touching to read such a letter and to realize how many fathers care so deeply about their daughters and how many husbands are moved by their wives. I applaud and encourage this partnership between men and women, for women's health. Empathy and understanding nourish everyone.

The reward from this letter came six months later, after I had recommended a doctor in Mr. K.'s area who treated his daughter with prescription Motrin. I was a guest on a radio call-in program and Mr. K. phoned to say that his daughter was no longer in any kind of pain. Her life and his had become joyous. She had been suffering for years and now she had no more problem. They had cried and celebrated together. He sensed a special closeness to her now and he thanked me profusely.

I felt a warm sensation when I heard him speak, and I can only say that it deeply gratifies me to share solid information that I know is right and to learn that people are spared the sorrow of suffering.

Would a Baby Ease the Pain?

All through my adolescence I had terrible cramps a week before and a few days into my period. I was put on Demerol and my doctor told me that the pain would go away after I had a baby. I went to work instead of having a baby and another doctor gave me Darvon. So I took painkillers a long time, and finally, I did get married and gave birth to two children. Now I'm thirty years old, and my periods are a little better, but I still have pain. Also, I find that I come down with colds and flu right around the time I menstruate. Is something wrong with me?
—H.U., Lake Placid, New York

Many women have said that doctors have told them that after they have babies they'll feel better. Sometimes after she has a child a woman feels more sanguine during her period because her uterus has relaxed, her cervix is more open, and the prostaglandin-containing blood exits easily. However, some women produce high levels of prostaglandins, and having babies is not going to change that. After the birth of her child, a woman who has high prostaglandins will begin to feel exactly as she did before her pregnancy. Menstrual cramps will return. Also, as a woman gets older, hormonal changes might bring on more pain.

Neither before nor after a woman has a child should she be treated with painkillers for menstrual cramps. This is not treating the cause of the problem. Again, drugs that will block the production of prostaglandins should help. Midol might be used at first, and if that doesn't have an effect on the pain, then over-the-counter Advil, Motrin, Nuprin, and Aleve are alternatives. These drugs are not sedatives, and you will not become fatigued with them, or with prescription NSAIDs.

As for the question of whether a woman is more susceptible to colds and flu around the time of menstruation, the answer is yes, she might be. Due to hormonal changes, a woman often experiences stress just before her period, and increased stress produces more steroids, hormones secreted by the adrenal glands. The steroids weaken the immune system, which normally fights disease, and a woman might not be able to fend off a rampant virus that's spreading the flu, herpes, or a seasonal cold. Vitamins, especially vitamins A and B_6, and good nutrition are important for strengthening the immune system at this time.

Is the Birth Control Pill a Safe Way to Stop Cramps?

My eighteen-year-old daughter's periods are irregular, but unfortunately, her menstrual cramps are not—they are constant, agonizing spasms that send her to bed. She has tried aspirin to no avail, and now the doctor is suggesting birth control pills. Isn't this a rather dangerous kind of a cure? Don't birth control pills cause cancer? I certainly want to see my daughter freed from her pain, but I don't want her to exchange cramps for cancer.
                                    —A.S., Fort Lauderdale, Florida

The association of birth control pills and cancer was reported years ago when birth control pills were relatively new and high levels of estrogen were used to make them. Today's birth control pills combine progesterone and estrogen hormones in much smaller quantities, and recent studies have shown that these newer pills are safe, especially if the woman who takes them is under thirty-five and a healthy nonsmoker with no history of diabetes or high blood pressure. There still is a higher incidence of phlebitis and blood clotting in women taking the birth control pill, but the contraceptive is not cancer-causing (see chapter 12).

The birth control pill will regulate this young woman's menstrual cycle and will also constrain the development of the endometrium, the uterine lining, that leaves the body as menstrual flow. There will be less blood during menstruation, and decreased prostaglandins, since they drop with the blood level. Without so many prostaglandins to cause cramps, the pain should subside or at least diminish. There are some women, however, who still suffer even though they are on the pill.

Over-the-counter and prescription antiprostaglandin NSAIDs (see pages 69 to 70) might be taken in addition to the birth control pill. In fact, while she's taking the pill, a woman knows exactly when to expect menstruation, and the time that she should begin to take a nonsteroidal anti-inflammatory drug or NSAID such as Motrin is much easier for her to figure out.

As long as a woman has her blood pressure checked twice a year, the pill is certainly safe, and a mother need not worry that her daughter will be increasing her chances of getting cancer.

The Pill and the Overweight Woman

I had incredible menstrual cramps along with irregular periods, so I went to my doctor and he put me on birth control pills. Everything was fine for a while, but three months ago I started to get cramps all over again, and they were worse than before. I know I'm overweight—5'4" and 150 pounds—and I wonder if that has something to do with it. I've often heard that if you are overweight you shouldn't be on the pill. Is this true? I'm only twenty years old and I don't want to do anything that's going to stop me from being able to get pregnant.

—M.J., Seattle, Washington

As long as a woman does not smoke or have diabetes or high blood pressure, even if she is overweight, she can take birth control pills. However, it is very important that her blood pressure be checked at least twice a year. Overweight women tend to have high blood pressure and this is one reason why they should try to lose weight. If a woman's blood pressure goes up, she must stop the pill immediately.

Her cramps could have become worse recently because women who are overweight have a lot of fatty tissue, which produces the hormone estrogen—which increases the thickness of the uterine lining during the menstrual cycle. So even though she is on the pill, the increased uterine lining could make her periods heavy again, boost the prostaglandins and, along with them, the pain.

She might try Midol along with the birth control pills two days before menstruation. If Midol doesn't ease the pain, she should try an over-the-counter NSAID or see a physician for a prescription. It is perfectly safe to take prostaglandin-blocking drugs in addition to birth control pills. However, I would also recommend that this woman try to lose weight. If she is thinner she will not have to worry so much about her blood pressure, her estrogen level will drop, and most likely her cramps will go away, too.

My Monthly Pain Is in My Head and Back

I don't have cramps the way everyone else does. I'm all right at the time of my period, and I only feel them slightly during ovulation. My main problems are headaches and backaches every month. I get a headache during ovulation and then about three days before my period. It's such a severe pain that I sometimes wonder if it's a migraine. I feel like King Kong is crushing my head in his hands and my eyes are about to explode. As soon as I start to bleed the headache stops, but then a backache takes over.

For the first two days of my period I have an excruciating pain at the base of my spine. My X rays show nothing. One doctor put me on Darvon, another suggested a partial hysterectomy, and

another said I have pain because of the way I'm built. I'm thirty-
three years old and I don't want a hysterectomy. What can I do?
There are so few days in a month when I feel good.
—Y.N., Tarzana, California

It is not uncommon for women to have headaches before their periods. Estrogen, the female hormone, increases before menstruation. Estrogen binds salt, which, in turn, binds water. Water tension pulls on the brain membrane and causes swelling and migraine headaches. A woman who suffers from headaches should cut down on her salt intake before her period, drink plenty of fluids to wash out her system, and she might even try diuretics (see chapter 4).

The headaches are coming from a hormonal imbalance before her period and during her ovulation. Birth control pills would regulate her hormones, so she might take them as long as she doesn't smoke or have diabetes or high blood pressure, and if she has her blood pressure checked twice a year. Also, vitamin B_6 has been known to offer some relief from premenstrual tension. I would suggest that she take at least 50 mg of vitamin B_6 every day to help her cope with the stress of her headaches and backaches. And on her most stressful days, she might double the dosage.

Nerves from the uterine area enter into the spine and often cause spinal and back pain. If a woman has a tilted uterus there is a definite pull on the nerves during menstruation. Birth control pills prevent a heavy buildup of the uterine lining and decrease the pressure on the uterine nerves to the spine. Painkillers don't treat the cause. For a doctor to suggest a hysterectomy without first examining this woman for a tilted uterus or prescribing medication that would reduce uterine pressure and menstrual flow is absurd. If birth control pills are ineffective, Danocrine (danazol), an antihormone, might end some of the pain and discomfort she is feeling. Danocrine must be taken every day and could be continued for months to curb the menstruation (see chapter 7).

However, if this woman exercises and keeps her body in shape, she might find that she will naturally lessen her flow and the pull on her nerves. Physically active women are known to have fewer aches and more moderate periods.

Are My Cramps from My IUD, or Are My Fibroids Acting Up?

I think my menstrual cramps are something out of the ordinary. I'm thirty-one, the mother of a nine-year-old son, and I've had a new type of IUD for a year. The pain that I get during my menstruation is new to me. I didn't have it before the IUD and I think the IUD might have something to do with it. My doctor doesn't want to give me birth control pills because I have fibroid tumors and he is concerned that the pill will make the tumors spread and grow. So I continue to use the IUD but I'm afraid that it's not staying in place. I have these fears of it going up into my uterus. The other night I had a dream about it. I need to know what's causing my pain.

—G.D., Detroit, Michigan

When a woman has menstrual cramps, it is always important for a physician to evaluate her condition carefully to rule out the possibility of infection from a poorly placed IUD, troublesome fibroid tumors, or any other serious pelvic disorders before he decides that the problem is primary dysmenorrhea.

Infection from an IUD will tend to spread even after menstruation, so if a woman continues to have pain and cramping after her period is over, she might have an infection in her Fallopian tube, where it could eventually lead to infertility. A doctor can tell if an IUD is well placed by using X rays or ultrasonography, the sound wave technique. If he suspects infection in the uterus or Fallopian tubes, he must then take a culture and treat the infection with antibiotics. If a woman has been assured that there is no infection and she continues to have cramping, a nonsteroidal anti-inflammatory drug (NSAID), might give her relief. Studies have shown that these drugs not only decrease cramps but also lessen the amount of uterine bleeding.

Her fibroid tumors might be causing the pain due to the decrease in their blood supply during menstruation. On the other hand, if bleeding becomes heavier than normal, a fibroid might have grown and broken through the wall of the uterine cavity, disturbing the uterine lining, which will bleed. Fibroids that are causing considerable discomfort and pain can be removed with an operation called a myomectomy, in which the surgeon can leave the uterus intact but take away the tumors. (Myomectomy is more fully described in chapter 15.)

Fibroids that are painful can be removed, and an IUD that persistently worries a woman can be taken out. However, a woman must always make sure that her doctor has carefully evaluated her case before he decides to make any medical moves. Cramps can be a sign of many different types of pelvic problems. If a woman has tremendous pain before menstruation, she might have pelvic endometriosis, as is discussed in chapter 7. A woman must gauge her body by herself, by understanding how it works. If the woman who wrote this letter is listening to her body and she feels the IUD is at fault, she might very well be right. She must ask her doctor for an evaluation and an explanation of her condition.

Drug Addiction or Hysterectomy?

My menstrual cramps make me feel as if I'm being cut with sharp knives without ever having had anesthesia. At first, doctors put me on birth control pills, but there's a history of breast cancer in my family, so I stopped them. I've seen many doctors and they always prescribe Percodan or Vicodin or Darvon for the pain, but I want to get rid of it, not sedate it. I'm thirty-one and I have two children now and I don't want to be walking around half asleep when they need me. The latest doctor I've seen wants to do a vaginal hysterectomy, but having recently heard you speak, I'm beginning to wonder if surgery is such a good idea. I need help now before I become seriously addicted to all these drugs I've been given. I've really come to rely on them for relief and I'm scared.

—R.C., Toronto, Ontario, Canada

Pain is the body's signal that something is wrong, and a doctor
needs to evaluate what the causes of the pain might be. In the case
of menstrual cramps, the cause can be a surplus of prostaglandins,
resulting in primary dysmenorrhea, or uterine infection, an IUD,
fibroid tumors, endometriosis (a condition in which the menstrual
blood is pushed back through the Fallopian tubes into the abdominal cavity)—all of which bring on secondary dysmenorrhea. A doctor must take his time to assess the problem, because painkillers may
not be appropriate.

The woman who wrote this letter is probably suffering from an
overabundance of prostaglandins and she might be helped by one of
the over-the-counter NSAIDs such as Advil, Aleve, Nuprin, or
Motrin, or an NSAID by prescription (see pages 69 to 70).

A hysterectomy should be the last possible treatment for any condition. A uterus is not just an unnecessary organ. The uterus and
ovaries might even have functions we don't know about today. They
do produce hormones, and if the uterus is removed the blood supply
to the ovaries is decreased and that might bring on other problems.
Ms. C.'s cramps, as described, are horrific, but medications such as
Danocrine tablets, Lupron injections, or Synarel nasal spray are
designed to lower hormones, relax the uterus, and stop menstruation
for a while. Any one of these medications would give her reproductive organs a rest, her body a chance to recuperate from her monthly
attacks, and might be an alternative for this woman. If the cramps
should recur, they will probably cause only minor discomfort that
can be curbed with antiprostaglandins (see chapter 7). If possible,
hysterectomy should be avoided forever.

Will Home Remedies Work?

*For the last six months I've had cramps every time I've gotten
my period. I'm twenty-three, and before now, my periods weren't
even noticeable to me. I guess something in my body has changed. I
don't like drugs and I don't want to take anything stronger than*

aspirin, which hasn't seemed to help me anyway. I'm a great believer in vitamins and fresh, natural foods. I'd like to know if there are any organic remedies or old-fashioned cures that might work. I know most doctors only like to recommend drugs, but I'm hoping you will be different.

—I.P., Shreveport, Louisiana

Heat is always helpful in relieving pain. If a woman places a heating pad on her stomach or underneath her back when she is in a supine position, the heat might relax the uterus and ease her cramps. Remember, there are muscles in the uterus that can contract and create a charley horse of the womb, and these might respond to warmth on the stomach. Nerves from the uterus enter into the spine and cause backache, so heating the back might calm the nerves.

A heating pad, however, is only one way to bring warmth to the uterus. Massage, a long soak in a hot tub, or a soothing liniment rubdown might naturally tranquilize the uterine muscles.

Alcohol and Pain. Recent studies in our laboratories have shown that alcohol has a definite relaxing effect on the uterine muscles. A mature woman who does not have extreme cramping might remedy her mild pain with a drink or two. She might even use a heat remedy along with a glass of wine. Naturally, I am not recommending alcoholic beverages to teenage girls, but a mature woman who knows her own body might be able to alleviate her pain with one or two glasses of wine.

Mind Control. Scientists have taught us that the brain creates its own opiate—a morphinelike substance called beta-endorphin, which affects the way a person is able to tolerate pain. Marathon runners who are pained and drained just before the end of a race are able to go that last half mile, it is believed, from a surge of beta-endorphins. The biofeedback movement has shown that people can learn to control their heartbeats and blood pressure, cure their headaches and insomnia, and so forth with their minds.

The ability of the mind to change the body chemistry with brain impulses and beta-endorphins is being proven again and again. If a person learns to relax—through yoga, meditation, reading a book of poetry, whatever suits her personality—it seems that beta-endorphins will do the rest. A woman who knows she will be suffering severe menstrual cramps might try to remove the pain herself by stimulating her beta-endorphins through her own forms of pleasure and relaxation. Some women feel particularly sexually responsive just prior to menstruation, and intercourse during this time might be nature's way of bringing beta-endorphins to the fore.

The first famous case of organic painkilling was that of the late Norman Cousins, a prestigious editor and writer who in the 1970s laughed his way out of a crippling disease with *Candid Camera* classics and old Marx Brothers movies: "I made the joyous discovery that ten minutes of genuine belly laughter had an anesthetic effect and would give me at least two hours of pain-free sleep. When the painkilling effect of the laughter wore off, we would switch on the motion-picture projector again, and not infrequently, it would lead to another pain-free sleep interval."[3]

Does Exercise Help?

I'm suffering from extreme cramping during my menstrual periods and my health club instructor told me that if I exercised more I wouldn't feel so bad. Is she right? Can exercise really make cramps disappear?

—E.R., Waco, Texas

Exercise can be naturally tranquilizing, and it is certainly a better painkiller than narcotic drugs. All women can benefit from personal fitness programs. As I mentioned before, an overweight woman has fatty tissue that produces excess estrogen, which, in turn, creates a thicker uterine lining, more bleeding, and, often, more cramps for her. It is always better to exercise and stay thin so that you keep your estrogen level down and you bleed only moderately.

I continue to recommend the following exercises, which fitness expert Olinda Cedeno shared with me years ago. The exercises should be done every day. At least, do them for the week before and during your period. Situate yourself on a floor mat or on carpeting. Here are Olinda's instructions:

Upper Back Stretch. Sit with your knees bent and legs crossed, Indian fashion (see figure 3-4). Clasp both hands behind your head and point your elbows out to the sides. Keep your chest raised, shoulders relaxed, eyes forward. Open your mouth slightly and breathe in for two slow counts. As you breathe out, pull in your stomach as much as you can, round your back, and drop your chin to your chest. Close your elbows together. Drop your chin farther into your chest, pull in your stomach tighter, and stretch your upper back. (see figure 3-5). Breathe in and rise up slowly to the original sitting position. Repeat the movement very slowly four times. On

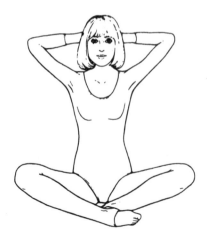

3-4 **Initial Position for the Upper Back Stretch.** Exercise for relief of menstrual cramps.

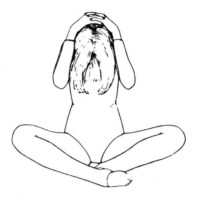

3-5   **Position Two for the Upper Back Stretch.** Exercise for relief of menstrual cramps.

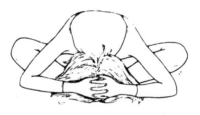

3-6   **Position Three for the Upper Back Stretch.** Exercise for relief of menstrual cramps.

the fourth round, instead of returning to the original position, breathe in and out and begin stretching downward, aiming the top of your head toward the floor. Continue to round your back and pull in your stomach. Open your elbows. Breathe in and out with the downward stretch until your head practically touches the floor (see figure 3-6). Relax your arms and hands on the floor. Breathe in and out, and with the head down, slowly roll up (see figure 3-7), vertebra by vertebra, to a sitting position.

Pelvic Tilt. Lie flat on your back with the vertebrae of your neck pressed against the floor. Bend both knees. Keep your feet flat and slightly apart. Keep your chin tucked and shoulders relaxed. Breathe

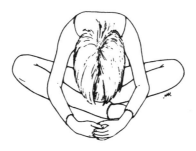

3-7 **Position Four for the Upper Back Stretch.** Exercise for relief of menstrual cramps.

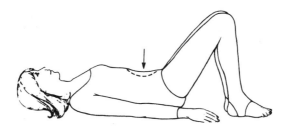

3-8 **The Pelvic Tilt for Relief of Menstrual Cramps.** The arrow indicates how the stomach must be pulled in as the small of the back is pressed against the floor.

in for two counts. As you breathe out, pull in your stomach, tilt your pelvis under, press the small of your back to the floor, and squeeze your buttocks as tight as you can. Hold for two seconds. Breathe out and relax. Repeat eight times. (See figure 3-8.)

Comfort Pose. For relief of cramps any time during your period, lie flat on your back. Bend both knees to your chest, relax your feet, and clasp each knee with a hand. Pull your knees down toward your armpits. Open your mouth slightly and breathe in for two counts, out for two counts. Breathe in and out for ten rounds or as many times as necessary for pain relief. Foot rotations increase circulation during the comfort pose. Point your toes, circle *outward* and flex five times. Point, circle *inward* and flex five times. (See figure 3-9.)

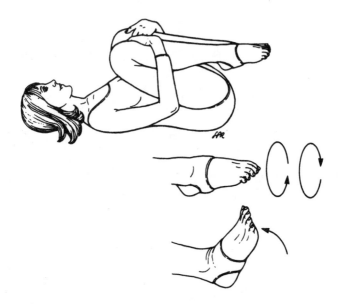

3-9   **The Comfort Pose for Relief of Menstrual Cramps.** Lie flat on your back with your
      knees pulled close to your chest. While in this position, point the toes of both feet and
      move each foot in a circular motion five times to the right (center drawing), flexing the
      foot with each rotation (bottom drawing). Follow these circular movements with five
      foot rotations to the left. Repeat these movements in cyclic fashion as many times as
      needed.

   These exercises work the stomach and lower back, and keep you
breathing deeply, to help you cope with menstrual pain. Menstrual
cramps are real, but so are the treatments for them.

4.

Premenstrual Syndrome—the Monthly Malady

THE WAY IT WAS

In the 1980s, when a woman I will call Helen visited my office, she told me she didn't know whether she was in the right place; maybe she should be talking to a psychiatrist instead of a gynecologist. She worked as a librarian and, befitting her position, Helen was an even-tempered, gentle, introspective person. Yet every month, approximately seven or eight days before her menstrual period began, she became "demonic," which is her word. She had tremendous difficulty coping with her life because everything, from the weather to a teenage boy who wanted reference books to the inflection in her husband's voice, seemed to irritate her.

Helen had already been divorced once, because after four years her previous husband had considered her to be "unreasonable and unbearable." She was afraid she might lose her second husband and also her job. It wasn't just her personality that underwent a transformation. Helen suffered physically, too, and because of this she had taken many sick days. But what could she do? A pulsating headache gave her double vision, and sometimes she couldn't even lie down and close her eyes because an accompanying backache was relieved only if she sat in a straight-backed chair for a while. All in all, she could hardly get through a day at home, much less at work.

"It's like being possessed," she said. "I know it's going to happen every month. I try to control my mind and my body, but the force is too much for me. I feel schizophrenic, as if I'm doomed. But then my period starts, and two days into it, I'm fine. I can't understand why the world looked so bleak, why my husband seemed so impossible, why I didn't like my job. Usually when I tell doctors about my pattern, they advise me to slow down. I know I'm not going to be cured by taking it easy with a vacation or meditation, or any of the two dozen suggestions I've received, so I'm here with you. My problem is physical, I think." Helen's problem was indeed physical, hormonal, and real.

Many women experience what today's enlightened doctors recognize as premenstrual syndrome, or PMS, which starts anywhere from two to fourteen days before menstruation and has a formidable list of symptoms. Here's a sampling: *feeling sad, hopeless, or self-deprecating; feeling tense, anxious, or "on edge"; marked lability of mood interspersed with frequent tearfulness; persistent irritability, anger, and increased interpersonal conflicts; decreased interest in usual activities; difficulty concentrating; feeling fatigued, lethargic, or lacking in energy; marked changes in appetite, which might be associated with binge eating or craving certain foods; hypersomnia or insomnia; a subjective feeling of being overwhelmed or out of control, and physical symptoms such as breast tenderness or swelling, headaches, or sensations of "bloating" or weight gain.*

When extreme, these symptoms help mental health professionals to recognize a severe PMS-related depression known as premenstrual dysphoric disorder, or PMDD, which affects a small percentage of menstruating women. For a psychiatrist to make a clinical diagnosis of PMDD, at least five of the above symptoms have to exist in the last week of the menstrual cycle and be nonexistent at other times. When the diagnosis is strictly followed, it reportedly affects 2.5 percent of menstruating women. Yet the total number of PMS sufferers might be as high as 90 percent of all women of reproductive age.

We know more about PMS today, however, because PMDD has sparked the interest of medical researchers. From a decade's worth

PREMENSTRUAL SYNDROME

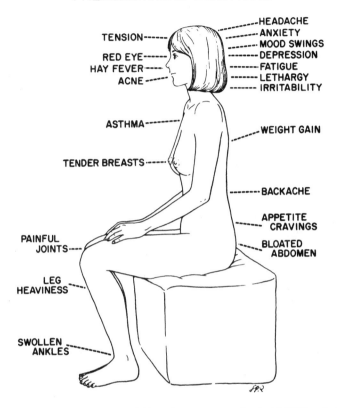

4-1   **Premenstrual Syndrome (PMS).** Typical symptoms associated with PMS are indicated. A woman might suffer one or several of these symptoms at the same time. The symptoms usually appear anywhere from two to fourteen days before the onset of the menstrual flow.

of investigations, we have learned how shifting patterns of the hormones estrogen and progesterone (see section "How Does Premenstrual Syndrome Begin?") might act on "receptors" in the brain and affect the release of your body's mood-regulating brain chemicals, the neurotransmitters. We have also discovered that calcium, magnesium, and certain vitamin supplements might bring relief to sufferers.

HOW DOES PREMENSTRUAL SYNDROME BEGIN?

A woman knows she has premenstrual syndrome (PMS) when, just like clockwork, the symptoms appear two to fourteen days before her menstruation and disappear shortly after she begins to bleed. It isn't likely that any one woman will experience every affliction mentioned earlier, but symptoms are known to combine in a variety of plaguing ways. A woman might be tired and depressed or have backache and nausea or become irritable and weepy. If she sees herself change month after month for a fairly fixed number of days, and she realizes that she can transform practically overnight, she suffers from PMS.

As I explained in chapter 3, the feminine cycle depends upon the ebb and flow of beautifully synchronized hormonal fluctuations. Before ovulation, estrogen, the first female hormone, is being produced by all the little egg cells in the ovaries. During ovulation, the Graafian follicle, the egg-of-the-month, bursts, ejects a mature egg cell, and leaves behind the cell formation called the corpus luteum, the producer of progesterone, the second female hormone. As a result of the increase of both female hormones, a soft spongy lining, a nest for a fertilized egg, builds within the womb. Of course, if the mature egg is not fertilized, the spongy uterine lining, which is made of glandular tissue rich in blood vessels, isn't needed. About fourteen days after ovulation, then, the unused lining will shed itself in the form of menstrual blood.

An imbalance of the two surging hormones was once considered key to understanding PMS, but that was before researchers discovered that many women with normal levels of estrogen and progesterone suffer, too. Now researchers feel that not only hormonal levels, but the way certain brain receptors—the action sites of nerve cells—respond to those levels, might cause PMS. Whatever inner workings eventually prove central to the syndrome, the fact remains that estrogen and progesterone are powerful forces within a woman's body.

There's a positive side to the estrogen/progesterone rush after ovulation. Estrogen increases the blood supply to the endometrium, the uterine lining that progesterone is turning into a bed for fertilization. Estrogen also makes a woman's skin smooth and blemishfree. Besides being the architect of the endometrium, progesterone relaxes the uterus, alters the cervical mucus, and can, in combination with estrogen, stimulate the sex drive. Just like a pregnant woman who, living with an increase of estrogen and progesterone for nine months, often feels sexier, a woman who has a high amount of female hormones after ovulation sometimes responds more sexually too. When these hormones are in balance, women usually feel wonderful. When estrogen and progesterone aren't in tune, when there's too much of one or too little of the other, certain symptoms connected to the premenstrual syndrome might arise.

On the downside, estrogen binds salt and salt binds water, so high estrogen can lead to water retention, which can cause swelling of the brain membrane. Then, the pulling of the nerve tissue surrounding

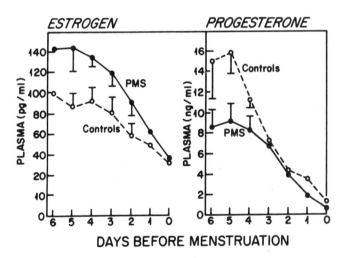

4-2 **Hormone Levels Before Menstruation.** In an early study of women with severe PMS, which has anxiety and mood swings as two of its main symptoms, the premenstrual estrogen levels are higher and the progesterone levels are lower, when comparisons are made with controls—women without PMS. Natural progesterone suppositories and tablets are effective in alleviating PMS symptoms in some cases.

the brain can result in headache, dizziness, and hypersensitivity to light, which are all symptoms of premenstrual syndrome. Also, a woman will feel heavy and bloated all over. She'll experience an added pressure in her abdomen and bowel area, and she might have gas pains.

The appearance of progesterone in the second half of the menstrual cycle might create a variety of symptoms. These symptoms will be more pronounced if there isn't just enough estrogen to balance the progesterone. There will be bladder pressure and bowel irritation from which gas and constipation might result. Progesterone might give a woman ravenous food cravings. She might long for sweets due to lowered blood sugar, and at the same time she might feel hot because her body temperature has risen. Women might develop allergic reactions and have little resistance to infection. Physical symptoms can become so severe that they upset a woman's mental health.

Progesterone can also make a normally energetic woman feel incredibly fatigued. For years, natural progesterone vaginal suppositories were recommended to alter a woman's hormonal balance and relieve her PMS. Many of my patients still find relief from PMS-related irritability, nervousness, and tension through progesterone suppositories or tablets; however, this treatment has *not* been shown to be effective in relieving PMS depression. One of the areas researchers are delving into is whether and how the female sex hormones affect the mood-regulating chemicals in your brain, particularly a neurotransmitter called serotonin. To date, no one has uncovered the hormonal interactions that result in PMS.

HOW BAD CAN IT BE?

When a woman's body goes into premenstrual syndrome, tension can build to the point of triggering irritability, lethargy, and depression. Sometimes a depression can be so intense that a woman doesn't get out of bed because she sees no reason to live. Suicides among women are known to increase during premenstrual days. At the other extreme, premenstrual women have succumbed to violent outbursts that have caused them to batter their own children. It has been reported that in the United Kingdom PMS can be considered a mitigating factor in a crime. And in France a woman who commits a crime while in the throes of premenstrual syndrome can plead temporary insanity. Like Helen, many women regularly feel as if they are becoming schizophrenic.

Even without creating a psychological side effect, however, premenstrual syndrome can drain a woman. The physical effects of PMS run the gamut: joint pains, backache, sinusitis, sore throat, glaucoma, conjunctivitis, styes, asthma, rhinitis (sniffles), acne, herpes, urticaria (skin rashes), migraine, epilepsy, syncope (fainting spells)—and this is only a partial list. Headaches alone can make a woman's whole body tremble.

Premenstrual syndrome is not a condition to be laughed at or considered weird. Millions of menstruating women are suffering pain, living with uncontrollable mood swings, and trying to cope. The syndrome invades their lives, breaks up their marriages, and undermines their ability to function in their homes or at their jobs. Until menstrual blood begins to flow, which is the time when progesterone and estrogen hormones diminish, many women don't feel well. They become themselves only after their hormones have reached a crescendo and then subsided. After that happens, they're fine—until the next time the monthly malady strikes.

HOW PMS WAS DISCOVERED

One of the first people to recognize the effects of premenstrual syndrome was Dr. Katharina Dalton, a British physician who in 1953 published the first paper in British medical literature on PMS. She wrote the paper with Dr. Raymond Greene, a noted endocrinologist who had been working on premenstrual syndrome at the same time.

Dr. Dalton's experiences with her own period led her to suspect that premenstrual changes had far-ranging effects. She herself got a splitting migraine each month before her period. In 1953, when she was called in on the case of a woman who had asthmatic seizures each month just before she menstruated, Dr. Dalton started to consider linking different symptoms with the premenstrual condition. Another case of asthma turned up, followed by a woman with a monthly migraine. Drs. Dalton and Greene interviewed eighty-seven sufferers in order to write their first paper, and the rest, as they say, is medical history.

Dr. Dalton became a pioneer and authority in the field of premenstrual syndrome. She was able to identify premenstrual changes as influences in criminal behavior, accidents, drug abuse, and death. Her work was applied to women in factories, schools, prisons, and hospitals, and for decades no one matched her dedication to the problem. Her books on premenstrual syndrome are widely known in the medical profession, and, as was mentioned earlier, her book *Once a Month* was the first of its kind, a breakthrough book about PMS.

Premenstrual syndrome hits the mighty and the meek, as Dr. Dalton points out when she describes the relationship of eighteen-year-old Queen Victoria to Albert in her book. Albert, a very rational man, could not find the logic in Victoria's unpredictable, emotional outbursts. She would hurl objects and scream at him, and no matter what he did—shout or keep quiet—he was wrong. Only Victoria's pregnancies gave him spells of serenity, and he looked forward to them because pregnancy, at least, he understood.

In the past men have not comprehended the turmoil that can ensue within women during their premenstrual days, and women, since doctors used to tell them that they were physically fine, did not connect personally disturbing, out-of-control times to their upcoming menstruations. Women now clearheadedly evaluate their premenstrual changes without fear that they'll be patronized or made to feel crazy.

Many forward-thinking doctors are doing their best to champion women by investigating the origins of premenstrual syndrome. One important study, headed by Dr. Peter J. Schmidt of the National Institute of Mental Health in 1998, reported that estrogen's hormonal activity *early* in the menstrual cycle might lead to PMS. In our book *PMS: Premenstrual Syndrome and You* (Fireside/Simon & Schuster), we explain that years ago studies showed that increased estrogen in the first half of the menstrual cycle affects PMS. Nevertheless, researchers continued to target the effects of progesterone *late* in the cycle. Dr. Schmidt's finding has shifted the focus back to estrogen. His study of fifteen women with PMS and fifteen women who were PMS-free highlighted the complex relationship between hormones and behavior, and showed that *estrogen might be just as potent as progesterone in promoting PMS.*

In recent years, doctors have started treating a percentage of women who have a severe PMS-related depression (PMDD) with antidepressants called selective serotonin re-uptake inhibitors, or SSRIs, brand-name drugs such as Zoloft, Prozac, Serzone, Paxil, and Luvox. In studies, these drugs raise levels of the mood-altering brain chemical serotonin and reduce PMS symptoms such as depression, mood swings, and cravings by more than half. Another antidepressant, Wellbutrin, is not an SSRI but has been prescribed for women with PMDD who appreciate its side effect as a weight reducer. However, these powerful medications should only be prescribed for women whose lives are seriously curtailed by PMDD. They are certainly not for everyone.

Lupron injections and Synarel nasal spray have been used to fight PMS but are also not highly recommended for everyone. Known as gonadotropin-releasing hormone (GnRH) agonists, they chemically induce menopause. PMS symptoms disappear but a woman becomes susceptible to conditions such as osteoporosis and heart disease.

I have always felt that the nutritional approach was the best first step to take in treating PMS. My PMS diet is detailed in our book *PMS: Premenstrual Syndrome and You.* For me a low-fat, high-fiber diet, vitamin supplements, and exercise (see pages 99 to 100) are a woman's best weapons for fighting PMS.

The most encouraging news is that calcium can bring relief to PMS sufferers. A 1998 study of over 400 women, headed by researchers at St. Luke's–Roosevelt Hospital Center in New York, showed that 1,200 mg of calcium carbonate a day cut PMS symptoms almost in half. Women have tried taking progesterone, estrogen, diuretics, vitamins, minerals, and herbs in efforts to treat PMS. I have personally advised these treatments for relief, and they seem to work for many women. Although the success rates vary from study to study, my patients often report good results.

The letters I've received have shown me that women are ready to fight for themselves, investigate extensively on their own, and use all their energies to overcome premenstrual syndrome. They write about their baffled spouses, their frightened children, and their own personal tortures. It's true that they can find some relief at this time, but women must demand improved treatments through continued research. After learning about the latest remedies from responses to the following letters, women might request new treatments from their doctors. First, however, a woman must recognize her symptoms to be able to judge the best treatments.

HOW CAN PMS BE RELIEVED?

"I'm Impossible to Live With"

I'm a talkative, optimistic, outgoing twenty-five-year-old woman for two weeks out of every month. For the other ten days to two weeks my whole outlook on life changes. I become moody and sullen. I don't talk much but when I do I'm usually negative. I'm so irritable that even if someone at work offers to buy me a cup of coffee, I growl and hiss. Also, my skin breaks out during those weeks. I gain at least six pounds, and sleeping becomes my favorite thing to do. I can't stand it. I've seen four doctors already and they've suggested everything—Zoloft, diuretics, and "the pill." I've tried diuretics but antidepressants and "the pill" don't seem safe to me. One of the doctors told me to exercise but I'm too sick for that. Is there anything you could suggest? I'm impossible to live with, and I feel I owe it to myself, my family, and my future husband, whoever he might be, to find a cure for these horrible two weeks.

—D.B., Terre Haute, Indiana

Please help me. Once a month I risk losing my husband and driving my children from home. I have seen my family doctor and all he does is give me vitamin B-complex. There have been times I wanted to take the whole bottle. I'm in despair for someone to help me. All my family and my husband's family say I'm going to have a nervous breakdown. I know something is wrong but I don't know what to do about it. I have turned my world into something that no husband or children would want. Please help me.

—R.H., Nashville, Tennessee

As I mentioned earlier, premenstrual syndrome is generally caused by hormonal activity, which can turn a woman upside down. Estrogen binds salt and salt binds water, so a high estrogen level can lead to water retention throughout a woman's body. This water-logged condition can create a sudden weight gain and pressure in the abdomen and bowels. The brain membrane swells along with everything else, and a woman's head begins to throb.

If a woman cuts down on salt a few days before she expects her symptoms, then she might be able to eliminate some of the water tension in her body. (By marking her calendar on the days that symptoms occur, a woman will be giving herself a guideline for the onset of the next month's syndrome.) While she's reducing her salt, she should drink a lot of water to wash out the salt that is already present. If she doesn't notice any relief and she still feels bloated, then she might try diuretics, such as spironolactone (brand name Aldactone), taken in the last two to fourteen days before a period.

It's difficult to determine from the first letter whether the diuretics helped Ms. B., but if you do turn to a diuretic to eliminate surplus water, be careful of your potassium level. Some diuretics will cause a woman to excrete too much potassium, enough to change her metabolism, tire her, and sometimes slow her heartbeat. In order to prevent potassium depletion, it's a good idea to eat bananas and drink orange juice, both of which are natural sources of the substance, while you're on diuretics. If a woman still doesn't feel like herself, she might want to visit the doctor to have her potassium level checked. He will be able to prescribe the exact potassium tablet dosage she needs.

Now if salt reduction and diuretics fail to make any alteration in the symptoms, the problem might stem from the progesterone that appears after ovulation. The increase in progesterone might be causing the depression in both women letter writers and giving Ms. B. her extreme fatigue and acne. It has been found that 100 to 500 mg of vitamin B_6 (pyroxidine) a day can bring relief to this situation. Women who have taken vitamin B_6 every day, or at least for two weeks of their cycles, have had less depression, more energy, and clearer skin.

Unfortunately, however, sometimes cutting down on salt and taking diuretics and extra vitamins does nothing to release a woman from the painful grip of her premenstrual syndrome. If the women who wrote these letters, or any women for that matter, try everything as outlined and still think they're impossible to live with, they might be helped by visiting a gynecologist or endocrinologist who has an understanding of PMS. No woman should feel that she has a stranger living in her skin for half of every month, and if a blood test shows a progesterone imbalance, it can be corrected with progesterone suppositories or tablets.

Women might experience PMS anytime during their childbearing years, right up until menopause. The syndrome is a sign that a woman's body chemistry, her hormonal balance, is somehow disturbed. She might be under stress, ill, have nutritional deficiencies, or be feeling the effects of age. Sometimes women encounter PMS for the first time after childbirth, after coming off birth control pills, or after tubal sterilization. Any event that affects hormonal balance can influence the onset of PMS.

I strongly feel that each PMS sufferer needs individualized treatment for relief. I begin by designing a natural approach to PMS relief, using nutrition, exercise, and vitamin—and sometimes herbal—supplementation before turning to medication. For me, the nutritional aspect is always the first consideration in treating PMS. (See our book *PMS: Premenstrual Syndrome and You* for an in-depth description of natural PMS relief.)

Most women need a minimum of 1,400 calories a day in order to function properly. I suggest distributing those calories over six small meals a day to help stabilize blood sugar levels and alleviate some symptoms. A woman's diet should include:

- whole-grain, complex carbohydrates such as whole-wheat bread, pasta, and cereals
- low-fat, high-calcium foods like nonfat yogurt, low-fat cheese, pink salmon (with bones), sardines, pinto beans, kale, bok choy, and broccoli
- essential fatty acids found in cold-pressed cooking oils such as sesame, walnut, or olive

You should avoid:

- sugar
- alcohol
- coffee and tea
- salt
- dairy products
- high-sugar fruits like raisins, grapes, bananas, cherries, dates or dried fruits
- high-carbohydrate foods like white bread, cake, cookies, doughnuts, pastries, and candy

I also recommend daily vitamin supplements starting with a vitamin/mineral multivitamin, and then additional vitamin E (400 IU), vitamin B-complex (100 mg), vitamin B_6 (200–500 mg), vitamin C (1,000 mg/time-released), and calcium 1,000 mg with magnesium.

(Some of my patients have also found relief by including herbal supplementation such as black cohosh.)

Regular, moderate workouts help decrease many physical and emotional symptoms linked to hormonal imbalance. At the start, I suggest a workout of twenty minutes, three times weekly, then increasing the time slowly, adding about three minutes to each session once a week for six weeks. Workouts should have a permanent place in every woman's week.

In creating individualized treatments I have found that sometimes, in combination with the natural approach to treating PMS, natural progesterone by prescription—either in vaginal suppositories (200 to 400 mg, once or twice daily or more if necessary); or in Crinone, a new gel (inserted two to four times daily); or in Prometrium tablets (100 mg two to four times daily)—brings relief of PMS irritability and nervousness. If you have difficulty obtaining natural progesterone in your area, you and your doctor can contact Madison Pharmacy Associates/Women's Health America Group at 1-800-558-7046; or Apthorp Pharmacy at 1-800-775-3582 (in New York: 212-877-3480).

It is only in extreme cases, when PMS symptoms include severe depression leading to PMDD, that a woman might need the SSRI antidepressants discussed previously, such as Zoloft, Prozac, Paxil, Serozone, and Luvox.

"Everyone Hates Me"

My doctor hasn't been able to help me. A week, sometimes two weeks, before my period I feel like no one wants to be around me. I am tired, dizzy, headachey, and very irritable. I'm sure everyone hates me until my period starts and I feel better. But then two weeks later, my awful feelings and paranoia begin again. I'm overweight, but otherwise I seem to be in good health. What can I do? Sometimes I'm so positive that nobody likes me I cry for hours.
—P.K., Brooklyn, New York

This is an extremely sad and poignant letter. No one has given this woman the support she needs to understand her condition and help herself. The headaches, dizziness, and fatigue she is suffering might be due to estrogen's hormonal activity. As mentioned earlier, she should cut down on her salt intake and drink plenty of water to wash out the existing salt. Daily dosage of vitamin B—particularly vitamin B_6—in 50-to-500-mg tablets might also help to counterbalance some of her symptoms, and diuretics might even be advised.

The fact that she is overweight is highly significant. Fatty tissue produces an excess of estrogen, so this woman obviously has an abundance of this hormone in her body. As her estrogen increases in the last half of her menstrual cycle, she is being overpowered. She must diet, exercise, and lose weight or the recommended remedies are likely to be ineffective.

Wellbutrin is an antidepressant that has been effective in relieving PMS-related depression while it helps curb appetite and contribute to weight reduction. This woman might ask her doctor about recommending Wellbutrin for her. She must begin to think positively, believe in herself, and try to slim down. If all this fails to help her improve significantly, she might well be a candidate for progesterone suppositories.

Will Having a Baby Help?

When I was a teenager I would get really unreasonable with my boyfriend and my mother at least one week out of every month. Sometimes in the middle of a nasty tirade, however, I'd stop because I'd get weak and dizzy. My mother thought there was something really wrong with me and took me to doctor after doctor. All the doctors said the same thing: "After you have children your hormones will change and you'll be fine." So I endured my adolescence, which I think was harder on the people around me than it was on me, and I married and gave birth to three terrific children in four years.

Now my problem is starting all over again. I don't seem to have changed at all, except now I have a husband and three children to cope with as well. After all those promises, what went wrong? Why did the doctors lie to me?

—A.G., Wheeling, West Virginia

Giving birth to a baby will not make a woman's premenstrual syndrome disappear. A doctor who tells a woman she can expect relief after pregnancy is either deluded or lying. Queen Victoria, as mentioned earlier, was serene during pregnancy, but only during pregnancy. A pregnant or breast-feeding woman lives with a steady hormonal balance in her body that makes her feel good, but after she gives birth or stops breast-feeding, her hormones return as if they had never left. A woman's hormonal activity before pregnancy will return after pregnancy. She will always be battling her premenstrual syndrome, and her best hope for relief will come from the remedies already discussed. On the other hand, she might be one of those women whose estrogen production changes as she gets older, in which case age might release her from her symptoms.

Is "the Pill" the Cure?

After I had my two children I went on "the pill" for seven years. I had lived with the horrible tension of premenstrual syndrome before my children were born, but with my pregnancies and then "the pill" I sort of forgot what the syndrome had done to me. Birth control pills made me feel wonderful. I would have been happy to live with them until menopause, but as I got older, my husband made me stop taking them. He got a vasectomy instead. I was fine for three months and then I began reliving the nightmare of my younger days. Headache, backache, a chronic cold, and a feeling of absolute doom for about ten days a month. I'm tempted to return to "the pill" in spite of its side effects for older women.

—E.C., Flagstaff, Arizona

Modern birth control pills contain a combination of estrogen and progesterone in amounts that vary widely from one brand of pill to another. Certain pills have a progesterone concentration that is too potent for some women and gives them acne and breakthrough bleeding. Other pills are designed to make estrogen the more powerful hormone. A doctor should be able to evaluate a woman and prescribe a pill that will be right for her, one that will not give her any discomfort.

For many years doctors thought premenstrual syndrome had decreased in women, but the fact was that many more women were on the pill and women who had been suffering from PMS felt better due to the steady hormonal level produced by the contraceptive. When "the pill scare" came, a great number of women discarded their supplies and turned to other forms of birth control. It was then that women who previously had been plagued by hormonal imbalance experienced their old symptoms once more.

However, reports on side effects had been based on studies of high-estrogen-containing pills. Studies have indicated that these side effects are greatly reduced if today's low-estrogen-containing pills are used (see chapter 12). A woman with severe PMS who sees a break in her misery and also needs contraception might ask her doctor for information about low-estrogen birth control pills. Since Ms. C. felt well when on the pill before, if her doctor finds no medical contraindications, she might resume taking it. This time she should be prescribed the lowest-estrogen-containing pill. Today we know that women over age thirty-five can continue to take the pill if they are nonsmokers and their doctors approve.

NOTE: If a woman with PMS starts taking a birth control pill and feels worse than she did before, she should try another brand with a different hormonal balance. If her symptoms never go away, she might be extraordinarily sensitive to the hormones in all pills and she should stop them immediately and altogether.

Migraine Misery

I'm forty years old and for the last six years I've been getting
terrible migraines a week before my period. The headaches are so
severe that I often have double vision too. Is there anything I can do?
—R.S., Montclair, New Jersey

Migraines come in several varieties. The classic kind is preceded by an aura—flashes of light and tingling sensations—before the headache actually begins. The common migraine is an escalating pain that doesn't have an introductory aura. A lack of food or sensitivity to certain foods can bring on a migraine, which might be considered a family trait.

In a class by itself, a premenstrual migraine is likely to be caused by hormonal fluctuations, and there are several treatments a woman might seek. Relief might come from a low-salt diet, the vitamin B group, progesterone suppositories, or birth control pills. All of these remedies have been described in this chapter. The prostaglandin-blocking drugs Motrin, Anaprox, and Ponstel, explained in chapter 3 might also be helpful.

If there is no letup, if none of these treatments work, a woman should make an appointment with a neurologist to determine what kind of migraine she has. A neurologist will look for hidden, underlying causes—disease or tumors. The source of the migraine might be something totally different than premenstrual syndrome. In fact, if it's a migraine not related to the menstrual cycle, one of several migraine medications—Imitrex, Zomig, or Maxalt-MLT—might remedy the situation.

Why Do I Feel I Can't Live Without Chocolate?

About five days before my period I find myself stocking up on
Sara Lee fudge brownies. That's how I know my period is coming. I
really don't have too many premenstrual worries, but this chocolate
craving keeps me a little heavier than I'd like to be. I stop at all the

candy counters and buy Snickers bars, Almond Joys, Mounds, Hershey's chocolate. I'm like a moth drawn to a flame, or better, a bear hooked on honey. Sometimes I bake chocolate cakes to get me through the week. When I tell my friends my period is making me a chocolate addict, they laugh. They say I should just admit I have a sweet tooth and forget it, but I know that most of the time I don't feel this need. Are they right? Am I crazy?

—F.M., New York, New York

Progesterone changes a woman's sugar tolerance so that her blood sugar level doesn't have far to fall before she feels a need, a bona fide craving, for food. Some women must have sweets, while others demand spaghetti. Desires might be different, but every woman who succumbs to a yen for a particular food can blame her urge and subsequent weight gain on progesterone. All the jokes about pregnant women wanting ice cream and pickles can be medically explained. Pregnant women have a high progesterone level, and just before menstruation, all women are also experiencing an increase in progesterone.

This woman is not crazy, but she has to be careful to control her craving or she'll become much too overweight. Usually the body's need for food can be satisfied by a small amount of the food craved, but she's going to have to be really strong. Progesterone is increasing her appetite so she'll need a great deal of willpower. A regular exercise regimen will also help to keep her slim and might decrease any other premenstrual symptoms, cravings among them.

Are Over-the-Counter Remedies a Hoax?

When I realized that I had tension and depression every month before my period, I began reading about premenstrual syndrome in all the books, newspapers, and magazines I could find. I tried everything I learned. I followed a low-salt diet, exercised, took vitamins B and E and zinc, but I was still a mess each month. Since I had seen ads for products designed to fight PMS, I bought one in the drugstore. I followed the directions but nothing happened. I don't understand. Is everything I read a lie? Or could my body just be different?

—D.S., Burlington, Vermont

The hormonal activity that causes premenstrual syndrome is still not completely understood. As mentioned earlier, Dr. Katharina Dalton had success in freeing many women from premenstrual problems by increasing their progesterone levels with natural progesterone suppositories. Many women still say that natural progesterone vaginal suppositories or tablets offer relief, but others have not been helped. Indeed, some scientists have concluded that progesterone is an ineffective PMS reliever. That does not mean that women should never try progesterone.

Likewise, in addition to fighting PMS with vitamin therapy, diet, and exercise, some women find over-the-counter products work for them, and some say they don't. I believe that each PMS sufferer has her own set of symptoms and must therefore have her own individual method of treatment.

Over-the-counter remedies usually involve herbal preparations such as evening primrose oil, which many women find extremely helpful. Two different types of over-the-counter products are Midol Maximum Strength PMS Formula and PMS Escape. The Midol product is basically a pain reliever with a diuretic, and might be most helpful for dealing with water retention and bloating. PMS Escape is a dietary supplement developed by Dr. Judith Wurtman, a researcher at the Massachusetts Institute of Technology. This powdered carbohydrate mix is designed to combat the depression, anger, and carbo cravings of PMS by raising levels of the calming brain chemical serotonin. Carbohydrates in foods such as whole grains might have the same effect and be cheaper—PMS Escape is $10 for an eight-packet box—but if the product works for you, I would not discourage its use.

I would like to suggest daily over-the-counter calcium carbonate supplements (1,200 mg) in combination with magnesium (600 mg) to Ms. S. In one study, calcium carbonate in that amount was shown to reduce PMS symptoms by almost half, as explained on page 96.

Would Yoga or Exercise Help?

My husband insists that yoga exercises can cure everything. He wants me to stand on my head before my period to improve my circulation and take away the heaviness I feel at that time. I believe in exercise, although I think jogging is too stressful to my knees, hips, and breasts, and I wonder if he is right. Would yoga help?
—A.T., Denver, Colorado

Exercise is very important and helpful in liberating women from premenstrual problems. It is known, for example, that competitive athletes and dancers have very little premenstrual tension. Exercise seems to steady hormonal secretions, the ovaries do not become overly stimulated, and there is less bleeding. Yoga is a stretching and relaxation technique, and I don't know whether that would have the same effect as strenuous exercise, which also affects the brain's mood-changing chemicals such as serotonin. However, if yoga is the fitness method that suits a woman's lifestyle, she should use it. PMS is such a debilitating condition that I strongly suggest that women open their minds to any possible means of natural therapy—transcendental meditation, relaxation, self-hypnosis. Some women have even found relief through acupuncture.

How About Calcium?

I've recently read that I could take over-the-counter calcium supplements for my PMS. Could a cure be this easy? Please let me know what you think.
—D.H., Middletown, New Jersey

I've always encouraged the natural approach to PMS relief, as described on pages 99 and 100, and in our book *PMS: Premenstrual*

Syndrome and You (Fireside/Simon & Schuster). I was therefore pleased when a 1998 study named calcium carbonate supplements effective for fighting PMS. Researchers found that four core symptoms of PMS (negative emotional effects, water retention, food cravings, and pain) were reduced by about half among PMS sufferers taking calcium carbonate (1,200 mg) daily for three menstrual cycles. The scientists speculated that calcium might work by inhibiting hormone released by a woman's parathyroid gland. I think all women with these core symptoms might try 1,200 mg of calcium carbonate in combination with 600 mg of magnesium daily for three months to see whether their symptoms are alleviated.

A Future Cure for PMS?

I thought I'd tried and heard everything about premenstrual syndrome since I've been struggling to overcome it for the last ten years. Now a friend says she is going to a psychiatrist who is giving her Prozac for premenstrual depression. Are there any other drugs that might be helpful? How close are researchers coming to a cure?
—J.B., Scarsdale, New York

A woman who is experiencing a severe depression that she thinks is related to her menstrual cycle should be carefully evaluated by a doctor. It is known that women can become so depressed before menstruation that they can take their own lives. Whether such a deep depression is brought on by premenstrual syndrome, or is a clinical depression unrelated to menstruation, or is a combination of an existing depression and premenstrual syndrome, is open to question.

Research is already being conducted on whether women with PMS-related depression might have genetic differences in the way their brain receptors respond to the female sex hormones, estrogen and progesterone. In recent years there has been a great deal of attention paid to how these hormones affect the brain's release of its mood-regulating chemicals, the neurotransmitters. Medications such as Prozac, Zoloft, Paxil, and Serozone, which affect the neurotransmitter serotonin, which has an uplifting effect on mood, have been prescribed for relief of severe PMS depression. I suspect that researchers will uncover the workings of other neurotransmitters that are affected by the ebb and flow of estrogen and progesterone, and that more medications will be targeted for PMS relief.

However, I see a future when PMS treatments are tailored to each woman. Today's researchers have spoken out about the complexity of premenstrual syndrome as it affects each woman. The fact that every woman who suffers does so uniquely is being more widely recognized. As this perspective takes hold, I believe that doctors will custom-design treatments for each PMS sufferer.

I feel that the natural approach to PMS relief is basic. I encourage all women to maintain a lifestyle that includes a healthy, well-balanced diet; exercise; and vitamin supplementation. After that, treatment can be tailored to fit a woman's symptoms. She might find relief with natural progesterone, or with diuretics, or with antidepressants. If a woman continues to suffer, she might need medication to stop her menstrual period completely for a while and give her reproductive system a "rest." Such a medication would be one of the GnRH agonists such as Lupron or Synarel. On the other hand, some women might benefit from oral contraceptives that can regulate their periods.

For me, the best news is the growing number of doctors who are tailoring their PMS treatments to the needs of individual women. I have successfully treated thousands of women with the "tailored treatment" approach, which takes into account personal symptoms, lifestyles, and needs. The results have been terrific. I remind the women in my care, however, that what works today might not work forever. As a woman matures or her lifestyle changes, she might need different forms of relief, but this is all part of the tailored treatment approach. A future cure depends on the physician who looks at each PMS sufferer as separate and unique.

5.

Unpredictable Periods

THE MENSTRUAL CYCLE—
YOUR BODY'S BAROMETER

As women's lifestyles and health habits are changing, so are their menstrual cycles. Many more girls today are experiencing menarche (the onset of menstruation) when they're ten or eleven, instead of at twelve, at thirteen, or even at the older ages that were more typical for first periods in the past. Also, once begun, menstruation extends longer in life than it used to, and it is not uncommon for menopause to be delayed until a woman reaches her late fifties.

In medical circles, it is thought that two of the main reasons for these menstrual changes are better nutrition and increased average weight gain. In spite of the endless appeal of junk food—french fries, chocolate malts, and burgers of all varieties—most people have become more health-and-nutrition conscious and are consuming quality foods and vitamins in abundance. So menstrual cycles—generally, over the years, and specifically, month-to-month—are reacting to healthier diets. Individually, women are experiencing more regular menstrual patterns. But there is still no "perfect" cycle.

Most women do not have exact twenty-eight-day menstrual cycles. In fact, the time span of cycles for any given group of women can realistically be plotted on a bell curve (see figure 5-1). Some women have their periods in fewer than twenty-eight days, while

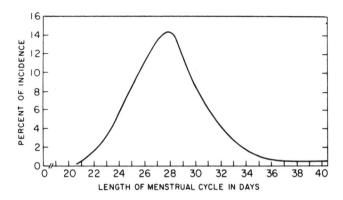

5-1 **Duration of the Menstrual Cycle.** The number of days from one menstruation to another varies anywhere from twenty-one days to, occasionally, more than forty days. The average length, as seen in the illustration, is around twenty-eight days.

others live with cycles that might take thirty, thirty-one, thirty-four, or more days from start to finish. Every woman usually knows what's "normal" for her, and she senses when "normal" goes haywire.

As explained in chapter 3, menstruation is the end result of a carefully orchestrated interplay between a woman's brain and her ovaries. Here is a biological phenomenon that shows how inseparable the mind, body, and senses can be. Everything is finely tuned. Hormonal systems are acting and reacting within. The cycle is supersensitive to changes inside and outside the body. It's known, for example, that certain female animals only have to *smell* their mates and they'll start to ovulate, while for others *seeing* their mates triggers ovulation. Obviously, "chemistry" is important in all of the animal kingdom, but humans have brains that play significant roles in their chemical reactions, and what can happen is amazing.

It is quite common for women who share dormitory rooms, apartments, even offices, to find that their menstrual cycles are in sync. And it also frequently happens that women who travel a lot have irregular or missed periods, and women who are under stress find themselves with erratic cycles. In fact, doctors see so much out-of-the-ordinary uterine bleeding that the different types have been categorized. *Amenorrhea* is the term used when menstruation has never occurred (primary amenorrhea) or has disappeared after months or years of normalcy (secondary amenorrhea). *Metorrhagia* describes heavy bleeding. *Oligomenorrhea* refers to infrequent or irregular bleeding, and *menorrhagia* defines the reverse problem— periods that come more often than once a month.

All these different types of what is medically recognized as "abnormal uterine bleeding" can usually be traced to events that are happening in women's lives that interfere with their cycles. What's ironic, however, is that sometimes a woman can worry so much about why her period has changed that her worry alters her hormonal secretions further and causes the menstrual mix-up to continue.

This nervousness exists because many women still have misconceptions about their monthly cycle. A survey conducted by Tampax in the 1980s showed a surprising lack of understanding about menstruation. The study, which still is the only one of its kind, found that:

- An astounding number (31 percent) of the women surveyed had no idea what was happening to them at the time of their first menstruations.
- About their first periods, 49 percent of the women interviewed felt pleased, had no problems; but two out of five, or 43 percent, stated that they were "frightened, confused, panicky, or ill."
- The menstrual cycle is a subject that most women do not talk about or only discuss with great difficulty. Only 35 percent of the women in the study felt that it was appropriate to talk about their periods at the office, while merely 33 percent felt menstruation could be a topic of conversation socially.
- A majority (87 percent) of Americans believe that women are very emotional when they are menstruating, and 35 percent believe that menstruation affects a woman's ability to think.

Such misconceptions and fears definitely contribute to stress and menstrual irregularity. The results of the Tampax report show how important it is to promote health education. If girls could be informed about their bodies before menarche, they might avoid menstrual problems when they are adults.

DEALING WITH UNPREDICTABLE PERIODS

Many women have written to me in states of complete confusion. They don't understand why their menstrual periods fluctuate so much and they're concerned that they might have serious physical problems. Most of the time, they are perfectly healthy. Their bodies are reacting to their environments or stress, however, and their doctors are not explaining the disturbances within their delicately balanced inner systems.

The aims of this chapter are to alleviate worry and misunderstanding and to give women insights into how to cope with unpredictable periods. With the questions from women who are living with their menstrual cycles askew, this chapter will help you to touch on your own problem—and solve it.

Don't Worry Until You're Married?

I am twenty years old and for the past two years I have not had my period. I've been to three doctors already and they all tell me the same thing. They say, "Don't worry until you're married and want a family." Not one of them was willing even to examine me. Needless to say, I'm not concerned about the future when I might be married. I am worried today. I did have my periods, irregularly, when I was younger and I took the pill for eight months to regulate myself. The trouble was that I gained thirty pounds, so I stopped taking pills. It was after I gave up the pill that my period disappeared altogether. Now I'm really scared that the blood is building up inside me and causing cancer. Why won't anyone help me?

—J.G., Portland, Maine

It is a basic human instinct to be concerned when you think you might be sick. It's ridiculous for a doctor to tell this woman not to worry until she is married. There are so many myths about menstruation, what it means in terms of health and womanhood, that most women will, naturally, begin thinking all sorts of things are going wrong. Even the Bible has added to the confusion:

> And if a woman have an issue, and her issue in her flesh be blood,
> she shall be put apart seven days: and whosoever toucheth her
> shall be unclean until the even. . . .
> And if a woman have an issue of her blood many days out of the
> time of her separation, or if it run beyond the time of her
> separation; all the days of the issue of her uncleanness shall
> be as the days of her separation: she shall be unclean.
> —LEVITICUS 15: 19, 25

There is nothing "unclean" about the menstrual flow. As explained in chapter 3, menstruation is a natural monthly cleansing of the uterus.

Of course, when a woman misses her period, her first thought is that she is pregnant. A pregnancy test resolves that suspicion, but if she isn't pregnant, then the concerns really mount, as they have with Ms. G.

Since Ms. G. had periods when she was younger, she obviously has all her female organs and no major physical problems. What she needs to do now is to learn to relax. She need not be overly concerned about uterine cancer—the disease is very rare in twenty-year-old women. The added body fat from her thirty-pound weight gain while she was taking the pill might have initiated her altered menstrual cycle. Then, her worries about the disappearance of her period might have caused stress, which might have blocked her brain hormones.

If a woman's brain hormones, LH and FSH, are not released, there will be no production of the ovarian hormones, estrogen and progesterone, and therefore no menstrual bleeding. She does not mention whether she is employed or attending college, but she might have a job or schoolwork that is causing her a great deal of anxiety, and that, again, would affect her brain hormones and her cycle.

It is not unhealthy for a woman to be without her period. But if Ms. G. wants, or feels a need to menstruate, she could take progesterone tablets such as Provera every day for five days to induce her cycle. Synthetic progesterone tablets are used either to stop prolonged menstrual bleeding or to produce an absent menstruation.

The progesterone tablets that a woman takes to start menstruation will relax her uterus, and if she has enough estrogen in her body, they will also build up the uterine lining, the endometrium. When a woman finishes with the progesterone tablets, this sudden, abrupt drop in the progesterone hormone will cause uterine contractions and a shedding of the endometrium. This uterine activity, two to five days after discontinuation of the tablets, will bring on her menstrual flow.

On the other hand, if a woman continues to take progesterone tablets, she will not have a period. However, even a woman who uses progesterone to forestall her cycle should also be ready to expect a menstruation when she finally stops the progesterone pills. This induced menstrual flow will cleanse her, and thereafter her cycles are likely to be regular.

Ms. G. might also be able to induce her menstruation in other ways. A strict diet aimed at returning her to the weight she was before she began taking birth control pills might bring back her periods, but she will probably resume her former menstrual pattern. However, she should remember that what she considers "irregular" might be "regular" for her particular body.

It is sad that all the doctors she consulted neglected to take the time to explain thoroughly the ebb and flow of her menstrual cycle. Menstruation is more to a woman than a sign that she has had the opportunity to be fertilized. Women who are not thinking about conception rarely relate their menstrual cycles to childbearing. The doctors' statement that she should not worry about regular menstruation until she gets married is extremely dismissive and insensitive.

Just because a woman is married does not necessarily mean that she wants to plan a family.

To many women, menstruation is a symbol of normalcy and well-being. To dispel all the myths and reduce fears of sickness when a period does not appear, women must know their bodies and understand themselves. With knowledge, concerns will come into perspective and missed periods will become less worrisome. The fact that a woman has skipped her period does not mean that her health is failing. Her body's barometer is most likely reacting to her environment.

Does It Matter That I Haven't Bled for a Year?

I began taking birth control pills a year ago when I was twenty-four and I stopped getting my period. Now I'm twenty-five and nothing has changed. My doctor says I'm healthy, but shouldn't I be concerned about not menstruating for so long?
                                        —R.J., Gadsden, Alabama

The birth control pill governs a woman's menstrual cycle. Some women who are on the pill stop bleeding because the pill is not allowing their uterine linings to build up as much as they had before. These women might have only light staining now and then, if anything.

If a woman totally loses her menstrual periods while she is on the pill, she should stop taking the contraceptive until she begins to bleed again. A renewed flow will show that the pill has not interfered with her body's normal hormonal fluctuations. Recent studies have shown that almost all women will resume menstruating when they go off birth control pills. And their menstrual patterns will be the same as they used to be. So if a woman had an irregular menstrual cycle before taking the pill, she will have her unpredictable period back again.

Now, if this woman stops the pill, waits a while, and still doesn't get her period, she should visit her doctor for an examination, and possibly for progesterone tablets. As mentioned in the answer to the previous letter, when a woman starts, and then stops, taking progesterone tablets such as Provera, a few days later uterine contractions begin and a period follows. A woman who does not bleed after taking Provera might first need to increase her level of estrogen with estrogen pills prescribed for two weeks, and then Provera for one week. After three weeks of hormone therapy, a woman should resume her period. A vitamin regimen that includes vitamins E, B-complex, and separate B_6 supplements might also help regulate a woman's cycle, whether she is on or off the pill.

My Daughter Has Never Had Her Period

I'm the mother of a fifteen-year-old daughter and I'm worried. She still hasn't gotten her period and she is embarrassed in front of her friends. I've been building up her confidence, telling her everything is all right, but lately I'm beginning to think everything isn't as fine as I've been saying it is. My period started when I was thirteen, and I remember being one of the last of my girlfriends to get it. My daughter is already two years older than I was and she still isn't menstruating. Is there something wrong with my little girl?
—G.G., Blair, Nebraska

A woman who has grown beyond her pubescent years without ever having experienced menstruation is living with *primary amenorrhea*—she has no period and has never had one. This mother is writing about her fifteen-year-old daughter, whom she should begin watching. If the teenager seems to be developing similarly to her girlfriends in other respects, if she has breasts and is not extremely fat or thin, then there should be no reason to worry. However, if her daughter does not appear to be growing at the same rate as her peers, then she might have a hormone imbalance or genetic problems, and a doctor should be consulted.

Since menstrual patterns are often inherited, and her mother started menstruating at thirteen, it is normal to expect that the teenager might have reached menarche by now. An athletic schedule, such as daily training in track, might delay merache, but it is possible that stress at school could be preventing the arrival of her menstruation. This concerned mother might try to talk to her daughter about her school situation or any other event that she thinks might be bothering the child. A discussion might help to relieve the tension.

Once this young woman passes her sixteenth birthday, if she still doesn't have a menstrual cycle, then it is time for her mother to bring her to the doctor. Primary amenorrhea can be caused by congenital malformations of a woman's reproductive organs. She could have been born without a uterus or a vagina, with ovarian abnormalities, or with a closed hymen that is preventing the blood from leaving the body. There might be chromosomal abnormalities or a malfunction in the brain hormones that initiate the menstrual process. Sixteen is the age at which all these possibilities should be checked by a physician.

After a medical evaluation, if all is well and a young woman has no physical problems, a doctor might want to prescribe hormones to bring on menstruation. Once triggered, a cycle often continues on its own.

Is It Dangerous to Bleed Only Two or Three Times a Year?

Since I started my menstruation I have only had periods two or three times a year. I'm twenty-seven years old and I've been to several doctors. They always suggest that I take the pill, which I did for a while, but I was afraid of side effects. I stopped the pill six months ago and I've only had one period since. I went back to the doctor and he said something about giving me shots, but I'm so worried something else might be wrong.

                                   —W.H., Stamford, Connecticut

This woman is living with *oligomenorrhea*, an occasional menstruation. She might have inherited *polycystic ovarian syndrome (PCOS)*, also called *Stein-Leventhal syndrome*, a condition in which the ovaries are slightly enlarged and they produce an excess of estrogen and testosterone, the male hormone, which is causing a general hormonal imbalance in her body. Brain hormones are not functioning properly and ovulation is off.

She should look at herself in a mirror to see if she has excessive body hair, which is one of the signs of polycystic ovarian syndrome. Does she have hairs on her face, around her nipples, or on her stomach? Perhaps she has hair growing upward from the pubic area toward her navel in a triangular fashion. Such a hirsute state signals an overproduction of the male hormone testosterone and the possible presence of the syndrome. On the next visit to her doctor, she might discuss the possibility of polycystic ovarian syndrome with him.

Birth control pills usually correct such a hormonal imbalance and regulate the menstrual cycle, but since this woman does not want the pill, she might be helped by taking the progesterone tablet Provera. Taken monthly, twice a day for five days, Provera, once stopped, can help induce menstruation. As explained earlier, progesterone, along with sufficient estrogen, helps build the uterine lining, the endometrium. After the tablets are stopped and the hormone is withdrawn, the uterus contracts and the endometrium is discharged by the body in the form of menstrual blood. Progesterone tablets, once stopped, might return a woman's monthly period to her, but often, in order to induce bleeding, the tablets must be taken routinely, month after month.

The fertility drug clomiphene citrate (Clomid or Serophene) has induced menstruation with success. A woman with PCOS who wants to become pregnant might be especially interested in trying clomiphene citrate. If she still fails to conceive, then ovarian drilling might help. This takes place during a laparoscopy, when ovarian tissue is punctured by laser or electrocautery to stimulate ovulation. Sometimes, a doctor advises exploratory surgery and a wedge resection of the ovary, when a portion of the ovary is removed to make it smaller and more efficient.

Ovulating and menstruating only a few times a year is not dangerous because there is no tissue buildup. In order for the endometrium to form, there must be ovulation, and Ms. H., the letter writer, ovulates only once very few months, when she bleeds. However, if she has PCOS, then due to the increased estrogen in her body, she might have a slightly higher than normal risk of breast cancer, and she should not forget her periodic breast self-examinations.

NOTE: *Do not expect a change in body hair when proper menstrual function is restored.* The hormones that might help regulate the menstrual cycle of a woman with PCOS will not change her increased hair growth. No hair-removal medications exist, and the ways to eliminate excess body hair are still electrolysis, waxing, depilatories, and shaving.

Is My Overweight Making My Periods Crazy?

I feel like a freak. I've been four years without a period and now it's as if my organs are dead. I'd like to have another child, a brother or sister for the daughter I had four years ago, but I haven't been ovulating. The doctors tell me I'm too heavy. After my daughter was born I weighed 150 pounds, but now I've gone up to 250. It just happened. I bloated up. I'm only twenty-five years old and I want to know what my weight has to do with my ovulation. Why am I not ovulating? Why can't I have any more children?
                                              —A.G., Tulsa, Oklahoma

For the past ten years my weight has been rising to the point I am at now—190 pounds. I'm thirty years old, married, and I'd like to have a baby but I'm having trouble conceiving because I only have three periods a year. Sometimes a period can last a whole month, and I'm never sure when I'm going to get the next one. I sure don't look forward to them because they're so incredibly heavy. I cramp and bleed in clots for weeks. I'm so tired that all I want to do

*is sleep but sometimes the pain keeps me awake. Doctors have told
me "It's all in your head," "Have a hysterectomy," "Lose weight." I
know the way my periods are is not in my head and I don't want a
hysterectomy because I want a child. Is my overweight making my
periods crazy?*

—T.C., Escondido, California

There's a very fine interaction between a woman's brain and her
ovaries that can be disturbed with a weight gain. When the body
becomes large, the hormones are diluted and they don't function as
they should. With her hormones under stress, a woman's menstrual
flow can stop completely or become irregular. Studies have shown
that increased fatty tissue in a woman's body is converted into the
female hormone estrogen. So an obese woman who gets her period
is likely to have an especially heavy one because the estrogen causes
the uterine lining, which will leave the body as menstrual blood, to
become particularly thick. Besides building up the endometrium, a
high level of estrogen also stimulates breast tissue and might lead
to breast cancer. There is also a chance that the uterine buildup
might bring on cancer of the uterus. An overweight woman is faced
with amenorrhea, but she is risking the possibility of a fatal disease
as well.

Why do women become overweight? The causes are both genetic
and environmental. About 33 percent of body weight is determined
by a person's genes. It is also known that certain people have an
increased size or number of fat cells in their bodies. Overweight
people, especially those who have gained and lost weight since
childhood, might have up to five times as many fat cells as people of
average weight. This oversupply of fat cells makes weight loss particularly difficult because pounds can be reduced only by decreasing
the *amount* of fat in each cell. On the other hand, emotional problems can be the cause of overeating, which results in weight gain. If a
woman also has a lack of physical activity, then she can put on more
pounds, often depression sets in, and a vicious cycle ensues. Missed
or heavy periods are signs that an overweight woman is in danger.

The women who wrote these letters should heed their body signals and try to lose weight. If they had normal periods before their weight gains, when they slim down they will regain their previous menstrual patterns. Of course, it is easier to say "Lose weight" than to do it, but a good way to start reducing is to eliminate red meat and starches. The physicians these women consult might suggest diets and exercise programs that fit their patients' individual needs.

The second letter writer, who inquired about her heavy periods, might also be helped with one of the over-the-counter or prescription NSAIDs, the prostaglandin-blocking drugs described in chapter 3. There is some evidence that heavy bleeding might be caused by high levels of prostaglandins in the uterus, and these drugs, which lower prostaglandin levels, might reduce bleeding for Ms. C. while she is on a diet.

In any case, losing weight is the first priority for both women, and for all women who are heavier than good health allows. Fat interferes with hormonal balance. These women want to become pregnant, to bear children, and their futures as mothers will have much better odds for success if they make their bodies fit so that ovulation and conception each have the chance to happen.

The Stress Factor

My first husband left me after two years of our horrible life together. Sometimes we wouldn't speak for weeks. He never treated me well and for me, the marriage was a long and stressful relationship. I had one abortion before and another after we married, which didn't help my emotional stability. I remarried, but my second marriage was just as bad and we separated. For a long time now, my periods have come every other month, sometimes I skip two months. I'm sure my stressful life is the cause of my menstrual problems, and I'm afraid of the blood building up when I don't have my period. I want my periods regular again. Could it be that something else is wrong with me?

—L.Z., International Falls, Minnesota

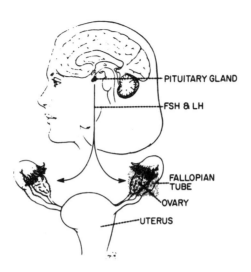

PITUITARY GLAND

FSH & LH

FALLOPIAN TUBE

OVARY

UTERUS

5-2 **How Brain Hormones Influence the Menstrual Cycle.** There is a close interaction between the brain hormones and the reproductive organs that control menstruation. There are releasing hormones in the brain that control the secretion of FSH and LH from the pituitary gland. These hormones will stimulate the ovaries to produce estrogen and progesterone, which, in turn, will stimulate the uterus to build up the endometrium (the uterine lining). It is the endometrium that is expelled as menstrual blood. If a person is under stress, the FSH and LH will not be released and menstruation will not occur. This absence of menstruation does not mean that blood is building up inside a woman. No menstrual blood is produced when the brain hormones are blocked. There is such a close interaction between the brain and the menstrual pattern that a group of women, living together and sharing similar experiences in a college dormitory, might find that their menstrual cycles are synchronized.

The hypothalamus in the brain masterminds the menstrual cycle. It is the hypothalamus that stimulates the secretion of the gonadotropin-releasing hormone GnRH, which in turn triggers the release of the brain hormones LH and FSH, and the cycle is set in motion. Any form of stress can affect the sensitive hypothalamus. College women who become very nervous before finals are known to skip periods, but when vacation time arrives and the pressure is off, menstruations resume their normal patterns.

Ms. Z.'s stress has not diminished, it seems, in years, and while her stress continues, her periods will probably be erratic. Women who go through divorces, start new jobs or marriages, or travel a lot can find themselves skipping periods. They need to stop, calm down, relax a bit, and listen to what their bodies are telling them. Their biological systems might react drastically if there is no respite. Women who push themselves too much risk nervous breakdowns, which can throw off hormonal balances to such extents that periods totally stop.

In order to tune her mind into tranquility and get her body working beautifully, Ms. Z. might try daily relaxation techniques to learn what it feels like to be calm. Just ten minutes of deep breathing or meditation can help a woman experience some peace. Of course, the best way to stop stress is to change the stressful situation in which you are functioning, but a person cannot always switch jobs or lifestyles so easily. Then, coping is the best way.

Ms. Z.'s problems do appear to be nearing an end. Her bad marriages are over, and she does not have to add any worries of illness to her concerns, because blood is not building up and causing cancer in her womb. Her hormones are not in balance enough to create the formation of a thick uterine lining. If she tries vitamin B-complex with extra vitamin B_6 to help regulate her cycle, does everything she can to calm her system—exercises, vacations, relaxation techniques—and still feels she is under stress, then she might seek counseling from a qualified psychologist or psychiatrist. But just being able to recognize your stress, as Ms. Z. has, is the first step toward banishing it from your life.

I Haven't Had My Period for Three Years; Could I Get Pregnant?

At first I was worried, but my doctor told me that he could give me hormone shots and it would start again. I decided not to take the shots because I saw no reason to bring on menstruation unless I wanted to get pregnant. Since I am not married, I do not want to have a baby. But I'm beginning to get a little nervous because I've recently met a man and started to have sex regularly. I haven't used any contraception because I've always thought I was probably infertile without the shots. Lately, though, I've been thinking that maybe I can get pregnant anyway. Do I need contraception?

—A.V., Durham, North Carolina

A woman who has experienced her menstrual period at one time, but not recently, has female organs that have stopped functioning for some reason. Perhaps this woman was stressed, or maybe she lost or

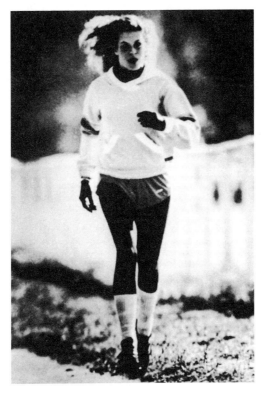

5-3 **Exercise and Women's Health.** Linda Schreiber, co-author of *Marathon Mom* (Houghton Mifflin), exemplifies how a woman can benefit from exercise. A mother of five, she found that the portion of the time she spent running gave her a return in efficiency, pleasure, and organization in her home life. We could all learn from Linda Schreiber, who has demonstrated how fitness can improve general well-being but still does not impair conception or childbearing. *Photo: Doug Paulding*

gained weight dramatically. Any of these situations might have caused her menstrual pattern to change. Sometimes a subtle shift in a woman's lifestyle goes unnoticed but it alters her hormonal balance. Then, if another shift occurs, her period might unexpectedly return.

Women who have become involved in romances and fallen in love have been known to have spontaneous ovulations. A wonderful relationship can certainly start the body functioning, and many women who have not had menstrual periods for years were amazed when they learned they were pregnant. Since Ms. V. certainly does not want to incur an unwanted pregnancy, I would suggest that she consult her doctor for a contraceptive that would be right for her.

On the other hand, a woman who has no periods and wants to become pregnant should make an appointment with an infertility specialist for an evaluation. If there is no problem other than amenorrhea, he can prescribe a fertility drug to induce menstruation. In fact, one fertility drug, Parlodel (bromocriptine mesylate), is being used by women who have amenorrhea in combination with high levels of the brain hormone prolactin, as determined by a blood test.

Galactorrhea, a leakage of breast milk, occurs when too much of the brain hormone prolactin is being produced by the pituitary gland. The result is a nipple discharge that might vary from barely noticeable—only occurring when the breast is pressed or squeezed—to an obvious leak. A woman who has missed several periods and also has a milky discharge from her nipples should see her doctor for blood tests to determine whether she is living with an excess of prolactin. If a prolactin imbalance is her problem, Parlodel will block the production of this hormone, stop her milk secretion, and reinstate her menstruation.

Could a Sluggish Thyroid Be My Problem?

I missed three months of my period and when my doctor checked me he found that my thyroid was underactive. He put me on birth control pills. I began to menstruate but now I'm off the pills and I'm not bleeding anymore. I'm wondering if my sluggish thyroid could be my problem? I'm also overweight.

—P.L., Hudson, Wisconsin

The thyroid gland is involved in stimulating the brain hormones LH and FSH, which trigger the menstrual cycle. So if a woman's thyroid is underactive, it will not be able to stimulate the brain hormones and ovulation will not take place.

This letter is a good reminder that the thyroid is very important in controlling a woman's menstrual cycle. A woman who has not had her period for a while might be given a thyroid test along with other hormonal evaluations. A low thyroid hormone production—hypothyroidism—can be corrected with thyroid medication, and once the gland is functioning properly, menstruation will probably recur.

The woman who wrote this letter is overweight, and her underactive thyroid might be the reason for her condition. If she takes the thyroid medication she might not only start menstruating, she might also find that she is able to slim down more easily.

Anorexia Nervosa

When I was thirteen I weighed 140 pounds—I'm 5'9"—and I started a diet to lose weight. Well, I got carried away and I went down to 98 pounds. I had anorexia nervosa. I lost my period and it never returned. Now I'm eighteen, I weigh 118 pounds, but I do not think my anorexia is over. I've been to several doctors who tell me I'm healthy and have no abnormalities other than I don't menstruate. I'm worried because maybe I'll never be able to have children.

—M.S., Baltimore, Maryland

Teenage girls who have eating disorders such as anorexia nervosa often feel out of control. They see life as something that happens to them. I hope Ms. S. is involved in family therapy. Conquering an eating disorder is easier if she and her family discuss family dynamics and everyone is open, aware, and supportive.

A young woman with anorexia is obsessed with becoming thin at all costs, usually through self-starvation. She might be using her emaciation as a cry for attention, or an emotional fixation might be driving her to reduce. In its extreme, anorexia can be fatal, so it is up to the parents to be sensitive to the weight loss of their teenage children.

Just as with weight gain, weight loss can put stress on the pituitary gland, prevent the brain hormones LH and FSH from being released, and arrest the menstrual cycle. I almost think this menstrual halt is nature's way of protecting an undernourished woman from adding more strain to her body.

It has been found that anorexic women often don't know that they are starving themselves. Looking in mirrors, they don't see themselves as shockingly thin—quite the opposite, many of them view themselves as too fat. They have trouble interpreting hunger signals, and psychologically, they feel victimized. It has been found that anorexics believe that everything they do must be to fulfill the demands of others. They feel personally ineffective, and the control they have over their bodies gives them a sense of power.

Treatment for anorexia nervosa must begin as soon as possible. The longer the disease lingers, the harder it is to overcome. Psychiatric counseling is needed to resolve the deeply rooted psychological problems that are causing the disease. There is also some evidence that vitamin B_6 might help to regulate the menstrual cycle at the same time. Once women can enjoy eating again and they gain weight, their periods will return and they will be able to have children. The 118-pound woman who wrote this letter is still underweight for her 5'9" height, and she should find a doctor who will recognize her problem and help her to increase her weight to the level at which her menstruation will return.

Could Jogging Affect My Menstrual Period?

Ever since I graduated from college and started working, I've been sitting behind a desk. At twenty-five years old, I felt myself getting out of shape. I started jogging a year ago and now I run five miles on weekdays and eight or nine miles on weekends. At first, my periods were lighter, and I liked that, but for the past two months they have disappeared completely. I also seem to have a vaginal discharge, which comes and goes, and I'm beginning to wonder what's going on. Jogging is supposed to make me healthy but it seems to be making me sick.

—S.C., Washington, D.C.

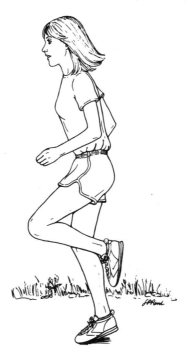

5-4 **Jogging and Menstruation.** Excessive physical activity such as jogging and strenuous dancing can lead to complete cessation of menstruation. Overexertion can result in weight loss and a blockage of the brain hormones that, in turn, might cause decreased and irregular menstrual bleeding. Serious female athletes have been known to become infertile and often have to reduce their exercise in their efforts to conceive.

Some exercise can enhance the menstrual cycle by alleviating stress and cramps and reducing the flow. However, excessive physical activity—such as jogging, cycling, or strenuous dance—can result in complete amenorrhea. Women athletes and professional ballet dancers are known to consider amenorrhea an occupational hazard. Periods probably stop because the constant exercise results in weight loss and a change in hormonal balance, which blocks the release of the brain hormones LH and FSH. Women who are physically active need high blood counts to carry added oxygen to their muscles, and a woman who is not menstruating is adjusting to this bodily need. Female athletes find the changes especially good for them since there is no menstrual fatigue when they are training and competing.

Ms. C. has no reason to worry. Menstrual absence is common to athletes, and the return of menstruation is practically a sure thing once physical activity is slowed down or stopped. She is not ovulating right now, so there is no buildup of her uterine lining, and that does not mean she is sick. It is perfectly normal for a woman doing as much strenuous exercise as she is to stop having ovulations.

Her vaginal discharge, however, might be due to a hormonal change inside her vagina. Since she is not ovulating, her estrogen level is lower, and a diminished estrogen level can dry the vagina and make it more susceptible to infection. And if she is wearing nylon jogging shorts, she is providing a hot, damp, airless climate in which germs can breed with ease.

This woman might attempt to restore a healthy vaginal environment by wearing cotton underpants and cotton shorts. If a change of attire does not alleviate her condition, she should consult a physician for treatment of her vaginitis. (For a more detailed discussion of vaginitis, see chapter 14.)

I Bled So Much I Thought I Had a Miscarriage

My period is normally like clockwork, but last month I was a week late and I had cramps, which I usually never have. I bled extremely heavily for three days. I couldn't get out of bed the first

*day at all. I've been trying to get pregnant and I think I might
have had a miscarriage. Could it be?*
                                              —T.P., Springfield, New Jersey

If this woman was under stress of some sort, anxiety might have
caused the lateness of her period. During this delay her uterine lining continued to develop. When menstruation finally began, her
flow was unusually heavy because by then the sloughed-off endometrium was much thicker and more vascular than it would have
been if she had had her period on time.

Since this woman was trying to conceive, there is, of course, a
possibility that she was suffering a miscarriage. Her period was a
week late. A conception that became defective—perhaps the fertilized egg did not implant itself properly in the womb—might have
taken place. Women who are completely in tune with their systems
can often sense whether they are pregnant. If this woman knows her
body, then she probably knows what happened.

Could a Fibroid Tumor Give Me Heavy Periods?

*My doctor says that my fibroid tumor is making me bleed
heavily and giving me pain each month. He wants me to submit to
surgery, but I don't like hospitals. Could you please tell me if there
are any other alternatives?*
                                              —L.B., Dugway, Utah

Fibroid tumors can grow in the middle of the uterine wall (intramural), outside the uterus (subserous), or in a position in the uterine
wall just below the surface of the endometrium, the uterine lining
(submucous). This last type of fibroid, which is called a submucous
fibroid, comprises only 5 percent of all fibroid tumors, but more
than the others, the submucous is the one that brings on the serious
problems. If it enlarges, it can break through the uterine lining and
cause very heavy periods. A D & C does not change the situation
because it will not remove the fibroid tumor, which continues to be

an irritant inside the uterus. The uterus cannot contract as it should to stop the bleeding because the tumor gets in the way (see chapter 15).

Some very recent preliminary studies have indicated that women with heavy bleeding could possibly cut down their blood loss by taking a prostaglandin-blocking drug such as Motrin or Anaprox (described in chapter 3). Either of these medications will lower prostaglandin levels and, in turn, will ease uterine contractions and lessen the bleeding. Progesterone tablets prescribed alone or in combination with an antiprostaglandin drug might also help relax the uterus.

If Ms. B. were prescribed the antiprostaglandin/progesterone combination she might reduce her bleeding and discomfort and avoid surgery. However, if the medications do not bring relief to her, she might require a myomectomy, an operation to remove fibroid tumors *only*. Once her tumor is removed, the bleeding should diminish. There is no reason to assume from her letter that she needs a hysterectomy. In fact, I would venture to say that a hysterectomy should not be performed except as a last resort. (For a more detailed discussion of fibroid tumors, see chapter 15.)

I'm Bleeding On and Off Every Two to Three Weeks; Do I Need a D & C?

It seems that every time I turn around lately I have my period. I'm bleeding on and off every two to three weeks; do I need a D & C? Do I have so much blood inside me that I should have it scraped out? Where is it all coming from?

—E.B., Boulder, Colorado

A D & C, *dilatation and curettage,* is an operation in which the opening of the cervix is gently and gradually enlarged with a series of specially rounded instruments called dilators. Then a small, spoonlike curette is inserted through the opening into the uterus to scrape out excessive tissue. A woman who needs a D & C usually bleeds very

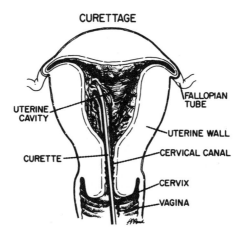

CURETTAGE

FALLOPIAN TUBE

UTERINE CAVITY

UTERINE WALL

CURETTE

CERVICAL CANAL

CERVIX

VAGINA

5-5 **Dilatation and Curettage (D & C).** This procedure is indicated for removal of excessive endometrial tissue, but it should not be used to cure dysfunctional bleeding. During a D & C the cervical canal is dilated—opened with metal rods of increasing diameters. A curette—an instrument with a sharp-edged open loop—is used to scrape excessive tissue from the uterine cavity.

heavily and has extremely long periods—indications that there is tissue built up that the uterus cannot get rid of by itself. The uterus cramps, the woman is in pain, and a D & C can help her.

This woman, however, does not bleed heavily. She has irregular bleeding, which indicates a hormonal imbalance, not a tissue buildup. A D & C probably will not change her condition at all, and women, in general, should avoid unnecessary surgical procedures.

She might need to have her menstrual flow regulated with a progesterone tablet such as Provera. She could take two tablets a day for five days. Then, two or three days after she has stopped taking the tablets her uterus will contract and a new bleeding will begin. Such a progesterone-induced bleeding is often referred to as a "medical curettage."

After treatment with progesterone tablets, this woman's menstrual cycle is likely to resume regularity. If the tablets do not work, then she might try birth control pills for a few months to regulate her flow.

Spotting

Every time my husband and I have intercourse I notice that I
stain afterward. I am not in any pain during sex so I don't
understand why I'm bleeding.
                                    —K.Q., Poughkeepsie, New York

A woman who spots after sex should immediately see a doctor. She might have a lesion or an erosion on her cervix, an active sore that is irritated during sex. There are also cases where spotting after sex has turned out to be a cervical growth—a cancer or a polyp. So a woman should make an appointment with her doctor to have a Pap smear and put her mind to rest that she does not have cancer. A cervical sore can be treated with medication or eliminated with electrocautery or cryosurgery, a freezing technique. A cervical polyp must be surgically removed.

If she has no cervical abnormalities, then her spotting might mean that her uterus is being irritated during active sex. In that case it is usual to experience some cramping and subsequent spotting.

Every so often during masturbation, orgasm, or for no apparent reason, a woman feels a cramp and notices a slight stain, which is usually the shedding of a few blood cells from the uterine lining. Sometimes an inadequate progesterone level during the last two weeks of a woman's cycle might result in mild uterine contractions that cause bleeding. Most of the time this type of spotting is not dangerous, but if it happens two months in a row, a woman should visit a doctor who could treat her condition with progesterone in the form of tablets or suppositories.

Anemia and Menstruation

I have heavy periods and cramping and I always have felt
incredibly fatigued while I am bleeding each month. My
gynecologist took a blood test and I discovered that I am anemic. I
have started taking twelve tabs of iron a day from the onset of my

flow until it is over, and I find that I feel much better and the
cramping recedes. I didn't even know that I had heavy periods
because women have no measurements for comparison, and I think
there are probably a lot of women like me who have severe anemia
and their doctors don't realize it.
                                        —A.W., Louisville, Kentucky

A woman might have heavy bleeding for a number of reasons. There might be a fibroid tumor that has broken through the uterine lining and is causing heavy bleeding. Some women don't coagulate well, which means that their blood does not clot properly, because they are taking aspirin or other types of anticoagulant medication. An IUD might be causing heavy bleeding, or a woman might be suffering from *adenomyosis,* a condition in which the uterine wall is exceptionally spongy and bleeding is particularly heavy.

When a woman bleeds heavily, she can become susceptible to anemia because the blood she is losing is not just extra blood she can afford to lose. During menstruation the endometrium, the glandular spongy lining of the uterus, the unused nest for a fertilized egg, is expelled. The uterus is cleansed and prepared for the buildup of another endometrium during the following cycle.

The menstrual flow will vary from woman to woman and sometimes from cycle to cycle. If an excessive amount of tissue is built up inside the uterus during one month, a woman will usually bleed more heavily because in order to expel the endometrium the uterus must contract more intensely. Since the activity in the womb is great, the uterus itself might lose blood too, and the result will be heavy bleeding that might cause anemia.

The uterus is supposed to squeeze like a tourniquet to prevent unnecessary blood loss, but if it doesn't squeeze properly, bleeding might emanate from the uterine cavity to which the endometrium is attached. A doctor might prescribe either a vitamin K and C combination that increases blood clotting factors and squeezes the uterus, or an Ergotrate-like drug such as Methergine, which also tightens the uterus. Ultimately, the menstrual flow is connected to the entire circulatory system and cannot be allowed to continue unchecked.

When a woman notices, because she is using an unusual number of pads or tampons, that her periods are heavy, or if she sees large clots in her flow, then she should visit her doctor. If she is also fatigued, she might be anemic and might need vitamin C and iron to strengthen her blood count. Depending on the cause of her bleeding, her doctor might suggest a D & C or prescribe the uterine-contracting drug Methergine. If the problem is an abundance of prostaglandins, the prostaglandin-blocking drugs Motrin or Anaprox might lessen the flow.

Can Vitamins Help My Period?

I have heavy bleeding and my doctor wants to do another D & C. The last D & C he did didn't cure me. I might need a hysterectomy. I think a hysterectomy would be an extreme way to alleviate my problem even though I have already completed my family. A dear friend told me that she read about vitamins controlling heavy bleeding. Doctor, please help me. Would vitamins work?

—F.J., Coquille, Oregon

Scientific evidence has shown that vitamin B_6 has had an effect on regulating menstruation, possibly because B_6 influences the signals from the brain that set off the menstrual cycle. In fact, in studies where women who were having trouble conceiving took vitamin B_6, they had an easier time becoming pregnant. So vitamin B_6 and vitamin B-complex, too, are natural menstrual regulators.

There have also been cases of women who have controlled heavy bleeding with vitamins, but this practice might not work for everyone. If this woman wants to try vitamin therapy to reduce her flow, she should know that the following combination treatment has been reported: 25,000 units of vitamin A three times daily taken with meals, 200 units of vitamin E daily, and 50 mg of zinc. These daily vitamins were taken every day for three months. After the vitamin therapy was begun, a blood test was given to make sure that the vitamin A was being absorbed. If pancreatic enzymes tested low, enzyme tablets were recommended to increase absorption. A woman who takes vitamins must be cautious about vitamin A, however. In high, long-term doses it can cause toxicity, but there have not been reports of bad effects from 75,000 daily units taken for a limited time. Every woman should check with her doctor and perhaps consult a nutritionist before embarking on vitamin therapy. Prolonged heavy bleeding is a symptom that should not be allowed to continue without medical attention.

BE YOUR OWN DOCTOR SOMETIMES

Menstrual irregularity causes so much silent concern—women worry that they are not in good health, that they are candidates for cancer, that they will never be able to bear children. Virtually all of these fears can be eliminated if women understand their finely tuned bodies. As explained in chapter 3, the feminine cycle has been portrayed as an almost supernatural occurrence, when in reality it is a beautifully organized ebb and flow of bodily hormones. Yet the intricacy involved in that ebb and flow is awesome. It is astounding that there are not more women suffering menstrual irregularities when you understand how many chances there are for things to go awry during the course of a monthly cycle. An ovulation can be interrupted by stress, physical exercise, travel, weight fluctuation, a change in lifestyle, sexual patterns, eating habits—so many events can influence menstrual patterns.

So, if a woman discovers that her period seems strange to her, that she flows differently, sporadically, or not at all—if she is not pregnant she should analyze the happenings in her life and take some time to be her own doctor. Everyone over twenty-five should maintain a steady weight. Has she gained or lost weight lately? Are there any changes in her daily routines? Has she recently suffered defeat or unexpectedly triumphed? Being promoted to president of her company can change a woman'smenstrual pattern as much as getting fired from her job. With all of these possibilities to consider, there is no reason to become immediately upset over an unpredictable period. If a woman is stressed, the B vitamins, deep breathing, stretching exercises, and any chosen tension-reducing outlet might aid in keeping her hormones balanced and her cycle "normal."

On the other hand, a woman who has prolonged staining, abnormal pain, or bleeding after intercourse should consult her doctor right away. These symptoms might signal serious problems, and a woman does not want to ignore them. This is her body and she alone is its protector.

6.

Toxic Shock Syndrome—
Are Tampons Really the Cause?

In the middle of 1980 the emergence of toxic shock syndrome (TSS) made everyone nervous and frightened. Fear about the ominousness of the disease spread as a horror story hit the headlines and terrified millions of people. The media's first reports were that menstruating women had died from toxic shock syndrome and that this fatal disease, which began with high fever, vomiting, and diarrhea, was somehow connected to the tampons that the dying women had been using.

Practically overnight, TSS became a sensational, highly publicized disease. The smallest hometown newspaper to the largest television network covered the story, and everyone was scared. Doctors' phones were ringing without pause as patients with coughs, chills, diarrhea, or slight fevers called to learn whether they could be victims of toxic shock. Rarely had a disease caught the public attention so quickly.

Doctors were nonplussed. What was the history of toxic shock syndrome? After over forty years of being safely used by women, why would the tampon suddenly be the instigator of disease? If women had a new, severe illness in common, why didn't gynecologists know about it? Toxic shock syndrome became the mystery of 1980.

Now we know that even when the TSS scare was at its height, the total number of cases, out of a population of over 50 million menstruating women, remained in the hundreds. And today it appears that 1 to 17 per 100,000 menstruating women might become victims of toxic shock syndrome. Children and men can also suffer the disease. And although the fatality rate has been noted at 5 percent, with immediate, intensive treatment the rate has been known to drop. But the mystery has not been solved. Where did toxic shock come from? How should it be treated? Dedicated researchers continue collecting clues.

THE BUNDABERG DISASTER

In 1928 in the small Australian city of Bundaberg, twelve children died very soon after having received injections against diphtheria. Five to twenty hours after they had been vaccinated, the children became sick with fever, vomited, and had watery diarrhea, and shortly thereafter collapsed in shock. In addition, several of the youngsters were found to have a red, strawberrylike skin rash.

It was a tragedy for the families of Bundaberg. They did not understand where the child-killing disease came from, but an investigation soon told them that the vaccine that had been used for the injections was contaminated with *Staphylococcus aureus (Staph. aureus),* a very potent and dangerous bacteria. These were the days before penicillin, so there would have been no hope for the children. Their disease, it was believed, was caused by a deadly toxin that was somehow liberated by the powerful *Staph. aureus.*

Some physicians who remembered the Bundaberg Disaster pointed out that the people who have been stricken by toxic shock syndrome have suffered the same symptoms as the twelve children in Australia. In fact, these symptoms of the disease have been shared by men, too, and whenever the symptoms show up, it is usually a toxin released by *Staph. aureus* that is to blame. There might have been much illness caused by this toxin over the years, but only in 1978 was the toxin-produced disease named: toxic shock syndrome.

THE FIRST DESCRIPTION OF TOXIC SHOCK SYNDROME

The disease of high fever, vomiting, and diarrhea eventually leading to shock and death did not receive much medical attention until November 1978, when Dr. James Todd, a Colorado physician, and his collaborators published a study in the prestigious British medical journal *Lancet*. In their study, they described a condition they called toxic shock syndrome—the phrase had never been used before, and it was probably not in Dr. Todd's mind that it would become an everyday expression. He was describing an illness that occurred without warning in children.

Seven children from eight to seventeen years old had a sudden onset of very high fever, headache, sore throat, watery diarrhea, and a red skin rash. These symptoms were often accompanied by severe kidney and liver problems. The children slipped into coma, and only after intensive hospital care did six of them survive. One child later died. The others, as they continued to recover, peeled on their hands and feet the way one might after a terrible sunburn.

Dr. Todd took a vaginal culture from only one patient, and in it he found the same *Staph. aureus* bacteria that had caused the Bundaberg Disaster. Then, researchers had something of a clue; at least they could make an association with the toxin that had killed children in Australia. Still, there was no connection made between tampons, menstruating women, and the disease until the last half of 1979 in Madison, Wisconsin, when it was found that six out of seven women who were hospitalized with symptoms similar to toxic shock syndrome were menstruating. The seventh patient had not yet begun to menstruate.

Further studies in Wisconsin prompted a reexamination of Dr. Todd's investigation, and it was learned that four of his study subjects were past menarche, two had had vaginal infections, three out of seven had developed the illness during menstruation, and all of these three had been using tampons.

And so there was a link between the *Staph. aureus* bacteria, menstruation, and—possibly—tampons, but these findings did not generate any major interest until the spring and summer of 1980, when more and more women succumbed to toxic shock syndrome.

In the ten years from 1970 through 1980, 941 cases of toxic shock syndrome were recorded in the United States, and almost half of them—408 cases—were reported to the Centers for Disease Control (CDC) in 1980 between January and October. The media initiated a tremendous alert, and medical researchers focused their energies on investigations that would tell them why the disease had suddenly begun to afflict so many people. Had the *Staph. aureus* bacteria altered? Had the human immune system changed? Before the real cause of the disease could be found, the number of TSS cases rapidly dropped. Why would an active disease abruptly slow down?

WHAT ARE THE SYMPTOMS OF TSS?

A danger of toxic shock syndrome is that its symptoms can at first seem to resemble the flu. In women, within five days of menstruation, usually on the third or fourth day before the onset, there is a sudden, high fever of at least 102 degrees Fahrenheit accompanied by severe vomiting and watery diarrhea. Dehydration can begin along with dizziness and a drop in blood pressure to below 90 systolic (normal would be 110 to 120). There is also a fine, sunburnlike rash that is most prevalent on the palms of the hands and the soles of the feet. About one to two weeks after the onset of the disease the skin will begin to scale and peel on the palms and soles especially, but at the beginning, a rash is the symptom to notice and so is a strawberry-red tongue and vagina. There might also be a sore throat, headache, and muscle pain.

A woman who is wearing a tampon should remove it, and menstruating or not, every victim should be rushed to the hospital within the first forty-eight hours of the disease to receive intravenous fluid to combat dehydration and build up her blood pressure. Antibiotics will also be administered. If a victim does not get immediate hospital care, she can lapse into a coma and her body can go into shock. There can be liver and kidney damage, her nervous system can be permanently impaired, and the shock can lead to death. Toxic shock syndrome usually lasts four to five days in the acute phase with one to two weeks of convalescence. Most deaths have occurred within a week, but with greater awareness and rapid medical attention, toxic shock can often be cured before life is lost.

IS IT ALWAYS FATAL?

As mentioned earlier, the death rate for toxic shock syndrome has been set at about 5 percent. In the eighties, an 8 percent figure resulted from the fact that victims of TSS often thought they had the flu, took aspirin, and stayed in bed. By the time their bodies went into shock and they were taken to hospitals, it was too late for doctors to save them. Usually they died within a week.

Today the death rate has greatly declined. Few of the already diminished number of cases of toxic shock syndrome are fatal. People who are ill with high fever, vomiting, diarrhea, and a body rash are admitting themselves to hospitals right away, and physicians are working fast. Using intravenous feeding to replace the fluid lost through diarrhea, vomiting, and fever, doctors are preventing the body from going into shock. Then, powerful antibiotics are effectively killing the disease. No one should think that toxic shock syndrome automatically means death. Fatalities are not the norm, but the key to survival is fast action and timing.

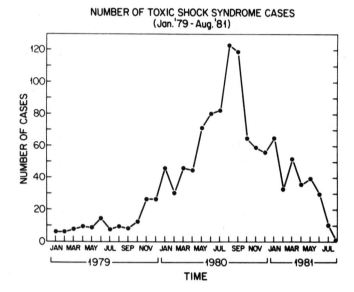

NUMBER OF TOXIC SHOCK SYNDROME CASES
(Jan.'79 - Aug.'81)

6-1 **Toxic Shock Syndrome.** The incidence of toxic shock syndrome increased rapidly during the summer of 1980 but dropped quickly one year later, according to statistics from
the Centers for Disease Control in Atlanta, Georgia. Although the incidence of
reported cases of TSS has declined, TSS is still an occasionally occurring condition
that affects women, men, and children. If a woman experiences typical symptoms of
TSS, she must immediately see a doctor.

WHO GETS IT?

The majority of the victims of toxic shock syndrome are menstruating women who are white and under thirty years old. Most of the
women who succumb to toxic shock are between the ages of fifteen
and twenty-five, with the average age being about twenty-three. A
woman who is over thirty only has about one-third the risk of contracting the disease as a woman under thirty. Perhaps during the
course of their lives older women have had time to develop immuni-
ties to the *Staph. aureus* bacteria. Just why younger women are the
more likely victims is still not clear.

Researchers have not been able to pinpoint specifics to determine
susceptibility. Studies have been done with TSS women and control

groups to test the number of times tampons have been changed, the brands used, the sexual patterns and partners of the women, their contraceptives, douches, and sprays. Although some variables that are discussed in the sections "Are Tampons Really the Cause?" (below) and "Is Any Form of Contraception a Cause?" (page 147) were discovered, there are no fixed conclusions to be drawn. Toxic shock remains fundamentally elusive.

One to 17 cases of toxic shock might occur in every 100,000 menstruating women, but even this estimate has varied. Toxic shock victims have been over sixty and under one year old; they have been nonmenstruating women, children, and men. The disease has taken hold during unforeseen infections—middle ear and throat infections, or an infection caused by a rusty nail that has pierced the skin. On these occasions, the *Staph. aureus* bacteria has had a chance to germinate and release the potent toxin that triggers the syndrome. Menstruating women might be the most frequent sufferers of this rare disease, but all types of people have been threatened by toxic shock.

ARE TAMPONS REALLY THE CAUSE?

Continuous research into toxic shock syndrome keeps demonstrating that neither menstruation nor tampons actually cause the illness. However, tampons might contribute to the development of the disease by giving the *Staph. aureus* bacteria a medium in which to grow. As the Bundaberg Disaster and the study by Dr. James Todd described earlier reveal, the disease is believed to be due to a deadly toxin that is produced by the bacteria and released into the bloodstream. As mentioned before, the bacteria can begin to multiply in infections that occur in various parts of the body. Nonmenstruating women, children, and men can provide the milieu in which the germ might thrive. Interestingly, however, *Staph. aureus* is present in about 10 percent of women during their menstruations, and it has been found in the vaginas of 73 to 100 percent of women with toxic shock.

Just how tampons might contribute to the proliferation of the bacteria and the subsequent liberation of the toxin is still a matter of guessing. Toxic shock syndrome seemed to increase with the introduction of new, superabsorbent tampons. A brand called Rely unfolded in the vagina and was so superabsorbent that it needed to be changed less frequently than other kinds of tampons. Women were becoming great fans of Rely, and a number of patients who were admitted to hospitals with toxic shock were, indeed, wearing Rely tampons.

Laboratory analysis was done to determine whether the material in the superabsorbent tampons was contaminated, but they were found to be sterile. It was then theorized that a superabsorbent tampon might have expanded to plug up the menstrual flow and create a pool of blood that, in combination with the blood-soaked tampon, created an airtight culture medium in the vagina in which the bacteria could flourish and the toxin could develop. Many theories required investigation before conclusions could be drawn, but Procter & Gamble, the manufacturers of Rely, didn't wait. They voluntarily withdrew their superabsorbent product from the market. Everyone was on toxic shock alert.

Reports confirmed that women who used different brands and sizes of tampons were also developing toxic shock. Rely was not the only tampon product that might have created the culture medium for TSS. It was postulated that tampons that remained in the vagina for many hours, especially those worn overnight, might be irritating the fine lining of the vagina and causing sores and abrasions that encouraged bacterial growth. Doctors suggested that women change tampons often, try not to let tampons stay in their vaginas beyond five hours, and wear pads overnight during their menstruations.

Tampon use dropped from 70 to 55 percent in the latter half of 1980, and toxic shock syndrome went into a decline. In all of 1980, however, toxic shock cases numbered 725 in a population of about 52 million menstruating women. The disease was, and is, rare. The sudden downward shift in cases after August 1980 might have been due to a change in the way women use tampons, the withdrawal of Rely, the awareness of women of toxic shock symptoms and their readiness to seek medical attention, more alertness from the medical establishment, prompt treatment, or all of these things. Researchers are still trying to learn whether a strain of *Staph. aureus* has changed in the last decade.

When a woman is menstruating, her body is stressed and less resistant to infection, so the bacteria and its toxin have little trouble taking hold. Since women who do not use tampons, nonmenstruating women, children, and men can become afflicted with TSS, tampons cannot be considered the source of the disease. A cause that is common to everyone has yet to be discovered, but until then, awareness is the best defense. A woman who thinks she has toxic shock symptoms should visit her doctor immediately and welcome the chance to receive hospital care.

NOTE: *Deodorant tampons pose no added damage.* No incidence of TSS has ever been directly linked to deodorant tampons. In fact, if they do not cause allergic reactions, deodorant tampons may be used in the same manner as the nondeodorant types. No tampon should be permitted to remain in the vagina for longer than six hours. A woman must understand her body, listen to its signals, and use her own good judgment when she begins her monthly use of tampons.

IS ANY FORM OF CONTRACEPTION A CAUSE?

Many under-thirty women, who form the majority of TSS victims, use no contraception at all. In one study of toxic shock sufferers, only 31 percent of the women were employing contraception, which is surprising since 70 percent of the women in America are contraceptive users. The conclusion is that contraception, rather than being a cause of toxic shock, might actually provide some protection against the disease.

Researchers have speculated that the birth control pill might help to defeat toxic shock more than other forms of contraception because the pill controls the buildup of the endometrium, the uterine lining that becomes the menstrual flow. Women on the pill have reduced monthly bleeding, and a light period means decreased tampon use and less likelihood of a heavily soaked tampon creating a culture medium in which bacteria might grow. At any rate, the important finding is that a large number of TSS women used no contraception of any kind.

WILL DOUCHING PROMOTE TSS?

Studies have been conducted to compare women's douching habits, the use of feminine deodorant sprays, and the incidence of toxic shock, and so far no significant connections have been found.

COULD A VAGINAL DISCHARGE LEAD TO TSS?

In Dr. James Todd's 1978 study, which named toxic shock syndrome, two out of seven patients had vaginal infections. In a follow-up study from Dr. Kathryn N. Shands and colleagues at the Centers for Disease Control, almost half—twenty out of fifty-two—of the women with toxic shock had vaginitis or a vaginal discharge. A selection of vaginal cultures from these women revealed the presence of *Staph. aureus*, the bacteria that promotes toxic shock. Although it cannot be said that the vaginal discharge brought on TSS, it seems logical that a woman with a persistent vaginal infection should visit her doctor and have a culture evaluated. Vaginal discharge and toxic shock have appeared together too many times to be dismissed.

DOES SEX INCREASE THE CHANCE OF TSS?

Sexual activity does not appear to influence TSS. Researchers have not been able to link either frequency of sexual intercourse, number of partners, or intercourse during menstruation to the onset of TSS. A woman might be worried about toxic shock, but she does not have to change her sexual habits in any way.

DOES TSS RECUR?

There is about a 30 percent chance that if a woman has had toxic shock syndrome one time she will get the disease again, probably within three months of her initial illness. Tampons do not cause TSS, but since they might provide a milieu in which bacteria can fester, a TSS woman should avoid tampons for a while and return to them only after her doctor has told her that all traces of *Staph. aureus* have disappeared from her body. Toxic shock symptoms might recur a second and third time, too, but the recurrences will be spaced further apart as a woman's immunity to the *Staph. aureus* bacteria builds. Eventually her body will fight off the disease, or the toxins will stop being produced, and she will no longer suffer.

WHAT IS THE TREATMENT FOR TSS?

Toxic shock syndrome can be cured with fast action. If a woman feels she is experiencing the symptoms of TSS, she should immediately see her doctor for a diagnosis. Once he identifies the disease, she must be admitted into the intensive care unit of her local hospital, where intravenous fluids can be administered to replace the fluid that she has lost through fever, vomiting, and diarrhea. The strain of *Staph. aureus* causing the illness will be isolated and the doctor will prescribe potent antibiotics to kill the bacteria. (Often the beta-lactamase-resistant antistaphylococcal antibiotics are the drugs used to fight TSS.) Hospital care must begin within twenty-four to thirty hours after the onset of the disease or a victim can go into shock and die. TSS is a serious, life-threatening disease that cannot be treated at home with over-the-counter remedies. In-hospital antishock measures are the only means to a safe recovery.

As research uncovers more facts, toxic shock syndrome will lose its remaining mystery, but research takes time. The women who have questions and fears today deserve the knowledge we can offer right now.

Are Tampons All Right to Use During Sports?

I'm on the swimming team at my high school and have to train every day. My mother became so worried about toxic shock when she heard about it that she didn't want me to wear tampons anymore. She told me to quit the team. I can't swim with those bulky pads. Now she has calmed down and I'm wearing tampons when I have my period but she has made me nervous about it. Are tampons dangerous when you swim?
                                                    —R.E., Pensacola, Florida

Toxic shock syndrome is not caused by tampons, although they might promote the disease by blocking the vagina and providing an environment in which the bacteria can flourish. The superabsorbent tampons that existed in 1980, because they expanded so fully within the vagina, seemed to offer a milieu that was especially conducive to bacterial growth. These tampons have been removed from the market, but that does not mean that a woman should have a lackadaisical attitude about other types of tampons.

A woman who is involved in sports and exercise can certainly use tampons, but she should take care to change them at regular intervals and switch to pads at night. For women who swim during their periods, a tampon is ideal. Even if a woman is having a light day, however, it is not a good idea to allow a tampon to remain in the vagina beyond six hours. Also, if a woman feels she is becoming ill with the symptoms of toxic shock syndrome—a high fever of at least 102 degrees Fahrenheit, severe vomiting, watery diarrhea, a fine sunburnlike rash that is most noticeable on the palms of the hands and the soles of the feet, possible sore throat, headache, and muscle pain—she should consult her doctor immediately. If a woman does not experience definite symptoms but she has a lingering vaginal infection, she should ask her doctor to examine a culture for TSS. Early detection is the best way to battle the disease.

Is It Safer to Use Cotton Tampons?

Until the toxic shock scare, I thought that tampons were made of cotton. I was surprised to learn that they had so many synthetic materials in them. I always think that natural is better than synthetic. Wouldn't all-cotton tampons be safer?
—M.Y., Raleigh, North Carolina

The original tampon was invented by Dr. Earle Haas of Denver. In an interview in the *Chicago Tribute*, Dr. Haas said that his product "never caused toxic shock. We never had any problem with it at all, because it was built just to absorb the fluid, not to block the flow." Dr. Haas sold his patent and rights to Tampax, which put tampons on the market in 1936.

Before 1977, tampons were made of rayon or a rayon/cotton blend. From 1977 on, 44 percent of the tampons sold were made of more absorbent synthetic materials—polyacrylate fibers, carboxymethyl cellulose, high-absorbency rayon-cellulose, and polyester foam. Tampax has reintroduced an all-cotton tampon under the brand name Tampax Naturals. It is advertised as the "first feminine protection made of 100% cotton" and is available in regular and super sizes. However, there is no scientific evidence to prove that the all-cotton tampon is safer than other kinds on the market. TSS is related to a tampon's absorbency more than its materials.

Although the rise in toxic shock seems to have coincided with the introduction of synthetic superabsorbent tampons, nothing has been discovered to prove that the materials used in these tampons were factors. The hypothesis remains that the fully expanded superabsorbent tampon, when left in the vagina for a long time, created an environment for bacterial growth. All-cotton tampons are not likely to be as absorbent as synthetic tampons, and in that respect they are probably less likely to clog the vagina, but whether they will make a difference in the incidence of toxic shock is not known.

Is a Sea Sponge Safer Than a Tampon?

The other day the women in my church group started talking about toxic shock and wondering whether the materials tampons were made from could cause the disease. Someone said that there were natural, organic sea sponges that could be used instead of tampons. Are these sea sponges safe?
                                        —D.H., San Bernardino, California

When the toxic shock scare happened, some women tried the sea sponge as a tampon substitute. The sponge is boiled first and then pressed into the vagina. After it is saturated, it is removed, rinsed, and reused.

Women thought the sea sponges might be safer than commercial tampons because they were natural and less absorbent. However, there has been at least one case of toxic shock with sea sponges and they are no safer than tampons. In fact, researchers at the University of Iowa have found microscopic particles of sand, minerals, bacteria, and chemicals in sea sponges. The FDA has classified the sea sponge in its "most hazardous" category. Sea sponges are too contaminated to be used internally, and women should not experiment with them.

How Often Should I Change My Tampons?

I'm confused about toxic shock and tampons. At first I thought I was supposed to change tampons often, but then I read that

frequent changes might cause cuts from the inserters. What am I
supposed to do? How often should I change my tampons?

—T.D., Maryville, Tennessee

At first it was felt that frequent tampon changing might cause vaginal irritations from the inserters, and abrasions might, perhaps, contribute to toxic shock syndrome. This theory has not held up under investigation. TSS is most likely due to the proliferation of the *Staph. aureus* bacteria, and tampons might create a situation in which the bacteria have a better chance to breed. Although super-absorbent tampons were probably more likely than other types to promote an environment hospitable to bacteria, all tampons are suspect.

The number of times a woman changes her tampons depends on her flow. If a woman always has a light period or if she is in the last day or two of her flow, she might not have to change her tampons frequently. This is the time when she must be most aware and not let a tampon stay inside her vagina for more than six hours. The longer a tampon remains within the vagina, the greater the chances that a bacterial milieu will be created. A woman should not become overly anxious about tampon changing, but she should not leave a tampon in all day, and at night she might switch to a pad.

My Tampon Is Falling Apart; Is That Dangerous?

I've recently found that when I remove my tampon there are
pieces of it still inside me. After my period one month I had a
terrible odor and I went to the doctor. He examined me and found
fragments of tampon material rotting in my vagina. Now I try to
douche and cleanse myself every month, but isn't it dangerous to
have tampons falling apart inside you?

—C.M., El Paso, Texas

Several women have mentioned recently that the synthetic fibers of their tampons were coming off. These fragments will not cause toxic shock syndrome because they are not blocking the vagina and creating the necessary environment for the development of the Staph. aureus bacteria. Generally, the vagina has the ability to cleanse itself, but if a woman experiences an odor that might be caused by tampon fragments, it would be appropriate for her to douche with lukewarm water alone or mixed with a tablespoon of vinegar. If a woman finds that the brand of tampons she uses regularly is shredding, she might try another brand.

Could a Broken Inserter Cause TSS?

A piece of the plastic inserter on my tampon broke off when I put in a tampon. I wasn't able to find the piece since I had my period at the time. I don't know what happened to it. Could this piece of plastic cause toxic shock?

—B.V., Valley Stream, New York

The tips of the plastic inserters on various tampons are bendable and should not be breakable. However, occasionally there might be a weak spot and a piece of the rounded tip might break off. The plastic material should not be harmful to the vagina. It does not make the vaginal environment a milieu for the bacteria related to TSS. This woman will not become sick from the plastic.

Most likely the plastic fragment came out during this woman's period when she was changing tampons, but if she is concerned that a foreign object might remain in her body, she should douche to cleanse her vagina. If her worry continues, she can make an appointment with her doctor for an internal examination, but there is no reason to believe that the inserter tip will cause any ill effects.

A HEALTH WARNING BEGINS

After the toxic shock scare of 1980, the government suggested that tampon products carry a health warning for toxic shock syndrome.

To this day, information on TSS is printed on the outside of tampon boxes and inside, on separate foldout sheets. Tampon manufacturers also maintain web sites with TSS updates. Women are urged to choose tampons that provide the minimum amount of absorbency needed to control their menstrual flows.

It is my feeling that tampons, used properly, are still safe for women. If a woman has used tampons for years and they have provided ideal sanitary protection for her, there is no reason for her to switch to pads. Toxic shock syndrome is a very rare disease, and death from it is even more rare. In fact, one leading researcher made an analogy about the woman who drives to the supermarket to buy a box of tampons. She has a much greater chance of losing her life on the road on the way to purchase the tampons than she has of dying from toxic shock syndrome if she survives the trip. However, if a woman notices any of the disease's symptoms during her menstruation, she should visit her doctor immediately. Awareness and action are the ways to conquer TSS for good.

7.

The Hidden Disease—Endometriosis

THE HIDDEN DISEASE—YOU MIGHT HAVE IT

Many of the more than 8 million American women who are suffering from endometriosis do not realize that they have it. For this reason, endometriosis has been named "the hidden disease." Even you might have it without knowing it.

Time and again, women feel the pelvic pain of endometriosis but they think that they are having menstrual cramps and they do not seek medical help. It is hardly their fault. Women have been conditioned to endure monthly menstrual ordeals, no matter how excruciating. Gripped by pelvic pain, they behave as they would with cramps. Women try to not let their abdominal discomfort, which they fail to recognize as endometriosis, interfere with the daily rhythms of their lives. Months and years go by, and sometimes, because women have not been alerted to the characteristic signs of this terrible disease, endometriosis slowly incapacitates each of their female organs. To stay healthy, every woman should learn all she can about endometriosis.

The typical endometriotic woman, although she might be a teenager or a homemaker, is more often a career woman who wants to establish herself in a field before she has a child. But then there is an irony to face. The stress of the marketplace that gives *ulcers to men* might be responsible for *endometriosis in women*, which is why the hidden disease was once referred to as "the career woman's disease." As women have multiplied in the labor force, endometriosis, with its pain, suffering, and subsequent infertility, has greatly increased.

During endometriosis, misplaced endometrial tissue from the uterus implants itself on pelvic organs and spreads throughout a woman's abdomen. Many afflicted women say that they feel like they are being "eaten alive" while they are facing repeated surgery, infertility, emotional traumas, and physicians who often do not seem to understand the agony that goes along with the disease. Women have been told either that their symptoms are "all in their heads" or that they must submit to surgery, which later on might prove unnecessary. Plagued by unrelenting endometrial pains, women of all ages have become seriously depressed and frustrated. But there is hope. Knowledgeable physicians and scientists who comprehend the situation are in a fight to defeat endometriosis.

Thanks to consistent, ever-mounting research, today the condition is much easier to spot in its early stages, and with quick detection, doctors have better chances of curing this painful disease. Women who are aware of the symptoms of endometriosis can now help their doctors reach a diagnosis early enough to curb this devastating condition.

WHAT IS ENDOMETRIOSIS?

Endometriosis is a disease in which the tissue that forms the endometrium, the lining of the uterus, spreads to the organs outside the womb. As explained in chapter 3, every month, during the last half of a woman's menstrual cycle—the two weeks that begin with ovulation and end in menstruation—the lining of the uterus grows rich in glandular tissue and blood vessels. Steadily, naturally, an emerging vascular layer turns the endometrium into a soft, spongy nest, a bed for a fertilized egg.

At this point, the endometrium exists to nurture fertilization, so if an egg is not fertilized, the body has no reason to keep this enriched lining. The cycle comes to an end. A woman's uterus begins rhythmic contractions that disturb the blood supply to the uterine lining and cause the unused endometrium to detach from the womb and leave the body as menstrual flow.

When a woman is healthy, the regular contractions of her uterus push the uterine lining, the sloughed-off endometrium, first through the cervix, the mouth of the womb, and then through her vagina. But a woman who gets endometriosis often has a constricted uterus and a tight cervix that do not let all the menstrual blood escape vaginally. Instead, a portion of the blood-filled uterine lining is pushed backward through the Fallopian tubes and sprayed out the tubes into the abdomen. Such a woman usually has a history of menstrual cramps.

Women with severe menstrual cramps have in their uterine linings high levels of prostaglandins, which can produce contractions similar to the ones experienced during labor and childbirth. In these women the chances are great that their blindingly painful contractions will push the endometrial tissue into places where it can run wild. Endometrial tissue that has been flushed into the Fallopian tubes and sprayed out into a woman's abdomen can implant itself on her ovaries, on the outside of her uterus, and in the cavity between the uterus and the rectum called the cul-de-sac. The tissue can begin to grow like a transplant on any of its new locations, and once that happens endometriosis has begun. It should be noted, however, that even if a woman does not have severe cramps, tissue can be pushed backward into the abdomen to cause endometriosis.

Each month, the fluctuation of the hormones estrogen and progesterone, which causes the production of the endometrium inside the uterus, is also having an effect on the endometriosis outside the uterus. The tissue thickens, bleeds, and since it has no escape, spreads throughout the abdominal cavity. Sometimes, as it expands and bleeds, the tissue breaks off in cystic chunks that implant themselves elsewhere and cause severe abdominal pain.

An endometrial mass spreading behind a uterus can pull and tilt the womb backward. The tissue can move into the ovaries and

ENDOMETRIOSIS

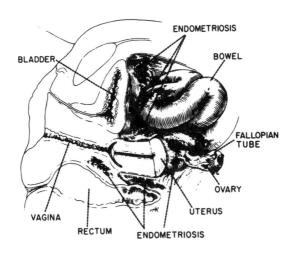

7-1 **Common Sites of Endometriosis.** Endometriosis is often referred to as benign cancer because it can spread to so many organs. This picture illustrates how the endometriotic tissue has traveled outside of the uterus—it has reached the area behind the uterus and in front of the rectum. Endometriosis can spread to the ovaries, the tubes, the bowel, and the bladder, causing pain, discomfort, bleeding abnormalities, and infertility.

Fallopian tubes, where it causes infertility. Endometriosis can even enter the bowel and create bloody stools and pain during peristalis, bowel movement. The tissue can penetrate the wall of the bladder, grow into the bladder, and then attach the kidneys and rectum. There have also been cases where endometriosis has spread to the lungs and—unbelievable as it might seem—the brain. If left untreated for years, endometrial tissue can even become cancerous.

Although pregnancy early in life might somewhat lessen the chances of getting endometriosis, many women will first develop the disease after childbearing, possibly at times when their lives become more stressful. Any woman who is living with a great deal of stress is a candidate for endometriosis, but if a woman can monitor her body for the distinct symptoms of the hidden disease she can possibly catch it at an early and curable stage.

The symptoms of the disease include a possible painful ovulation two weeks before menstruation, severe cramps during menstruation, and a deep abdominal pain on one side or the other or an unspecific abdominal pain before or after menstruation. Other signs are infertility and pain during sexual intercourse. (Many women who are infertile and are told they have no physical defects might, indeed, have endometriosis.) During the course of the disease, pelvic pain caused by pressure on a woman's organs and nerves slowly intensifies.

Doctors are not sure why endometriosis attacks some women and not others. Why are certain women with menstrual cramps spared? Why are women without menstrual cramps victims? There is some evidence that the disease might be hereditary, and a woman who keeps watch over her body should remind her doctor to check for endometriosis if anyone in her family has had the disease, if her menstrual pattern alters during stressful intervals, or if any of the above symptoms begin to nag at her sense of well-being.

WHY DOES ENDOMETRIOSIS OCCUR?

Papyrus records from 1600 B.C. show that the Egyptians might have been the first to document symptoms of endometriosis, but for approximately 4,000 years thereafter very little medical attention was paid to the disease.

In 1860, Dr. C. Von Rokitansky described a tumor that had endometriotic characteristics, and in 1867, a Dr. Cullen of Baltimore, Maryland, wrote about endometrial tissue within the uterine wall. According to the British, the word *endometriosis* was born in 1922, when a Dr. Blairbell of Liverpool used the term for the first time in a medical report. Americans claim otherwise. They say that in 1927 the famous Dr. J. A. Sampson of Albany, New York, invented the word.

Whether or not he is the originator of the term *endometriosis*, Dr. Sampson is nevertheless well-known for explaining the existence of the disease. His "tubal reflex and implantation" theory—the backward flush of endometrial tissue through the Fallopian tubes and into the abdominal cavity as described in the previous section—is highly regarded and has been confirmed in monkey studies. The uteri of monkeys were opened so that their menstrual flow bled right into their abdominal cavities, and when this was allowed to happen all the monkeys developed endometriosis.

Certainly, Sampson's "backward flush" theory is the most likely explanation for why endometriosis occurs, especially for why it so often turns up in stressed women with severe menstrual cramps. However, *women without menstrual cramps can also have the disease,* and there are even cases in which men have developed endometriosis in their bladders following prolonged treatment with the female hormone estrogen for prostate gland cancers. These circumstances give credence to other theories: (1) that endometriosis is genetic; (2) that it is spread through the lymph and circulatory systems; and (3) the embryonic theory, which holds that endometriosis exists in the embryo as dormant tissue and hormonal fluctuation during adult life activates it.

It seems likely, however, that although some endometriosis might be of embryotic nature, and some endometrial tissue might be spread throughout the body by the circulatory system, the majority of cases of endometriosis are probably caused by the backward flush of the uterine lining. In fact, many doctors have chosen to use the Sampson theory as a way of explaining the disease to the growing number of women who are suffering from endometriosis today.

Before the advent of the women's movement and the days of career first/children later, many more women became pregnant while they were in their teens or early twenties. With more pregnancies during their reproductive years, women experienced fewer menstrual cycles, and endometriosis was a much rarer disease. Early pregnancy might have reduced the possibility of endometriosis because from childbirth on the cervix, the mouth of the womb, is more relaxed and menstrual blood flows more easily from the uterus. When tension is minimized in the female organs, there is less likelihood that the endometrium will be trapped internally. Uterine muscles will not tighten with the kind of intensity that creates severe menstrual cramping.

Another reason endometriosis might not have been as common years ago is that after women bore children early in their lives, they breast-fed the infants, and not long after breast-feeding they became pregnant once more. This cycle continued for most of their menstruating lives. With so many pregnancies and so much breast-feeding, a woman considerably decreased the number of menstrual periods that would provide her with opportunities for the development of endometriosis. It is interesting that today, among groups of women who still believe in early childbearing and continue to have large families, endometriosis is rarely seen.

In fact, years ago it was thought that endometriosis struck only middle-class white women and that women in minority ethnic groups were not susceptible to the disease. We, of course, know differently today. Any menstruating woman can get endometriosis. Doctors in the past just did not realize that many middle-class, white, career women married later in life and had only one or two children, and that their stressful lives and pregnancy patterns made them victims of the disease. As millions of women changed their lifestyles and chose to delay—or, as is increasingly the case, forgo—childbearing, endometriosis crossed all barriers. It exists in women of all races, ages, and social stations.

The disease has been linked mostly with women who have dysmenorrhea, severe menstrual cramps. A dozen or so years ago, when women's lifestyles were obviously beginning to change, women's cramps might have been held in check by the birth control pill. The pill would have prevented a heavy buildup of the endometrium and there would have been fewer uterine contractions and less tissue to move into the abdominal cavity. However, the pill scare brought a drop in the number of women taking birth control pills, and many women are again living with menstrual cramps and the possibility of getting endometriosis.

It seems that the figures on endometriosis are being pushed upward by the fact that today there are fewer pregnancies, fewer women on the pill, and lifestyles are often more stressful. Once women are under stress, their bodies secrete more steroid hormones from the adrenal glands. The steroid hormones then lower the amount of immune antibodies that a woman produces. Since immune antibodies are needed in full force to reject any foreign tissue, as well as to kill infections and viruses, a stressed woman with reduced antibodies will obviously have a hard time protecting herself against endometriosis.

Healthy women who are not stressed are usually able to reject endometrial tissue that might be pushed backward into their abdomens during severe menstrual cramps. But that pervasive nemesis, stress, makes women lose their capacity to ward off wayward endometrial tissue. Stress weakens the immune system, which would normally fight off the onset of endometriosis; a body weakened by stress usually has trouble fighting off illness. With the power of the immune system diminished by stress, the displaced tissue implants itself on pelvic organs and takes root like a transplant the body has accepted.

Lately, there is a theory that a woman's immune system might be affected by exposure to industrial pollutants such as dioxin or polychlorinated biphenyls (PCBs). Some studies suggest that countries with high levels of PCBs have the greatest number of endometriosis sufferers. However, the link to pollutants has yet to be proven. One study comparing blood levels of toxin in eighty-six women with endometriosis and seventy endometriosis-free women showed no significant difference. Long-term investigations should bring results soon.

Nothing about endometriosis is clear-cut except the fact that it is a *terrible disease* that can tilt the uterus and grow into the ovaries, tubes, bladder, bowel, rectum, and kidney—and even invade the lungs and brain. An endometrial tumor is like a fungus that spreads out of control. It brings on infertility and torturous pain, and can lead to repeated surgery. It must be stopped before it causes all these horrendous problems or, worse, results in cancer.

IS THERE A CURE?

It is not impossible to stop endometriosis after it starts, but it is not easy. A woman who has suspicious pelvic pain or a mysterious mass that her doctor cannot seem to define will probably need an exploratory operation called a laparoscopy. It is difficult to confirm endometriosis through magnetic resonance imaging (MRI) or ultrasound. Small areas of endometriosis might be missed completely. A large mass might be spotted using these diagnostic techniques, but the only way to know that a mass is endometriosis is through surgery or biopsy.

During a laparoscopy, a doctor makes a small incision in a woman's navel and inserts a specially designed periscope that enables him to view her pelvic organs. He might spot endometrial implants right away. If he sees ovarian cysts, he can aspirate fluid from them and test the liquid for endometriosis.

A laparoscopy is usually performed in an ambulatory facility in a hospital or in a freestanding clinic. Although it is a good diagnostic tool, it is not foolproof. A surgeon will be able to see large masses of endometrial tissue, but if the endometriosis is minimal, or within other tissue, or behind the uterus, it might elude his view.

This possibility of hidden endometriosis might not concern a competent physician who believes in his ability to diagnose pelvic endometriosis from a woman's history and his own clinical examination. A capable doctor who conducts an internal examination has the skill to feel the tender or painful growths of endometriosis behind the uterus or on the tubes and ovaries, and his expertise can often help a woman with her diagnosis. In fact, a woman might seek out a second opinion from just such a gynecologist—a specialist in endometriosis who has the sensitivity to diagnose and treat her.

After a good doctor performs a laparoscopy, when a woman is diagnosed as having endometriosis, she should begin treatment immediately. For many years, because endometriosis seemed to bypass women who had conceived, doctors suggested that the best treatment for endometriosis was pregnancy. Now, not only do knowledgeable doctors consider pregnancy a ridiculous way to curb the disease, but it has been found that women who have suffered from endometriosis, although they might feel better during the nine months of gestation, often face recurrences after their children are born. Pregnancy is not a cure, although many doctors encourage women with endometriosis who want children to try to conceive when they're younger because the possibility of infertility will increase as they get older.

Another form of treatment for endometriosis has been the birth control pill. The pill contains the hormones estrogen and progesterone, which create a sort of pseudopregnancy and prevent the endometrium from developing to any great extent each month, so the pill arrests the disease. However, it does not eliminate it. The feminine hormones continue to fluctuate and to stimulate the endometriosis so that the tissue remains alive. Although the birth control pill is useful in preventing the development of endometriosis, it *will not cure* the disease once it has started.

A state of pseudopregnancy to fight endometriosis can also be achieved with injectable progestin (Depo-Provera), and with oral progestin (medroxyprogesterone), or progesteronelike medication (Megace).

The only FDA-approved drugs for treating endometriosis, however, are Danocrine (danazol), a synthetic derivative of the male hormone testosterone, and the gonadotropin-releasing hormone (GnRH) agonists, a breed of hormone suppressors found in drugs such as Synarel (nafarelin) nasal spray and Lupron (leuprolide acetate) by injection. Both Danocrine and the GnRH agonists block the release of the brain hormones FSH (follicle-stimulating hormone) and LH (luteinizing hormones), from the pituitary gland, which set the menstrual cycle in motion. A woman's ovaries are not stimulated to release an egg so there is no ovulation and estrogen and progesterone hormones do not increase. When a woman does not ovulate and her female hormones remain low and do not fluctuate, there is no buildup of the endometrium and no chance for endometriosis to grow. Of course, there is no menstruation either, and a woman is in a state of pseudomenopause.

Another important mechanism of action of Danocrine is the blockage of hormone receptors in the endometriosis. Therefore, even if small amounts of estrogen and progesterone are present in the bloodstream, these hormones will be prevented from stimulating the endometrial tissue, which will gradually disintegrate.

Danocrine is my first choice of treatment for endometriosis. The drug is really an antihormone, because it is able to stop the spectacular ebb and flow of the feminine hormones estrogen and progesterone, which, while they're orchestrating the menstrual cycle producing the endometrium within the uterus, are also rejuvenating the endometriosis. The hormones trigger the production of a monthly blood supply necessary to the tumorous growths of the disease. When a woman takes Danocrine tablets every day for several months, she is curtailing her hormone production and thereby preventing the endometriosis from getting the renewed supply of rich blood vessels it needs for survival. The endometrial tissue dies and, like all dead tissue, is slowly reabsorbed by the body and disappears.

I like Danocrine because in addition to its direct effect on the pituitary gland, unlike GnRH agonists, it blocks receptors in the endometrial tissue and helps to destroy the disease more effectively as well. In addition, Danocrine can be taken in tablets; GnRH agonists are destroyed by stomach acids and are available only as nasal spray or by injection. Danocrine also has fewer side effects. While Danocrine's side effects can include weight gain, fluid retention, acne, decreased breast size, vaginal atrophy, and hot flashes, within a few weeks of stopping the drug these side effects disappear. Side effects of the GnRH agonists are bone loss and heart disease, however, and medication for one or both of these conditions might be needed afterward.

EFFECT OF DANOCRINE

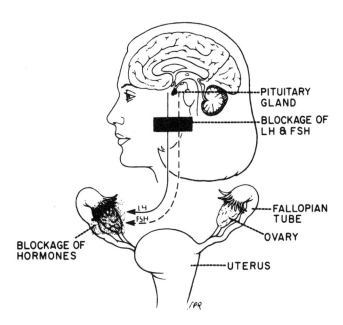

7-2   **Effect of Danocrine (danazol) on Endometriosis.** The reason Danocrine is so effective is that it has several mechanisms of action. First, it blocks the brain hormones FSH and LH, a blockage that stops menstruation and prevents estrogen stimulation of the endometriosis. Danocrine also blocks hormone receptors in the endometriotic growths, which disintegrate and disappear. Therefore, this drug can result in a complete reabsorption of the endometriosis without the need for surgery. Danocrine will revert all of a woman's symptoms and restore her fertility.

It is now recommended that if a woman with widespread endometriosis needs surgery she be placed on Danocrine or GnRH agonists for three months prior to the operation to allow the drug to melt away the more advanced stages of the disease. If this is not done, surgery might be extremely complex and risky. When Danocrine or GnRH agonists have not been used prior to surgery, doctors have accidentally cut into the bladder, bowel, and other organs. Women have awakened in recovery rooms and found themselves in horrifying conditions.

Exploratory surgery should be performed as a treatment for endometriosis only when a woman has large masses that must be removed. However, a physician should not attempt extensive surgery with the goal of removing the disease totally, because he will never be able to succeed. A surgeon cannot remove every bit of endometriosis in a woman's body. After surgery, the disease might come back. A woman's doctor might tell her that he has cut, burned, or laser-vaporized endometriosis away, but if a woman is not placed on Danocrine or GnRH agonists after her operation, the disease can return. A complete "pelvic cleanout," a hysterectomy in which both ovaries and tubes are also removed, is the only surgical procedure that can really terminate endometriosis, but such a drastic operation must be viewed as a castration. A woman who has had such a "pelvic cleanout" will not be able to produce hormones of her own anymore and of course she will never be able to bear children.

Before endometriosis grows into larger masses, it's a good idea to have laparoscopy surgery. During a laparoscopy, the extent of the disease can be evaluated, the ovaries and Fallopian tubes assessed, and visible endometriosis can be removed through excision or endometrial ablation (destruction of the disease through laser-vaporization or electrocautery). Afterward, a woman should receive Danocrine or a GnRH agonist for several months to prevent reappearance of the disease.

QUESTIONS ABOUT ENDOMETRIOSIS

Endometriosis is a major cause of infertility. Too often, women have chalked up their abdominal pain to the "normal" pain of menstruation when they have had endometrial growths spreading throughout their bodies. Women must become aware of the symptoms of endometriosis in order to quash this dreadful disease early. Women who have not been aware have lived in despair and unhappiness. Their letters express the physical pain and emotional suffering that have ruined their marriages, divided their families, and scarred them in every way.

Why Don't Doctors Understand?

My husband and I have spent our life savings trying to find help for our eighteen-year-old daughter. In two years she has been in and out of hospitals fifty times. She describes a pain in her side that feels like a hot poker jabbing at her day and night. Doctors have said that she has endometriosis and a bladder problem. After she had an operation for a ruptured cyst, they told us that other cysts were tiny, nothing to worry about, and that the endometriosis was barely there. Then why is she in so much pain and anguish? She is always in the hospital so that one doctor or another can "have a look," and we own enough medication to go into the pharmaceutical business. Here's what happens: One doctor prescribes hormones. Another doctor says that hormones will kill her. A third doctor thinks that hormones are the only thing that can help her. What do we do? Some doctors say her pain is emotional, all in her head. One gynecologist looked right at her and said, "It can't hurt that badly. You have to learn to live with pain." She has been handed prescriptions for tranquilizers and painkillers, which she is afraid to take because she doesn't want to become addicted. We all want to cure her problem, not hide it. Besides hormone pills, tranquilizers, painkillers, she has received countless X-ray treatments. She has severe headaches, leg cramps, kidney problems, a constant discharge, spotting. Yet none of the so-called medical experts we've seen have come to any agreement. Nobody seems to know what to do. Where do we turn? Please help us.

—H.J., Bakersfield, California

Cramps used to be a part of my life. I never thought much about them until college, when they became so intense I couldn't study for exams. I went to a doctor when I was nineteen and he admitted me to the hospital for an exploratory and told me I had endometriosis. Then he told me I needed major surgery to burn it all out. I had the operation but a year later the endometriosis came back. The doctor put me on the strongest birth control pill, which I took nonstop for six months. I was supposed to increase my dosage each time I noticed a sign of menstruation and as a result I was taking four birth control pills a day. I gained thirty pounds, and finally I had a three-month period. I was very sick and the doctor said I only had one choice—hysterectomy. I was twenty-one years old when all my female organs were removed. It has been almost two years now and I've just started to get used to the hormones I will have to take for, I guess, the next thirty years. That's the physical part of my problem, but there's an emotional part too. My fiance left me after the operation and I found out that other men are not interested in me when they hear about my surgery. I've become depressed and I've gained twenty-five pounds. I've tried getting help and advice from different gynecologists, but they tell me my mental state has nothing to do with my operation and they dismiss my problems. No one should have to live like this or be treated this way.

—N.K., Columbus, Ohio

These women have learned that many doctors do not know how to relieve the suffering caused by endometriosis. The teenager in the first letter seems to have minimal disease that her doctors are not able to see during exploratory surgery. Although it is not mentioned in the letter, she probably had a laparoscopy, an operation in which a specially designed periscope is inserted through a small incision in a woman's navel to afford a view of her pelvic organs. The endometriosis might have spread inside other tissues or it might be growing behind her uterus in areas hidden from a doctor's sight.

During a pelvic examination, a sensitive physician will be able to feel the lumpiness created by displaced endometrial tissue behind or to the side of a woman's uterus. A competent doctor is also aware that no matter how little disease might be evident, the suffering can be extreme. Even minimal disease can cause relentless, stabbing pain. Endometrial tissue that has implanted itself outside a woman's uterus can begin to press and pull on her nerves and organs. The tumors enlarge like rolling snowballs and slowly join the bowels. The tissue can grow into a woman's Fallopian tubes, block them, and cause sterility. Endometriosis can surround and compress organs until they can no longer function.

The eighteen-year-old woman in the first letter has been shuffled in and out of hospitals for years and still she has met no one who has evaluated her with compassion and comprehension. Her pain is real, but at this point her emotional experiences might be overriding her physical condition and scarring her for life. She is probably afraid to trust anyone in the medical profession even though there *are* understanding doctors who know how to treat a woman with endometriosis.

Before this woman undergoes any further surgery she should visit a large medical center for a consultation with an infertility specialist or an endocrinologist who is willing to treat her with the drug Danocrine (danazol), discussed earlier. For emotional support and advice, she might also contact the Endometriosis Association International Headquarters: 8585 N. 76th Place, Milwaukee, WI 53223; 800-992-3636; www.endometriosisassn.org; (E-mail) endo@endometriosisassn.org.

This young woman has time to find the right treatment while she still has her female organs. The woman who wrote the second letter is not as fortunate.

A woman whose doctors suggest that she undergo surgery for endometriosis should always seek a second opinion. Ms. K. trusted her doctor, and he proceeded to ravage her body. Endometrial tissue spreads like fine sand inside the abdomen. It travels behind and around pelvic organs and there is no way a doctor can burn it all away.

Surgery for endometriosis can be more complicated than cancer surgery, and if necessary, it requires the skill of a leading microsurgeon, who operates with the aid of magnification, using special fine instruments and bloodless techniques. Before submitting to surgery, a woman should make an appointment with an infertility specialist or an endocrinologist at a university hospital or a metropolitan medical center where physicians have become more familiar with the hidden woman's disease. Surgery is only helpful if there is a large tumorous mass of endometrial tissue that can be scooped out during an operation, but, as was explained earlier, Danocrine or GnRH agonists should be given before and after surgery to melt away as much of the tissue as possible.

Birth control pills might prevent the advancement of endometriosis, but they will not eliminate the disease that already exists. This woman was put through a heartrending ordeal with surgery and birth control pills before she underwent a hysterectomy at the young age of twenty-one. A hysterectomy is not the treatment of choice for endometriosis. Ms. K. was put in a menopausal state before she had the opportunity to try Danocrine, the drug that might have cured her. By living with synthetic hormones for so many years of her life, Ms. K. is now increasing her susceptibility to breast cancer. Her profound sense of despair is perfectly understandable. She, too, might be helped by contacting the Endometriosis Association at the above address and sharing her experiences with women who have had their own personal horrors generated by the disease.

Both of the women who wrote these letters have been victims of unnecessary surgery. Sometimes, when endometriosis is causing continuous spasmodic pain, a woman agrees to anything to find relief. Women with endometriosis must guard against knife-happy surgeons who have little understanding of the disease. A woman should never sign a consent form for a hysterectomy until she has discussed her case with at least two reputable medical experts who have extensively treated endometriosis in women. She should never visit a physician without being escorted by a spouse or a loved one who can help her gain perspective on the doctor's advice, and above all, she should remember that no surgery should be advised until there has been an attempt to curb the disease beforehand with medication.

Her Intuition Saved Her Baby's Life

I had pain for all my adolescent years, from thirteen until I was twenty, when I found a doctor who operated on me. He fixed a tilted uterus and removed endometriosis, and told me I could get pregnant, since my husband and I wanted a child. The pain returned after we moved to a new town. I went to another doctor, who said the endometriosis was all over and I needed a complete hysterectomy at age twenty-two. He said I would never get pregnant anyway. I refused and went on painkillers. It seemed my endometriosis was really growing and affecting my period. My doctor insisted I have a hysterectomy but I kept saying "No." Then instinct told me to take a urine sample to another doctor and I learned that I was pregnant. I didn't have a tumor, I had my little boy, who was born six months later. Thank God I didn't have a hysterectomy. How can doctors be such quacks?

—W.A., Virginia, Illinois

This woman was a typical endometriosis patient, yet she was in pain for seven years before she found a doctor who could make a diagnosis. When that doctor corrected her tilted uterus, he increased her chances for conception. The second doctor was completely misinformed. It is possible for a woman with endometriosis to become pregnant after the proper infertility surgery alone, but if the disease is detected early, if the proper medication is prescribed, and then surgery is performed, chances for conception are much better.

Fortunately, this woman followed her intuition and refused to submit to a hysterectomy. Her doctor prescribed painkillers that could have harmed her baby, but from what she writes, her baby is healthy. Ms. A.'s son is living proof that every woman should *listen to her body.*

Is a Hysterectomy the Cure?

When I was nineteen years old my doctor operated on me to remove a cyst from my ovary but during the surgery he discovered endometriosis and removed my right ovary and tube. Then the doctor put me on birth control pills because he said he wanted to create an artificial pregnancy. The pills made me fat and depressed and they didn't help because a year or so later I had a cyst on my left ovary. This time the doctor did a total hysterectomy and at the age of twenty-one I was put on estrogen replacement. I have tried avoiding estrogen because I heard it could cause cancer, but when I don't take it I have headaches and a dry vagina. Over the last five years I have tried three different kinds of estrogen—one grew hair on my face, one gave me acne, and one made my breasts hurt. Is there anything else I can do? I almost wish I still had the problem with endometriosis rather than all these hormone problems!

—N.S., Odebolt, Iowa

I had three hysterectomies to cure my endometriosis. First, I had a hysterectomy and I was left with part of my uterus, one ovary and tube. The endometriosis got worse instead of better and ten months later I had another hysterectomy to remove my cervix. Then three months after that, when my pain returned, the doctor performed surgery to take out everything he left behind the first and second time. I'm thirty-two years old and I feel like I am ready for a rest home. Is hysterectomy the only way to treat this disease?

—W.P., Fairbanks, Alaska

Two years ago I had an operation and my doctor cut out the endometriosis on my left side. He put me on Danocrine, four pills a day, but now I have stopped the medication. The trouble is, every time I get my period I am in pain. I take codeine but my doctor says that if my period continues to be bad he might have to give me a hysterectomy. I am twenty-nine years old and I have a five-year-old daughter. I don't mind not having any more children if a hysterectomy will make the pain go away. I am at the end of my rope and I don't know what to do.

—F.J., Albany, New York

It is appalling to learn that a hysterectomy was performed on the twenty-year-old woman who wrote the first letter. A woman who has a hysterectomy in her twenties will be placed on hormones for the next twenty or more years, and when given in high doses, replacement hormones can increase a woman's risk of breast cancer.

NOTE: *A hysterectomy is not a cure for endometriosis*—it should be viewed only as a last resort. A hysterectomy that includes the removal of both ovaries is like a castration. After this operation, a woman will never produce her own hormones again, and she will never be able to bear children.

When *no other treatment is available* to a woman who has extensive endometriosis, and more than one doctor has told her that a hysterectomy is the only way she will be able to function in life, then a complete "pelvic cleanout"—which includes removal of both ovaries and tubes—is necessary or her endometriosis will return. A "pelvic cleanout" is an extremely drastic operation, however, and a woman should always search for another route to relief before submitting to this surgery.

If a hysterectomy is unavoidable, a woman should select her surgeon carefully. One has to wonder about the competence of the doctor who cared for Ms. P., who wrote the second letter. Without ever prescribing Danocrine, Lupron, or Synarel to shrink her endometriosis, he performed surgery after surgery. He did not seem to realize that modern physicians are doing everything possible to save women's organs.

The woman who wrote the third letter should not become so frustrated and distraught that she surrenders her reproductive system to a surgeon's knife. Unlike the women in the first two letters, she still has time for alternatives.

Ms. J.'s problem might be menstrual cramps and not endometriosis, and she might be helped by prostaglandin-blocking drugs such as Motrin or Anaprox (see chapter 3). However, in her letter she does not mention the length of her Danocrine treatment. She should have used the drug for at least six months. Perhaps she did not take Danocrine long enough to eliminate all of her endometriosis and the pain she is suffering is not menstrual cramps but a recurrence of the disease. It is perfectly safe for her to begin taking Danocrine again, this time for six to nine months, to wipe out her endometriosis as best she can. In fact, a woman might return to Danocrine whenever endometriosis flares up.

After treatment with Danocrine, if there are no signs of endometriosis that a doctor can detect, an under-thirty-five-year-old woman who does not want to become pregnant might be placed on birth control pills to prevent a recurrence of this hidden disease. The pill will reduce the buildup of a woman's uterine lining, lessen her menstrual flow, and thereby give endometriosis little chance to attack.

Neither of these options requires surgery. If it is found that adhesions—the fibrous bands that form during endometriosis and "glue" a woman's organs together—are causing her pain, there is a possibility that this woman might need an exploratory laparotomy to remove them. But I see no reason why Ms. J. should be facing a hysterectomy at age twenty-nine.

My Doctor Cut into My Bowel During Surgery

Four years ago, when I was twenty-seven years old, I had such pain in my abdomen that I went to my doctor to find out what was wrong with me. He said I had a cyst on my ovary and endometriosis, and he operated on me. He removed my ovary and told me I was going to be fine. He said he was sure I could get pregnant. Well, my husband and I tried and tried but I never conceived. Then the pain in my abdomen started all over again. The doctor kept telling me not to worry but I knew something was wrong again. I had to lie in bed with a heating pad on my stomach before and during my menstruation. Finally, when I reached the point where I could hardly walk, the doctor examined me and said that my endometriosis was back and I would need a hysterectomy. I was twenty-nine years old and he admitted me to the hospital. The surgery took six hours and when I woke up I found I had been given a colostomy and my bowel was being drained into a plastic bag outside my stomach. My doctor said that my case was unusually difficult. In order to free the endometriosis a cut was made in my bowel and a surgeon was called in to perform a transverse colostomy to drain the bowel so the cut could heal. Two months later I was readmitted to the hospital for another operation to close the opening. I still have severe abdominal pain and I think I have been mutilated by a doctor who did not know what he was doing. Have you ever heard of cutting into the bowel during a hysterectomy? Or is cutting the bowel a fancy way of removing endometriosis?

—E.M., Sun River, Oregon

This woman's hysterectomy was performed in spite of the fact that Danocrine, Lupron, and Synarel have been proven to be effective treatments for endometriosis. Yet Ms. M. was never offered a chance to try a drug that might have given her relief and helped her to conceive with her remaining tube and ovary. Now she will never be able to bear children.

Her physician told her that her case was "unusually difficult," but skilled surgeons see cases like hers all the time. Her gynecological surgeon should have called in a surgical specialist to help him free the bowel before he cut into it. Endometrial tissue and adhesions can bind down the bowel and complicate surgery for a doctor who is unaccustomed to operating on women with extensive endometriosis.

An infertility specialist at a university hospital or a large medical center would have had more experience and he might have suggested one of the endometriosis-fighting drugs to her. If prolonged drug treatment had not dissolved her endometriosis, then the specialist might have recommended surgery. Still, he probably would have suggested a drug before surgery to remove the advanced stages of her disease and make his job easier. Had her own doctor prescribed medication for her for three months before the scheduled hysterectomy, the endometrial tissue binding her bowel might have disappeared. She might have been spared the trauma of a colostomy if her doctor had been more informed.

As it is, this woman had her bowel drained outside her stomach, she underwent a second operation after her hysterectomy, and she is still left with pelvic pain. Also, nothing can remove the horror that must have seized her when she saw her bowel being drained. Hers is surely a distressing account, and it emphasizes once more the need for all women to seek out knowledgeable medical specialists who routinely care for and cure endometriotic women.

I'm a Prisoner of Endometriosis

In the course of three years I've been hospitalized five times for laparoscopies and twice for intravenous therapy. I have always had intermittent pain and have been told I have bladder problems and gas pains. The first laparoscopy showed adhesions and endometriosis. The doctor cauterized the endometriosis and said my adhesions were from an infection. He considered the endometriosis cured and put me on antibiotics for infection. When the antibiotics didn't work, he put me in the hospital for intravenous therapy. My pain never went away but the doctor kept insisting that I had an infection and he did another laparoscopy. He said he saw nothing and gave me painkillers. After that I went to one highly recommended doctor after another for my pain. None of them ever read the previous reports on me. I was back in the hospital every time another gynecologist wanted to take a look at my organs. Each doctor said he saw nothing. One thought I had an atypical infection. I even went on intravenous therapy again. My pain was so unbearable I moved back with my mother. For three years I was unable to work. Finally, I found a doctor who told me that my endometriosis had never gone away. He prescribed a low-dose birth control pill and now I feel as I've been released. The pain has subsided. If only someone had helped me sooner. All these years, while I've been treated for infections and bladder problems, I've been a prisoner of endometriosis.

—H.G., Glaston, South Carolina

Endometrial tissue disrupts the smooth surface of a woman's organs and adhesions, fibrous bands that can bind the uterus, the tubes, and the bowel, begin to develop. Ms. G.'s first doctor wrongly diagnosed her adhesions as signs of infection unrelated to endometriosis. The conclusion started a tragic chain of events for her.

Endometriosis can implant itself in a woman's body and never be seen. Sometimes the disease infiltrates other tissue and is invisible to the eye of a surgeon. The woman spent thousands of dollars, underwent operation after operation, and still did not get any answers until a sensitive doctor, without even doing a laparoscopy, told her she still had endometriosis.

Usually a skilled physician can detect endometriosis during a pelvic examination and a woman can be spared the anxiety of a hospital stay. A woman must know the symptoms of endometriosis—painful ovulation two weeks before menstruation, severe menstrual cramps, a deep abdominal pain before or after menstruation, painful sexual intercourse, infertility—and she must insist that her doctor seriously listen to her complaints. Even if a doctor says he cannot find a reason for a woman's pain, she should know that endometriosis might be the source of her suffering. Many doctors who call themselves gynecologists are not board-certified, and many surgeons are not trained in the physiology of a woman's organs, so the possibility of endometriosis does not occur to any of them. These doctors treat symptoms without looking for causes.

Once a woman realizes that endometriosis might be attacking her body she should look for a doctor—an infertility specialist or an endocrinologist at a university hospital or a large medical center—who has a reputation for treating women with this disease. Every woman should aim at establishing the right partnership for her own health care.

How Can I Be Saved from Needless Butchery?

I have been having especially painful intercourse so I went to the doctor, who said I had growths on the back of my uterus. After ruling out an ectopic pregnancy, he told me that I probably had endometriosis but to be absolutely sure of his diagnosis I had to have exploratory surgery. He wanted me to agree to a laparoscopy and possible laparotomy. I was shocked to hear that the "usual" way to diagnose the nature of these growths is surgery. This seems drastic to me. There must be an alternative. I think any time a person must undergo surgery there is a threat to life. How can I be saved from this needless butchery? What are my choices?

—S.E., Mechanicsville, Virginia

Even though it is exploratory, laparoscopy must be considered a form of major surgery since the operation, most often, is done after a patient has received general anesthesia. Still, in spite of the surgical risk, many doctors like to perform laparoscopies to confirm a diagnosis of endometriosis. Laparotomy, however, is not a routine way of diagnosing endometriosis. During a laparotomy a surgeon makes an incision in a woman's abdomen and explores her organs with his hands. I doubt that a laparotomy will be in store for this woman, and in fact, she might not need exploratory surgery at all if she seeks a second opinion from an infertility specialist or an endocrinologist at a large medical center.

There are many doctors at busy urban medical centers who are treating endometriosis regularly. Since women with the endometriosis visit such centers all the time, these physicians have become very familiar with the disease. They are able to study a patient's medical history, examine her, and make a diagnosis without ever going near an operating room. Specialists are aware of the latest research and findings and they are more likely to prescribe a medication such as Danocrine, Lupron, or Synarel to a woman with endometriosis than to operate on the disease immediately. A good doctor will use surgery as a last resort rather than as a first step.

How Do I Know If I Have Endometriosis or a Pelvic Infection?

I'm thirty-seven years old and for the past four years, since I had my second child, I've been wearing an IUD. For the last two years I have had a sharp pain in my side two weeks before my period and I feel like I have gas pains too. I also get cramps, which I never used to have. My doctor doesn't seem terribly concerned, but I read a magazine article about endometriosis and I think I have the symptoms. Do you think my problem is endometriosis or some other kind of disease or infection?

—J.K., Wilkes-Barre, Pennsylvania

Often when a woman goes to her doctor with an abdominal pain he will say she has an infection without thoroughly evaluating her, and he will prescribe antibiotics. If a woman's problem really is endometriosis, the antibiotics will not help her at all. Her pain will continue.

This woman has pain *before* her period, as well as menstrual cramps, so the chances are more likely that her trouble is endometriosis. When a woman has a pelvic infection her pain is usually worse *after* menstruation because the pumping contractions of her uterus can draw in bacteria from the vagina to the Fallopian tubes and her tubes can become inflamed.

If a woman has pain after menstruation, she should have a blood count taken to see if there is a rise in white blood cells, which would signal infection. Certainly an IUD should be removed immediately, and if symptoms and blood count point toward a pelvic infection she should be placed on antibiotics right away.

Ms. K. has borne two children, but having children will not make her immune to endometriosis. Her life might have suddenly become stressful, and stress is the harbinger of endometriosis. Her doctor might want to perform a laparoscopy to diagnose the condition since her pain patterns do seem to signal a presence of the disease. First, however, he might try to determine the spread of her endometrial growth with a pelvic examination. If he feels the granular nodules and senses that endometriosis is about to overrun this woman, he might treat her with Danocrine for several months to stop her menstruation and give her body a "pelvic rest."

When the organs are relaxed, irritations have time to heal. Deep abdominal pain can also be caused by dilated veins, similar to varicose veins, in a woman's pelvic organs, and a Danocrine-induced rest will give this situation time to change for the better. So far, medical experts have found that Danocrine is perfectly safe. If this woman's doctor has not considered the drug, she might want to suggest its use.

Sex and Endometriosis

For almost a year I had been unable to have intercourse. I went to a doctor who performed a laparoscopy and told me that I had moderate endometriosis. Besides the pain during intercourse I also had backache, moodiness, dizziness, and I was always tired. He put me on Danocrine for three months and I felt pain-free for three months after that. Now the pain is back when I have intercourse, but I want to become pregnant. The doctor suggests that my husband and I keep trying to conceive for a few more months and if nothing happens, he will consider me an infertility patient and perform surgery to cut out the endometriosis. Is there anything else I can do to improve my sex life before I have to face an operation?

—L.O., Trenton, New Jersey

A woman's pleasure during sex might suddenly turn to pain when her partner thrusts his penis against internal organs that are sites of her endometriosis. Painful sexual intercourse, which is medically known as *dyspareunia,* can happen at any stage of the disease, and every woman should recognize this particular discomfort as a sign of possible endometriosis.

Sexual intercourse can hurt no matter what the extent of the disease. Only a minimal amount of tissue might be pulling on nerves, but

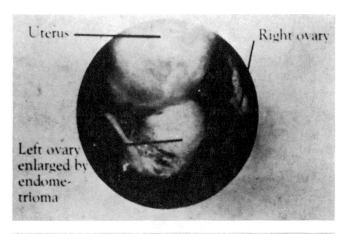

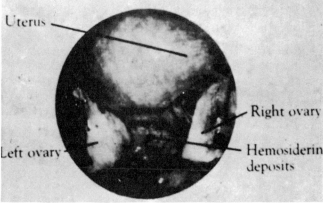

7-3 **The Effect of Danocrine Therapy on Pelvic Endometriosis Is Demonstrated.** These photographs were obtained during laparoscopy before and after Danocrine treatment. The top picture shows extensive endometriosis with the ovary completely adhering to the back portion of the uterus. During a repeat laparoscopy, after six months of Danocrine therapy (bottom photo), the endometriosis has disappeared and both ovaries and tubes are free. The only signs of endometriosis are the small brown spots (hemosiderin deposits) located beneath the ovary.

it might be growing in a spot that is directly affected by sexual activity. A woman must tell her doctor about the symptoms, as Ms. O. did.

Ms. O. visited a doctor who diagnosed her endometriosis and treated her with Danocrine (danazol), but her therapy lasted only three months. The extensive studies I have done on the effectiveness of Danocrine have shown me that treatment for *at least six months* is necessary to produce an optimum cure for endometriosis. A woman who takes Danocrine for six months, nine months, or longer will be giving her abdomen an extended "pelvic rest" when she will not be menstruating. Then her body will have the time it needs to reabsorb endometrial tissue that is dissolving with the daily help of Danocrine.

Right after the drug has been stopped, a woman's pelvis should be clean and her body should be in good shape for conception. Women with endometriosis have very high infertility rates, but many victims of the disease become pregnant right after prolonged Danocrine treatments. I suggest that this woman be treated with Danocrine again, for at least six months, and that immediately after she stops the medication she try to conceive. As she takes the Danocrine tablets her endometrial tissue will begin to shrink, her pain will gradually disappear, and she will start to enjoy sex again.

Have a Baby

About a year ago I became ill with severe abdominal pain and periods that arrived with killer cramps. My doctor gave me an internal examination and said I had a mass on my right side the size of an orange, but he didn't know what it was. He admitted me to the hospital, performed a three-hour laparotomy, and told me I had endometriosis. His suggested treatment was pregnancy. My husband and I are both twenty-five and we wanted to save money and buy a house before we had a baby. I don't want a baby right now, but my doctor didn't blink an eye when he said I should have one. He didn't even ask me if I was ready to raise a child. I can't believe that pregnancy, which I consider the beginning of a lifetime commitment to another person, is the way to cure disease. Please tell me there are other treatments. Could doctors really be so chauvinistic that they push us into pregnancies without any thoughts about our lives and our emotions?

—T.Z., Madison, Wisconsin

I am twenty-seven years old and three years ago I began having what I called my monthly stomachaches, sort of upper abdominal cramps. I can't tell you how badly they hurt. Sometimes I'd be incapacitated for two days. My gynecologist said he was "99 percent sure" that I had endometriosis. He told me that the disease could cause infertility and that pregnancy was the cure for it. My husband and I stopped using birth control and within three months I was pregnant. I believed the doctor when he said pregnancy was going to cure me, but my monthly stomachaches continued during the nine months, and they never let up, not even when I breast-fed my baby boy and I wasn't menstruating. It has been three years now and we live in a new town. My current doctor says there is nothing else I can do. He insists that I don't have endometriosis, because my pain is high in my abdomen and I have no discomfort during intercourse. My pain has made me permanently depressed. I am not enthusiastic about making any plans for the future. I consider myself a sickly person and I'm afraid that someday I just won't be able to cope at all. I'm writing in the hope that you might have some advice for me.

—P.C., Berrien Springs, Michigan

If a woman does not want a baby, it does not make sense for a doctor to suggest pregnancy to her as a cure for endometriosis. Certainly, as the woman who wrote the first letter suggests, pregnancy-as-treatment is a chauvinistic approach. And as the woman who wrote the second letter explains, pregnancy is not necessarily even an effective way to find relief.

Many women who have endometriosis have suffered various kinds of pains throughout their pregnancies. Sometimes, as a growing fetus swells a woman's uterus, the expanding womb causes the adhesions, the fibrous bands that develop during endometriosis, to stretch and pull painfully on her nerves. If stretched taut, the adhesions might also break and increase the pain. At the same time, as an enlarging uterus pushes against organs that already have pressure from endometriosis, pain stabs a woman again.

Pregnancy was thought to cure endometriosis because after childbirth a woman's uterus and cervix are relaxed organs that are less likely to cause a backup of endometrial tissue. Research has shown us, though, that although pregnancy loosens up organs, halts the menstrual cycle, and stops the diseased tissue from spreading, it does not affect already-rooted endometriosis. The endometriosis that was within a woman before pregnancy is often still thriving afterward. The estrogen and progesterone hormones that endometrial tissue needs for survival are present in her body during pregnancy at levels sufficient for the disease to remain intact. Even if a woman has been fortunate enough to be without endometriotic pain during her pregnancy, after childbirth she might feel the pain once more.

Moreover, as explained earlier, pregnancy is no longer considered a cure for endometriosis. Although the progress of the disease might be halted—and the woman might even feel better—during her pregnancy, the already rooted endometriosis remains and begins to grow again after the pregnancy.

Endometriosis can travel to a woman's upper abdomen, kidneys, lungs, and even her brain. Ms. C., the writer of the second letter, might, indeed, have endometrial growth in her upper abdomen. Painful intercourse is not required as a symptom to verify the disease. Not every woman with endometriosis has difficulty during intercourse.

Both of these women could probably benefit from treatments with Danocrine, Synarel, or Lupron, drugs that work to deaden endometrial tissue so that it can dissolve and be reabsorbed by the body. If their present doctors are unfamiliar with the drugs, or are adverse to prescribing them, these women might want to switch to specialists who treat endometriosis at university hospitals or large medical centers.

Can Tranquilizers Help?

My painful menstruations began when I was ten years old. My mother took me to the pediatrician and he prescribed tranquilizers

*for me. My periods became heavier and heavier and the pain never
really went away. By the time I was fifteen I had been hospitalized
four times for pain and vomiting. I didn't want to take tranquilizers anymore but the doctor said I was overly sensitive to pain and
I was "making myself sick." He felt that the tranquilizers would "ease
my hysteria." I demanded to see a psychiatrist, who said nothing
was wrong with me, but he gave me tranquilizers whenever I
complained of pain. Nothing changed. I took tranquilizers off and
on and I was always in pain. At eighteen, during a routine physical
at school, I was accused of being pregnant by the examining doctor.
This was impossible but he sent me to another doctor, and finally
I ended up with a surgeon who performed a laparotomy and
discovered extensive endometriosis. He followed up the laparotomy
with a bilateral salpingo-oophorectomy [removal of both ovaries]—
and now I take Premarin. A year has passed, though, and I still
have cramps. My doctor is baffled and I'm afraid after all that has
happened to me, I'm going to be put back on tranquilizers again.
I'm shocked at how little doctors seem to know about endometriosis,
and how much grief they cause women.*

—E.B., Columbia, Maryland

Devastating. This unfortunate young woman received treatments that never should have been recommended. Girls are menstruating much earlier than they used to in previous decades. As a
result of these early menstruations, and exposures to family stresses
that used to be hidden from children, adolescent and preadoles-
cent females are turning up with endometriosis in much greater
numbers.

Most pediatricians have very little knowledge of endometriosis.
They are not in the habit of diagnosing the disease and, apparently,
it does not occur to them that this condition would appear in a
youngster. Tranquilizers should never have been prescribed. This
young woman's doctor did not understand the disease, and her
mother should have sought a second opinion when the physician
suggested tranquilizers for a ten-year-old.

When a daughter is suffering from pain before or during menstruation, a parent should try to have a compassionate conversation with the young woman. She might be under emotional stress that she is afraid to reveal. A parent should ask questions and elicit a daughter's feelings. If a young woman has the chance to unburden herself without reprobation, she might become less susceptible to endometriosis. A mother or father can save a child of theirs from the horrors that Ms. B. experienced and is still experiencing.

No one took Ms. B.'s symptoms seriously, and she was not properly treated for endometriosis when the disease was in its early stages. Over the years, endometrial tissue had a free rein in her body. Then she fell into the hands of a surgeon who castrated her under the guise of curing her. He removed both of her ovaries when she was only eighteen. Would he have cut off the testes of an eighteen-year-old boy who had a pain in his groin? His action was barbaric.

Before she even reaches her twentieth birthday, Ms. B. is taking Premarin, a drug used for menopausal women. The hormones in Premarin will stimulate endometriosis again and in a few years she might wind up in the hospital to have her uterus removed. Her story is tragic.

My Doctor Stretched My Cervix; Is That Good?

Five years ago I began cramping before and during my menstruation. The doctors I visited said my pain was psychosomatic. About eight months ago, after an auto accident, my cramps got to the point where I could hardly walk. I went to a doctor who put me in the hospital for a laparoscopy and then told me that I had endometriosis on the right side of my uterus. He stretched my cervix but the pain did not go away. There is always an ache on my right side. Now he says I have to have my cervix stretched again. Does a small cervix cause endometriosis? I don't understand.

—R.T., Colonia, New Jersey

Physicians who are not up-to-date might still believe, as doctors used to, that menstrual cramps can be caused by a "too tight" cervix. In the past, to ease a woman's suffering, a doctor would often stretch her cervix during a so-called dilatation, a procedure in which surgical rods in larger and larger diameters are inserted through the cervix into the uterus. However, after dilatation, a woman's cervix would heal exactly as it was before, or it would be even tighter because scar tissue had formed. Obviously, stretching a woman's cervix did not relieve her menstrual cramps.

As explained in chapter 3, we now know that menstrual cramps are caused by the high level of prostaglandins secreted by a woman's uterine lining. Cervical stretching does not change prostaglandin production. Also, to my knowledge, there are no cases in which a stretched cervix has prevented the onset of endometriosis. And once the disease has implanted itself and is growing in a woman's abdomen, stretching the cervix is a total waste of time. After a doctor has diagnosed endometriosis, he should begin immediate treatment with Danocrine medication.

Every day, this woman's disease has a chance to progress further. I suggest that she look for a doctor who has kept abreast of the latest findings in the field of gynecology.

Can Depo-Provera Injections Cure Endometriosis?

The pain I get from endometriosis is so familiar to me. It starts high, shoots down toward my vagina, and throbs until I want to scream. My doctor started giving me injections of Depo-Provera every six weeks and I thought I had found salvation. The pain diminished! But now I find that other things are bothering me. I'm tired all the time, I'm bloated, and I've gained ten pounds that I can't seem to lose. If I knew that Depo-Provera was the best way to get rid of my pain I wouldn't complain, but I really would like to feel better. Do I have any choice, or is Depo-Provera my best bet?
—S.I., St. Paul, Minnesota

Depo-Provera, a long-acting synthetic progesterone given by injection, is released slowly and remains stable in a woman's body for six weeks. A woman will not menstruate while she is on Depo-Provera, which, since it inhibits ovulation, is 99 percent effective as a contraceptive. As a treatment for endometriosis, however, Depo-Provera can be helpful, but it is not the first-choice method of attack. Like progesterone tablets, Depo-Provera keeps the hormone progesterone at a steady level in a woman's body, and by its very presence progesterone maintains the blood supply that feeds the endometriosis. So, although Depo-Provera might restrict the rampant growth of endometrial tissue by inhibiting ovulation, it does not destroy the existing clumps of disease.

NOTE: *Neither progesterone tablets alone, nor oral contraceptives, will wither the tissue.* Any time one of the female hormones is present, endometrial tissue survives.

Hormone-containing birth control pills will have the same effect as Depo-Provera. When it comes to fighting endometriosis, the FDA-approved drugs are favored. Without inflicting severely debilitating side effects, the drug Danocrine will cause endometrial tissue to shrivel up and die because Danocrine will stop hormone fluctuation, inhibit ovulation, and also block the estrogen and progesterone receptors in the endometrial tissue. As the woman who wrote this letter testifies, the side effects of Depo-Provera are extreme fatigue and weight gain. By cutting down on salt and taking vitamin B-complex with extra vitamin B_6, she might combat her tiredness and control her weight problem.

However, if a woman cannot tolerate Danocrine, or if she has breakthrough bleeding, I would recommend an injection of Depo-Provera. The treatment of choice is an FDA-approved drug, but Depo-Provera, in spite of its lesser effectiveness and side effects, is the second-line drug.

Do Birth Control Pills Cure Endometriosis?

*I began having interminable, agonizing pain in my lower left
pelvic area a year ago and my doctor diagnosed my endometriosis.
Since then, he has treated me with birth control pills. I am now on
my fourth kind, since one by one they begin to give me problems like
weight gain, acne, water retention, and depression. I'm thirty years
old and my doctor says I will have to stay on oral contraceptives
until menopause. The idea of birth control pills for another fifteen
to twenty years scares me. He also said something about doubling
up on the pills this month to stop my menstruation entirely for a
while. Will glutting my system with birth control pills really cure
my endometriosis? Each time I put a pill in my mouth I wonder
what I might be doing to myself.*
—H.N., Philadelphia, Pennsylvania

When young women who have menstrual cramps take birth control pills, they are protecting themselves against developing endometriosis. As explained earlier, birth control pills contain levels of estrogen and progesterone hormones that limit the monthly buildup of a woman's uterine lining, the endometrium, and moderate her flow. A reduced uterine lining affords less opportunity for the onset of endometriosis. However, once a woman has endometriosis, the pill is not the treatment of choice.

Research continuously proves that the pill will not cure endometriosis. Past findings from the National Institute of Child Health and Human Development (NICHD) reiterated that oral contraceptives, the most commonly prescribed treatment for endometriosis, might not be the most effective therapy. As mentioned in the "Is There a Cure?" section of this chapter, the estrogen and progesterone hormones in the pill support the blood supply that keeps the displaced endometrial tissue alive in a woman's abdomen. The NICHD study confirmed that the pill supports the diseased endometrial tissue—and that with the birth control pill, endometriosis remains intact. NICHD researchers suggested that the best way to tackle endometriosis was by suppressing ovarian function (thereby eliminating fluctuation of estrogen and progesterone) and arresting menstruation, and that this is most successfully accomplished through the use of Danocrine, Lupron, or Synarel.

Some doctors have in the past attempted to stop menstrual flow by asking their patients to double up on birth control pills, to sometimes take three or four pills a day when they have signs of breakthrough bleeding. The basic principle—that inhibition of a menstrual flow will alleviate the growth of endometriosis—is sound, but trying to carry out that principle with birth control pills rather than with Danocrine is misguided, since birth control pills cannot eliminate the disease.

Any woman who is taking the pill for endometriosis should know that it is not an effective cure. Scientific studies have proven that with Danocrine especially the cure rate for endometriosis is high. Also, the pregnancy rate for endometriotic women who want to conceive climbs after these women have received Danocrine treatments.

Is Danocrine a Miracle Cure?

My infertility sent me to a Dr. Getwell who performed a laparoscopy and announced that I had a large mass of endo-metriosis on my right ovary, and then told me to get pregnant. Pregnancy was the only way to cure the disease, he said. I failed to conceive after months of trying, and my intercourse was becoming painful. I telephoned Dr. Getwell because I was scared that I wasn't getting pregnant and I wouldn't be cured. He yelled at me and shouted that I should not bother him unless I was pregnant— this was after I had already paid him at least $2,000 for surgery and office visits. Then a neighbor told me that her doctor treated her endometriosis with a drug called Danocrine. After making an appointment to see her doctor in three weeks, I learned that several other friends had been helped by this medication. Is Danocrine a

*miracle cure? How does it work? Why did Dr. Getwell say that
pregnancy was the only cure?*

—T.T., Mishawaka, Indiana

As explained earlier, pregnancy does not cure endometriosis. And
as far as medications go, neither estrogen nor progesterone tablets,
birth control pills, nor Depo-Provera injections have been approved
by the government as effective treatments for endometriosis. After
extensive studies in the United States and abroad, Danocrine,
Synarel, and Lupron acquired FDA approval as treatments of choice
for endometriosis.

Danocrine (danazol) was a breakthrough drug synthetically
derived from the male hormone testosterone. As explained earlier
(see pages 164 to 168), danazol, which is the generic name for the
drug, blocks the release of the brain hormones LH and FSH, which
set the menstrual cycle in motion, thereby preventing ovulation,
which in turn prevents the growth of the uterine lining and the
nourishment of the endometrial tissue. Danocrine also blocks the
hormone receptors in the endometrial growths so that if estrogen
and progesterone are in the body, they will be unable to stimulate
this tissue. Without nourishment, the endometrial tissue gradually
shrinks, dies, and is reabsorbed by the body. It is important to
remember that in many cases GnRH agonists are effective alternatives to danazol.

The side effects of danazol vary. A woman might gain five to six
pounds while she is on danazol, and she might notice that her skin is
slightly oily and occasionally she might see an acne blemish.
Danocrine is eliminated from the body very quickly so there is
hardly time for long-term side effects to take root. The hundreds of
endometriotic women I have treated with Danocrine have tolerated
the drug very well. Side effects of GnRH agonists include hot
flashes, headache, bone loss, and heart disease.

If there is anything negative about the endometriosis-fighting
drugs it is that they are expensive, but many medical insurance plans,

and even Medicaid, have paid for the treatments. In the long run, the price of these drugs might be cheaper than years of doctor visits and operations. Ms. T. has already paid Dr. Getwell two thousand dollars and she still feels terrible.

A woman with endometriosis will usually have to take an FDA-approved drug every day for at least six months for the treatment to work. Many doctors start with a 200-mg Danocrine tablet four times a day—two in the morning, two in the evening—but recent studies have shown that a woman with moderate endometriosis could be given a 200-mg tablet three times a day—one in the morning, two in the evening. In fact, endometriosis in its early stages might only require a 200-mg tablet twice a day. Lupron is given as single injection, once a month for six months. Synarel nasal spray, one spray in each nostril, twice a day.

I have seen hard and painful endometrial tissue, which has cemented a woman's organs and pulled her uterus backward, soften and dissolve with one of these drugs. Not every woman is cured, however. No drug can cure all the people all the time. Still, they are remarkable medications, and it would be wonderful if they could someday make surgery for endometriosis a memory.

If surgery for endometrial masses cannot be avoided (see pages 170 to 172), drug treatment is still essential. A woman should be placed on one of the FDA-approved drugs for three months prior to her operation to melt away the more advanced stages of the disease, and after surgery prolonged drug treatment is recommended to prevent a recurrence of the endometriosis.

The discovery of Danocrine, Lupron, and Synarel was news that should have spread like wildfire among members of the medical profession, but unfortunately, many doctors were unaware. Women who inform their doctors will be helping themselves and other women who suffer from endometriosis to find relief.

Will I Grow a Beard or Go Through Menopause If I Take Danocrine?

This month my doctor told me that I had endometriosis. A friend of mine had endometriosis and she was treated with Danocrine. I mentioned the drug to my doctor and he said that Danocrine was a male hormone that would make me grow hair and go through menopause. He did not want to prescribe it. My friend has no complaints about the drug. What's going on here?
—K.C., Forest City, North Carolina

All hormones—male and female—share similar chemical structures. Danocrine has a synthetically created structure more akin to testosterone than estrogen, but it certainly is not a male hormone.

I have treated hundreds of women with Danocrine, and the side effects have not been severe or debilitating. Weight gain is the main unwanted reaction. Every patient gained five to six pounds when she began taking Danocrine tablets. Sometimes it is a good idea for a woman on Danocrine to counterbalance her weight gain by reducing her salt intake and eliminating her extra fluid with a diuretic.

Usually after three or four months on Danocrine (danazol), most women begin to drop the added weight and feel better, but that initial leap in poundage is a sure thing. Other side effects are minor and unpredictable. Some women experience oilier skin and occasional acne blemishes. Other women notice vaginal infections, which might occur because the estrogen hormone is staying at a low level.

Actually, blood tests have shown that women on Danocrine have the estrogen and progesterone levels of women who have just completed their menstruations. It is usually during the first few days after menstruation that a woman feels her best, and this postmenstrual sense of well-being has no similarity to a menopausal state. A woman on Danocrine stops menstruating, but in no way does her body go through menopause. None of the hormonal dips that accompany the change-of-life are prompted by Danocrine. In fact, women on Danocrine, partly because they are now completely pain-free, often feel in such good spirits that they don't want to stop the therapy. An increase in hair growth is extremely rare, and women on Danocrine usually look as great as they feel. However, if a woman is extremely worried about hair growth, Lupron or Synarel—the GnRH agonists—might be better suited to her.

When Endometriosis Spreads to the Bladder

I've had horrible menstrual cramps ever since my teens. After different doctors told me that my pain was "all in my head," I gave up on the medical profession. Now I'm twenty-six and the waves of pain across my abdomen are ten times worse than they used to be. Sometimes I'm bedridden for two or three days before my period starts, and when I do begin to flow, the pressure on my bladder is so constant that I run to the bathroom all the time because I think I have to urinate. Recently I noticed that when I do urinate during my period, the blood that I thought was coming from my menstruation is really blood in my urine. What does this mean?
                                                    —K.D.,Youngstown, New York

As yet, this woman has not been diagnosed as having endometriosis, but her symptoms do seem to indicate that the disease has invaded her body. She has a history of menstrual cramps, severe abdominal pain, pressure on her bladder, and bloody urine.

Endometrial tissue can implant itself outside a woman's bladder, and if left untreated, it can penetrate the wall of the bladder and continue to grow inside the organ. The diseased tissue in the bladder will bleed just like the uterus does during menstruation and bloody urine will result. If this woman's doctors had investigated her complaints of cramps, they might have discovered her endometriosis in its early stages, before the tissue had traveled into her bladder. In her present condition, treatment will probably require medication and surgery.

I have observed several patients with advanced endometriosis that moved into their bladders and caused them to urinate blood. A number of these women have been successfully treated with Danocrine Once the disease has entered the bladder, however, it usually cannot be completely destroyed by the drug. Surgery is often needed. One woman in my patient group underwent a nine-month Danocrine treatment followed by surgery to remove the portion of her bladder that was replete with endometriosis. After surgery, with her endometriosis eradicated, she became pregnant, gave birth to a healthy baby, and was delighted. Every woman's story should end so happily.

It is important for a woman to find a physician who will treat her for endometriosis when the disease is in its early stages. Unfortunately, the woman who never encounters a skilled, compassionate physician might have to prepare herself for two-arm treatment with Danocrine and surgery if the disease spreads into her bladder.

Surgery for removal of endometriosis in the bladder is very tricky, and a top urologist should be sought. After endometriosis implants itself on the outside and inside of a woman's bladder, only a gynecologist/urologist team can cure her.

If the endometriosis had been spotted during Ms. D.'s teenage years, she might not be suffering so much today. Every woman must aim for rapid detection of endometriosis as soon as she notices symptoms. Menstrual cramps and severe abdominal pain, as this woman describes, are two definite signs of trouble. The disease is spreading and all women must be alert.

Could I Have Endometriosis in My Lungs?

After my doctor diagnosed my endometriosis, he operated on me twice to cut out the diseased growths. Then he put me on the birth control pill. Well, I've been off the pill now for four years and I have pain on my right side in my abdomen, and also on the right side of my chest. I went to the hospital last month with a collapsed lung and one doctor said something about endometriosis in my lungs. Is this possible? Could I really have endometriosis in my lungs?

— L.Y., Harlan, Kentucky

Endometriosis has been found in the bladder, the kidneys, the lungs, and even the brain. There are several theories that attempt to explain how the disease manages to travel so far from its normal sites. In the "How Does Endometriosis Occur?" section of this chapter, the Sampson theory, which describes the backward flush of endometrial tissue through a woman's Fallopian tubes and into her abdominal cavity, gives some understanding of how the disease can take root. Another theory holds that endometrial tissue originates in different spots within the body during embryotic life, and when the child becomes a woman hormones stimulate her tissue and it begins to grow. Thus, endometriosis might flourish in rare places.

Other scientists feel that endometriosis could be spread by a woman's bloodstream to areas outside her abdomen. This hypothesis seems more reasonable than the embryotic theory, but whatever the reason for the expansion of endometriosis, the unbelievable spread of the disease is real. Each month, as this woman's uterus sloughs off its lining, the endometrial tissue that has attached itself to her lung sheds, too. Then her lung collapses.

I have treated two patients whose lungs have been attacked by endometriosis. One woman's lung collapsed at occasional intervals. The other woman's lung collapsed each month when she had her period. One woman took Danocrine for nine months, and the other for a year. In both cases, the endometriosis dissolved. One woman had a recurrence of the disease but she returned to Danocrine and has not felt the pain of endometriosis again.

Ms. Y. might benefit from a similar extended Danocrine treatment, but she must remember that any time she has a twinge of endometriotic pain, she should visit her doctor immediately. If caught early, endometriosis will not have a chance to advance so far.

Can Vitamins Cure Endometriosis?

When my daughter was twenty-five years old I watched her suffer in despair from endometriosis. She sometimes wept for days

and when she would visit the doctor she would beg for a hysterec-
tomy. I prayed for a cure and one day I read that vitamin E had an
effect on reproductive organs. I didn't know anything about vita-
mins but I insisted that my daughter try massive doses of vitamin
E. She did so reluctantly but a miracle happened. Her pain subsided
and now she is a healthy thirty-year-old woman. Her doctor
examined her and said, "Sometimes these things take time to work
out." She didn't tell him about the vitamin E because she didn't
think he would believe her. Anyway, I am passing the word to you
in the hope it might help other women end their suffering.
—V.L., Los Angeles, California

Endometriosis is such a terrible condition that every possible
form of relief should be tried while doctors make their determined
efforts to eliminate the illness.

We do know that certain vitamins might influence bodily functions. The B vitamins, which affect neural transmissions that orches-
trate menstrual flows, have been used to regulate periods. Ms. L.'s
daughter took massive doses of vitamin E, and there have also been
cases of women who overcame endometriosis with high daily doses
of vitamin B-complex, vitamin E, and selenium.

It is important for a woman to continue a health habit that works
for her. Vitamins will not harm a woman with endometriosis, and
although we do not have scientific proof that vitamins will cure the
disease, maybe they will do some, as yet undocumented, good.

CAN ENDOMETRIOSIS LEAD TO CANCER?

There is a cancer called *adenocarcinoma of the endometrium* that can
develop within a woman's uterine lining and can often be cured with
a hysterectomy. In the past, women on estrogen replacement therapy
without progesterone became more susceptible to this endometrial
cancer, which is activated by high levels of estrogen. Now, since the

same glandular tissue that forms a woman's uterine lining is the source of endometriosis, the diseased endometrial tissue is liable to become cancerous, too, if it is overly stimulated by estrogen. For this reason, estrogen tablets should not be used to treat endometriosis.

Rarely, however, does endometriosis become cancerous. I have seen a few sad cases of endometrial cancer that spread with the tissue to all parts of the body. Cobalt or radiation treatments had to be given and the women eventually died. In other instances, of course, women with endometrial cancers have been cured.

All this just proves, once more, that endometriosis is a serious disease that every woman must try to recognize in its earliest stages. The sooner endometriosis can be detected, the greater a woman's chances of banishing the dreaded disease from her system.

INFERTILITY AND ENDOMETRIOSIS

A woman with pelvic endometriosis is going to be much less fertile than a woman who does not have the disease, but the reasons why are elusive. Due to the nature of the disease, endometriosis might generally interfere with the overall ovulation mechanism. In some cases, endometrial tissue seems to form a shelf around an ovary so that an egg cannot reach the Fallopian tube. There are also times when endometrial tissue appears to collect inside the Fallopian tubes and obstruct the passage of the monthly egg.

An endometriotic woman should consult an infertility specialist at a large medical center for advice and treatment. The doctor will conduct a complete workup to check her for ovulation abnormalities and thyroid problems, and will X-ray her uterus. When it has been determined that endometriosis alone is causing a woman's infertility, she should receive the appropriate treatment to increase her chances of conception.

Endometriosis is one of the leading causes of infertility, but if the disease is diagnosed and treated at an early stage, there's a good chance a woman can become pregnant. At the start of its development, endometriosis does not usually destroy the fimbria, the finger-like extensions of the Fallopian tubes that in effect grab ovulated eggs, the keys to conception. (Pelvic inflammatory disease [PID], however, can destroy the fimbria and leave you with little hope.) When a woman with endometriosis is treated with one of the endometriosis-fighting medications—Danocrine, Lupron, or Synarel—she is making progress to regain her fertility. Many women have conceived immediately after having taken a medication for a prescribed length of time, and those who have not become pregnant have resumed treatment for an additional six to nine months, which further enhanced their fertility.

The possibility of conception is even greater if drug therapy is combined with a laparoscopy, the surgical procedure mentioned earlier, performed on an outpatient basis. In a couple of hours, you're home. A small incision is made in your navel and a thin, telescope-like, lighted instrument is passed into your abdominal cavity. A doctor can see and remove endometrial growths as well as adhesions (scar tissue) that have formed as a result of the disease. Sometimes medication is given after surgery, which might increase your chances of fertility. However, the most important thing is to learn how to recognize endometriosis early.

To keep a woman healthy and fertile, endometriosis should be detected in its early stages and treatment should be started as soon as a diagnosis is made. A woman must become alert to the symptoms—possible painful ovulation two weeks before menstruation, severe menstrual cramps, a deep abdominal pain on one side or the other or an unspecific abdominal pain before or after menstruation, and painful sexual intercourse—to prevent endometriosis from advancing so far that it causes hard-to-reverse infertility.

In the next chapter, endometriosis and infertility are discussed in answers to letters from endometriotic women who have tried to conceive. Some of the women have succeeded while others remain hopeful and determined—all of them are courageous.

THE PROGNOSIS IS HOPEFUL

The increased incidence of endometriosis, so torturous and disabling, need not cause women to return to the early childbearing patterns of their parents and grandparents. A knowledge of the disease and its causes can help prevent its development. Some doctors have helped women discover endometriosis with the aid of a pain map. A pain map indicates areas of pain on a paper grid of the female body and thereby enables a physician to chart the extent of the disease. The doctor can then use MRI, transvaginal ultrasound, or the most definitive diagnostic tool, laparoscopy, to identify and classify a woman's stage of endometriosis. The revised American Society for Reproductive Medicine's classification of endometriosis (1996) allows for four stages of the disease, from minimal to severe, depending on the size, location, and range of the endometrial tissue and adhesions.

We are still fighting the war on endometriosis. There is no absolute cure yet, but many battles have been won. Researchers are continually working on new medications to inhibit the disease. Other hormonal medications might join the GnRH agonists Lupron, Synarel, the injectable implant Zoladex, and Danocrine (danazol) to halt the spread of endometrial tissue. Some of the possible drug therapies include GnRH antagonists, which are similar to the GnRH agonists but with quicker results, and mifepristone, better known as RU486.

I am optimistic about the future for endometriosis sufferers, for the same reason I feel good about the future for PMS sufferers—doctors are starting to tailor a woman's treatment to fit her individual situation. The natural healing approach is being used along with medication and surgery, and women are being advised about the benefits of diet, herbs, exercise, and vitamin supplements to conquer endometriosis.

8.

Why Can't I Get Pregnant?— Understanding Infertility

TRYING TO HAVE A BABY

Diane leaned back on the sofa and watched Barbara coo to her new-born baby as the infant nursed on her mother's breast. Diane's eyes moistened. She blinked quickly, breathed deeply, and willed away her tears. Heartache was mixed with the happiness Diane felt for her best friend. Diane and her husband, Joe, had been trying to conceive for five years, and Barbara had hardly tried at all. Barbara just didn't use her diaphragm for one month and she was pregnant.

Envy consumed Diane. She couldn't help herself. Doctor after doctor had told her everything was all right, but for her and Joe, sex had become a chore. Every month the anxious wait to see whether or not her period would come ended in a menstrual flow and a depression. Why couldn't she become pregnant? Why wasn't she already a mother? She should be nursing her own baby instead of watching Barbara breast-feed.

Such frustration and bewilderment! One wishes that Diane were not so typical, but her feelings are shared by millions of infertile women. Envy at seeing the newborn child of a friend or relative is common, and most infertile women *know* that their reactions are not unique. However, sometimes no amount of knowledge can stave off the emotional impact of infertility. Once-happy marriages are saddened, but husbands and wives who begin to despair should know that their sorrows can often be lifted. With patience, understanding, and the proper care, more than 70 percent of the 6.1 million U.S. couples, 10 percent of the childbearing population, suffering with problems of conception can be helped. Men and women who fight off feelings of failure and find the right infertility specialists often become the loving, happy parents they dreamed they'd be.

Even an average, healthy, young couple will not always conceive when they have sexual intercourse on the woman's fertile days. Although pregnancy takes only one strong sperm and one egg, the sperm might not be in the perfect shape each month, or an egg might not be fully matured, or the sperm might not be chemically compatible with a particular egg-of-the-month. In the best of circumstances, the average couple will take about nine months to a year to conceive. Of course, the older the partners are, the longer it will take them to achieve pregnancy.

One of the reasons infertility is increasing is that as the culture has changed people have postponed childbearing, and fertility decreases as men and women grow older. In both men and women, the optimum years for conception are those between the ages of twenty-two and twenty-six. Of all women who try to become pregnant, only about 25 percent who are over thirty-five and 22 percent who are over forty succeed.

Contraception, venereal disease, pelvic infections, and most particularly endometriosis can affect a woman's fertility. The mind/body connection cannot be overlooked, either; personal problems, stress, and pressures might have physical effects on a man or a woman. Tension can make a woman's Fallopian tube squeeze out the egg before it has the chance to complete its journey to the uterus. There are many stories about couples who have adopted children after years of being unable to conceive, and then suddenly things change and they become pregnant. Often, these postadoption pregnancies occur because tensions have disappeared.

Infertility always used to be considered a woman's problem, but science now has discovered that 40 percent of all infertility cases are related to the male, 40 percent belong to the female, 20 percent are due to couple problems, and sometimes couples have no discernible troubles. Between a man and a woman who love each other, the question "Why?" becomes poignant and dreadful. Infertility, which so directly affects emotions, can be a draining issue, but many physical causes can be sought out and corrected when the right doctor is in charge.

WHEN INFERTILITY IS CAUSED
BY THE MALE

Many men are infertile because they have low sperm counts, sperm with poor motility (movement), or sperm with strange morphology (structure, shape). When observed under a microscope, sperm are supposed to have straight, forward movements in order to swim through the uterus to the egg. Sometimes if there are abnormalities in the sperm cells, they don't travel well. There is the time-honored joke that as a man gets older his sperm swim "backward." An older man often does have "thin, tired" sperm, but a young man can have "limp" sperm, too.

Excessive use of alcoholic beverages, cigarettes, caffeine, marijuana, and drugs such as cocaine, barbiturates, and amphetamines can affect a man's fertility, as can medications for ulcers, high blood pressure, and other conditions. Men can have weak sperm from jogging in nylon shorts that constrict the testicles, and can destroy their sperm for at least two days when they soak in hot tubs—heat is a real sperm killer.

Sometimes infertility occurs because men have too much intercourse and their sperm become thin or because they lose interest in intercourse. Many men say that they would like to raise children but they're subconsciously against the idea. They're worried about becoming fathers and they create psychological barriers that prevent good ejaculations. Some men, when they have been infertile for a long time, cannot perform under pressure. In the movie *Divorce, Italian Style*, Sophia Loren would call Marcello Mastroianni home from work on her fertile days but he just could not perform and he became a target of her "castration." This is a good time to mention that fertility, potency, virility, and performance are not necessarily connected. Many men who have low sperm counts are potent sexual athletes, while many men with high sperm counts have diminished sex drives. A sexy man might not be a fertile man, and vice versa.

Also, when a man is overtired, malnourished, overweight, stressed, or jetlagged, he might not produce an adequate number of healthy sperm. Illness with high fever can also affect sperm production and motility. These problems, however, are usually temporary. More serious is the presence of an undescended testicle, which can damage the testes and decrease sperm production, or the absence of the vas, the duct that carries the sperm from the testicle to the penis.

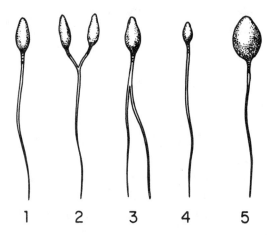

8-1   **Sperm.** Sperm (or spermatozoa) are microscopic organisms with heads and tails that enable them to swim rapidly on their own, like baby tadpoles. A sperm head contains all the genetic materials to give the father's characteristics to the baby. Only normal-looking, healthy sperm, like the one illustrated on the left (1), would be able to fertilize a woman. If the man is producing abnormal, odd-shaped sperm with two heads (2), two tails (3), small heads (4), or large heads (5), he will be infertile. If his sperm's motility (movement) is slowed, infertility will also occur.

A common cause of male infertility is varicocele, a bulging of the veins near the testicles. When a man has varicocele, his veins do not carry the blood from the testes and sperm motility drops. The testicles grow outside a man's body because sperm can only be perfectly produced in a temperature about one degree lower than body temperature. That's why in summer the testicles hang lower and in winter they are closer to the body. If a man wears tight pants or nonporous nylon underwear in a hot climate, he is increasing his chances of infertility. If he has varicocele, too, it is highly unlikely that he will help to conceive a child.

If a couple feel that they are infertile, the man should have a complete physical examination with a sperm analysis. Many men with varicocele undergo surgery to remove the varicoselike veins near the testicles. Sometimes a sluggish thyroid is the cause of male infertility and the problem can be corrected with thyroid hormone medication. Additional vitamins, particularly the B vitamins, have been known to increase sperm production. There could be many causes of a couple's infertility, but it is only fair and logical that if a woman is about to undergo testing, her mate should also be tested. (See also "Should I Have a Sperm Count?" on pages 248 to 250 of this chapter.)

WHEN INFERTILITY IS CAUSED
BY THE FEMALE

There are myriad reasons why a woman many be infertile. A vaginal infection that kills sperm before they enter a woman's uterus obstructs conception. A vaginal infection from an IUD, which might have gone unnoticed at the time it occurred, could have resulted in a damaged Fallopian tube that is causing a woman to experience ectopic pregnancy or overall infertility. Also, a veneral disease could have injured the fimbriated ends of a woman's Fallopian tubes. These fingery ends that look sort of like octopi catch the egg-of-the-month and start it on its way to the uterus, but if the ends lose their fine, grasping qualities, pregnancy will not have a chance.

One of the main causes of female infertility, however, is endo-metriosis, the devastating disease described in chapter 7. During endometriosis, endometrial tissue that should have been sloughed off as menstrual flow is flushed backward through the Fallopian tubes and sprayed out into the abdomen, where it implants itself on a woman's pelvic organs. As the endometrial tissue grows, it can press, squeeze, and strangle the tubes, ovaries, and uterus, and can cause serious infertility. The presence of only a minimal amount of endometriosis is often the hidden source of a woman's fertility crisis.

Then there is the delicate, but precise, hormonal balance that must be maintained in order to make a woman's body the perfect home for a fertilized egg. The female hormones alter the cervical mucus during middle-of-the-month ovulation. The cervix turns, opens, and the mucus gives the sperm a medium in which move-ment through the cervix to the uterus is facilitated. In order to have this mucus change, a woman must have a proper ovulation with its accompanying hormonal fluctuation, but the hormones that trigger ovulation must be in sync *before ovulation* to create a balance of the female hormones *after ovulation*.

Often an infertile woman does not have a regular ovulation because the hormones that trigger ovulation are not ebbing and flowing as they should. A sluggish thyroid or an ovarian dysfunction might be affecting the hormonal balance that is necessary for ovula-tion to occur. These are physical problems that need to be tackled. In the emotional sphere, stress can result in improper ovulation. Sometimes the pressures of life, plus the stress caused by the couple's longing to have a child, mix up ovulation patterns. Tension inhibits the release of the brain hormones that signal the start of the men-strual cycle, and ovulation either does not occur or is incomplete.

Relief from stress might come from a demystification of the ovu-lation pattern with the use of a basal body temperature (BBT) chart (see pages 216 and 217), and over-the-counter ovulation predictor kits. A kit allows a woman to test her urine for the natural surge in luteinizing hormone (LH) that precedes ovulation. Testing begins around Day 11 of her menstrual cycle and continues until ovulation

CERVICAL MUCUS

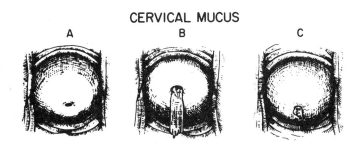

8-2 **Cervical Mucus.** There is a distinct change in cervical mucus throughout the menstrual cycle. Immediately after the menstrual period the cervix is pointed backward and there is no or only minimal cervical mucus, as illustrated in A. In all the drawings, the round, smooth, protruding cervix is viewed through a dilated (opened) vagina, the pleated area surrounding the cervix. Just before ovulation, in the middle of the cycle, the cervix turns forward as shown in B. The cervical canal opens at this time and makes it easier for the sperm to enter into the uterus. The cervical mucus becomes abundant and a woman feels wet. The mucus turns so thin and slippery that it can be stretched between two fingers (see figure 3-2). This "stretchability" is an indication that a woman is about to ovulate; she is in her fertile stage. After ovulation, as the progesterone increases, the mucus again becomes scarce and thick, as in C. The cervix closes once more and turns backward.

occurs. The B vitamins, especially vitamin B_6, when taken in doses of 50 to 300 mg daily, have been shown to aid in the alleviation of stress and the promotion of pregnancy. A woman should also remember to remain supine, with her hips slightly elevated by a pillow, for at least half an hour after intercourse in order to trap the sperm within her womb.

Experienced infertility specialists can help a woman by administering fertility drugs or ovulation-inducing medication. If she and her husband cannot conceive alone, artificial insemination with her husband's sperm might bring them their baby.

WHEN THE INFERTILITY PROBLEM IS SHARED

Infertility, although it might originate within either a man or a woman, can also be the result of a shared problem. A couple might not be able to conceive because they have poorly timed sexual relations.

A woman might be a "morning person" and her husband a "night person," and their conflicting sleep patterns might decrease their sexual intercourse. Sexual intimacy might also be interrupted by far-flung work and family obligations that separate the two people. Couples might only get together at times that are not conducive to conception. A woman might not be ovulating during the occasion when she is having intercourse with her mate.

Couples might not know that in order to conceive they should have intercourse during a woman's ovulation, which is the time when the egg-of-the-month escapes from the ovary, approximately thirteen to fourteen days before the start of a woman's menstrual flow. Misunderstanding of the menstrual cycle can cause a couple to think they are infertile when they are merely misinformed.

It is also possible that a woman's cervical mucus and her husband's sperm are incompatible. The woman's body might reject the man's sperm in a rare immune response that is another shared cause of infertility. Researchers in the field of immunology are working on ways to solve this problem, while recognizing that the biggest shared difficulty might be emotional.

If both partners have completed infertility workups and the results fail to show any reasons for their inability to conceive, emotional stress can permeate their sexual times together. Honesty and open communication are the best antidotes to a couple's extreme frustration. When faced with infertility, a man and a woman must pool their emotional and medical resources and not hesitate to lean on and love each other.

IT'S ALL RIGHT TO CHANGE DOCTORS

Sometimes two pairs of eyes and ears are better than one. A couple who have been counseled by an infertility specialist for months or years, who have been tested and told that everything is excellent, and who are still childless, should feel perfectly justified in consulting another doctor. In one case, a woman I will call Sandra was tested by her doctor for thyroid function and he interpreted her test as normal. Sandra remained infertile for almost five years until she brought the test to another doctor who told her that her thyroid value was only slightly inside the normal level. He prescribed thyroid medication along with the ovulation-inducing drug Clomid and in two months Sandra became pregnant. Her infertility problem was the result of a minor physical malfunction that was easily corrected. Her first doctor, however, did not spot the problem as a problem.

Every doctor must be given a fair chance to counsel a couple and evaluate each partner. A doctor who is sensitive and understanding can often draw out the emotional difficulties and pressures that have been suppressed, and sometimes during the counseling phase alone couples become pregnant. Husbands and wives feel released because they have found someone who will help them, and their shared personal "chemistry" seems to change.

If a physician does not devote time to counseling a couple's problem, and he repeatedly tells an infertile husband and wife that they are fine, the couple should seek another opinion. University medical centers and teaching hospitals usually staff infertility specialists who are the best in their fields, and a couple might make an appointment at one of these hospital complexes.

The subject of infertility provokes far-reaching questions about emotions, physical health, family relationships, self-image—the list goes on and on. As mentioned before, circumstances can be changed for more than 70 percent of all infertile couples. Men and women really must learn all they can about the causes of infertility, and they must fuel themselves with optimism and pledge each other support.

QUESTIONS ABOUT INFERTILITY

When Should I Be Considered Infertile?

I am twenty years old and my husband is twenty-four. We had been trying to conceive for a year with no luck. I went to my

*gynecologist and he said I should wait another year and stop
worrying. I waited a few months and then demanded he give me a
more thorough examination. The doctor sent my husband for a
sperm analysis and he told me to wait until after my next period
and have my tubes X-rayed. I did this and he said everything was
OK. Months have passed and it has now been almost two years
since my husband and I started trying to have a baby. I know I am
young, but how much longer do I have to wait to hear that I am
infertile? My doctor has not tested my thyroid or studied my
ovulation. Why can't I make him test me now? Isn't two years of
heartbreak enough?*

—F.K., East Stroudsburg, Pennsylvania

According to Dr. Charles Westoff, a fertility expert at Princeton
University, a woman in her early twenties has a 20 to 25 percent
chance of conceiving during any given month that she and her husband try to start a family. In her late twenties, a woman's chance of
conception drops to 15 to 20 percent. In her early thirties, a woman's
odds are 10 to 15 percent and in her late thirties she has only a 9
percent chance of becoming pregnant during a month of trying.

Given a year, the chances of achieving pregnancy are 95 percent
for the youngest women, 85 percent for the late twenties age group,
75 percent for women in their early thirties, and 65 percent for
women over thirty-five.

Generally, if a woman under thirty has not conceived after having
tried for a year, she can be considered infertile. A woman who is
between thirty and thirty-five would be considered infertile after six
months of failed conception, and a woman over thirty-five should
probably seek medical help if she has not become pregnant after
three months. Since an older woman needs more time to become
pregnant, her treatment should be sought sooner than a younger
woman's.

Ms. K., the twenty-year-old woman who wrote this letter, has
been trying to conceive for two years and her doctor does not seem
to have given her an in-depth workup at all. In my estimation, it is

time for her to seek help from an infertility specialist at the teaching hospital or university medical center that is nearest to her. A good gynecologist is not necessarily a practiced infertility specialist. Ms. K. and her husband need to be examined and evaluated by an expert. At the same time that they are inquiring at a teaching hospital or university medical center, they might request the name of other infertility specialists by calling the national HelpLine of RESOLVE, the National Infertility Association, at 617-623-0744.

Ms. K. and her husband should also understand the proper time for conception. A 1980s population survey conducted by Tampax showed that 40 percent of the women surveyed thought that they could become pregnant while they were menstruating, and 57 percent of the men assumed that they could impregnate menstruating women. A woman can never become pregnant while she is menstruating. The perfect time for conception is just before ovulation, about two weeks before a menstrual period. Sometimes a woman will misinterpret middle-of-the-month spotting for a menstrual flow, and when she learns that she is pregnant she thinks that conception occurred during her period. She is living with a misunderstanding. In spite of what you might read in the popular press, there is no conception during menstruation.

A highly skilled infertility specialist at a teaching hospital or university medical center will educate a couple about their bodies and search for the cause of their infertility, sometimes at less cost to the couple than a physician who is in private practice. Husbands and wives who are suffering from problems of conception should, without hesitation, make appointments with physicians who staff first-rate institutions.

I've Had Every Test Imaginable; Could the Hot Tub Cause My Infertility?

I've been trying to have a baby ever since I was thirty-two. Now I'm thirty-six and I'm worried about all my lost time. My husband's sperm has tested out fine. I've kept basal body temperature charts

and I've had every test imaginable—postcoital tests, uterine biopsy, laparoscopy. I've even been artificially inseminated twice, but with no results. My uterine biopsy showed a possible weak ovulation and I've been taking a fertility drug for a year. Lately, though, I've been starting to suspect the hot tub. My husband and I use it about four times a week. We usually avoid it during my ovulation, but could it be possible that somehow soaking in the tub is making us infertile?
                                            —G.R., Santa Rosa, California

Even though the emotional residue of an abortion or a miscarriage can disturb a woman for some time, the fact that she has been able to conceive is a positive sign. The odds are that a woman who has never been pregnant is going to have a more difficult time achieving conception. Ms. R., at age thirty-six, has never become pregnant so her situation is slightly less optimistic than if she had conceived.

Since Ms. R. mentions the tests she has undergone to find out the cause of her infertility, she has presented an opportunity to describe the *infertility* workup that helps a doctor find clues to a woman's lack of conception.

Initially, a woman will be given a complete physical examination, after which the doctor will hand her basal body temperature (BBT) charts on which she can record her ovulation patterns for a couple of months. A BBT chart is a good way to get a complete picture of a woman's monthly cycle. However, an over-the-counter ovulation predictor kit can gauge the onset of ovulation more precisely. Doctors often recommend use of both ovulation monitoring methods. Yet, recent studies have found that *a woman and her partner should have intercourse just before, and during, ovulation to conceive,* and the kits are a boon to scheduling.

As for BBT charting, it begins on the first day of the menstrual cycle, which is the first day of bleeding. A woman takes her temperature—an oral reading is fine—as soon as she awakens. Usually a woman's morning temperature is 97.5 before ovulation. At ovulation, her temperature either drops slightly or remains the same. A day or two after ovulation, the reading jumps one degree to 98.5, where it remains until immediately prior to menstruation, when it drops. In fact, the first sign of pregnancy is a temperature that remains at the higher level.

Intercourse should be followed by a postcoital test. A woman reports to her doctor within hours of intercourse. He takes a sample of her cervical mucus. By observing the mucus under a microscope, a doctor will be able to see if the sperm are surviving in the medium. He is checking the compatibility of the man's sperm and the woman's mucus.

While ovulation monitoring is going on, a doctor should take a blood test to check the woman's thyroid function. She will have to fast for six to eight hours before the blood sample is withdrawn, but this test is very important. So often, a sluggish thyroid is found to be the cause of a woman's infertility.

After he judges a woman's BBT charts a doctor might still want to perform a uterine, or endometrial, biopsy. From a few days before up to the first day of a woman's menstruation, a doctor will insert a small catheter into her uterus and withdraw cells from the uterine lining. Analysis of these cells can indicate whether a proper ovulation is ensuing month after month.

To digress for a moment, Ms. R., the woman who wrote this letter, says that her uterine biopsy indicated a possible weak ovulation. There's a chance that she does not produce enough progesterone, the female hormone that supports pregnancy, in the two weeks following her ovulation. She might well be treated by daily progesterone. Natural progesterone is available in tablets as Prometrium, as a vaginal gel called Crinone, and in suppositories specially prepared by pharmacists. With progesterone, her ovulation pattern could change for the better.

A woman's infertility workup might also include follow-up tests such as a hysterosalpingogram, an X ray of her uterus and tubes. If dye easily flows from the Fallopian tubes, they are probably functioning normally and are not obstructed. The X ray will also show whether the uterus is shaped perfectly and positioned properly. If a

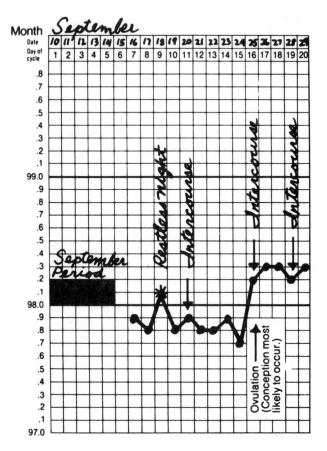

8-3 **Basal Body Temperature (BBT) Chart.** The basal body temperature is a temperature taken the same time every day as soon as a woman awakens in the morning. This very important procedure is used to determine whether a woman ovulates and when she is most fertile. The BBT is low for the first thirteen to fourteen days after menstruation. It often drops immediately prior to or during ovulation, which will be the time when a woman is most fertile. After ovulation, progesterone will be produced in the ovary and will increase the temperature approximately one degree. If the temperature remains high for more than two weeks a woman might be pregnant. If the temperature is low during the two weeks following ovulation, a woman might have inadequate progesterone production and might need treatment in order to conceive.

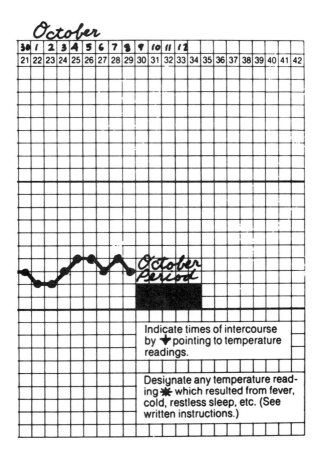

October

Indicate times of intercourse by ↓ pointing to temperature readings.

Designate any temperature reading ✱ which resulted from fever, cold, restless sleep, etc. (See written instructions.)

hysterosalpingogram pictures a woman's reproductive system as beautiful, and months pass and she still does not conceive, then a laparoscopy might be in order.

As explained in chapter 7, a laparoscopy is an exploratory operation. A surgeon makes a small incision inside a woman's navel through which he inserts a specially designed medical periscope that enables him to observe a woman's organs. He looks for abnormalities of the ovaries or Fallopian tubes, or the presence of endometriosis. Sometimes after a woman undergoes a laparoscopy, for some unknown reason she becomes pregnant. I have seen many women conceive after this surgery. Perhaps just moving the organs somehow stimulates them to function properly.

At any rate, Ms. R., aside from a possible weak ovulation, does not appear to have any physical dysfunctions, but her suspicion about the hot tub might prove true. A man who sits in a hot tub can kill his sperm for at least two days. In fact, there are certain cults in Japan that use the hot tub as a form of contraception. To increase their chances of conception, this couple should dismantle the hot tub for a while, increase their B vitamins, and continue to have a healthy sexual life. Ms. R. might also ask her doctor about treatment with progesterone tablets, gel, or suppositories to enhance her ovulation.

Could Eight Years on the Pill Make Me Infertile?

I took birth control pills for eight years, from age twenty to twenty-eight, when I started trying to get pregnant. I haven't used any contraception for three years and I still haven't been able to conceive. I've been to two doctors and had every test in the book. Neither of the doctors could find any reason for my infertility. At this point, I'm blaming the pill. What do you think?

—S.B., Boston, Massachusetts

In recent years, birth control pills with low hormonal content have been found to have fewer negative side effects than the initially pre-scribed birth control pills with high hormonal levels. Widely used for over a decade, the pill is considered to have a positive influence on fertility. The pill rests the ovaries, reduces menstrual bleeding, and paces a woman's hormonal flow so that her monthly cycle does not strain her organs. When a woman wants to conceive, her repro-ductive system, after years of lessened activity, is usually in fine shape for fertilization.

Most women resume regular menstruation and become quite fertile after they stop taking the pill. If a woman had no history of elevated blood pressure, abnormal bleeding, or other circulatory problems while she was taking birth control pills, then she should have no trouble conceiving. A woman who misses periods while she is on birth control pills should stop them immediately to allow her cycle to correct itself. It might take several months before menstruation resumes if she has skipped periods while on the pill, but then her former cycle should return. A woman should also remember that if she had irregular menstrual periods before the pill, she will have the same irregularity after the pill.

Even if the pill has caused problems for a woman, once her normal menstrual pattern returns she should be fertile. It is difficult to know from this letter why Ms. B. is infertile, but her eight years on the pill are not likely to be the cause.

What Is Polycystic Ovarian Syndrome?

I am twenty-five years old and I have been married for three years. My husband and I want to have a child very much, but three doctors have diagnosed me as having polycystic ovarian syndrome. I have an irregular menstruation and an elevated estrogen level. My current doctor has suggested the fertility drug Clomid. Could you tell me more about PCOS and, if I do get pregnant, will Clomid harm the baby?

—I.L., Milan, Indiana

Polycystic ovarian syndrome (PCOS) is usually a hereditary condition that in the past was called Stein-Leventhal syndrome (see the next letter). The ovaries become slightly enlarged and their surfaces develop hard shells. During normal ovulation, an egg bursts from an ovary and enters a Fallopian tube. When a woman has PCOS, the hard outer shell surrounding her ovary imprisons the egg and a normal ovulation cannot occur. The egg can't get out—it becomes a fluid-filled sac, a cyst inside the ovary. As more and more eggs are locked within the ovaries, more and more cysts develop and the ovaries become larger and larger. About 10 to 15 percent of all women have polycystic ovarian syndrome. They live with irregular periods and they have exceptionally high amounts of estrogen produced by their larger ovaries.

It is difficult for a woman with this syndrome to become pregnant because her inhibited ovulation causes infertility. Once in a while, an egg might break through the ovarian shell and a woman might become pregnant, but this conception will be by accident. The condition stops a woman from being able to plan intercourse for pregnancy because she does not know when, or if, she might be ovulating.

Clomid (clomiphene citrate), a fertility drug taken in 50-mg tablets once or twice, or occasionally three or four times, daily, is one way to reverse the condition. A five-day treatment with Clomid is started on the fifth day of menstruation, and as soon as the drug is taken, it begins to act as an anti-estrogen agent, blocking a woman's estrogen production. As the estrogen hormone drops, a woman might experience hot flashes, body aches, and some tightening of the chest.

Once Clomid is stopped, estrogen levels leap so high that they trigger the release of the brain hormones that set the menstrual cycle in motion. This is when ovulation usually occurs successfully. It is clear that the best time for a woman with PCOS to try to conceive is three to five days after she finishes her Clomid treatment.

To determine the best time for conception, a woman might also use an over-the-counter ovulation predictor kit. The chance of having twins is only slightly higher than normal with Clomid, which leaves a woman's body by the time of conception and does not harm the developing embryo.

Some women with PCOS are also glucose intolerant or insulin resistant. Overweight women with PCOS are more likely to develop type II diabetes. A number of diabetes treatments have been used, but a most encouraging study of women given d-chiro-inositol, a drug derived from natural components in certain fruits, vegetables, and B vitamins, showed improved insulin activity followed by improved ovulatory function.

NOTE: *Other types of ovarian cysts, not related to polycystic ovarian syndrome, can also be present in a woman's body.* For example, when there is an incomplete ovulation, an egg can form a cyst that might well disappear in a month or two. If a cyst does not disappear after a few months, a woman might need surgery to remove it. A single ovarian cyst usually does not affect fertility, but certain kinds of cysts are potentially cancerous, and surgery, followed by a lab analysis of the cyst, will be able to give a woman an understanding of the kind of growth she has. (For more information about ovarian cysts, see chapter 15.)

Could All the Hair I Have on My Body Be Connected to My Infertility?

I'm not gorgeous but I'm not exactly ugly either. I've won three beauty contests. I entered them, though, because I wanted to prove to myself that the hair I have on my chin, belly, and breasts would not prevent me from succeeding in life. I went to a psychiatrist for over a year before I would let a boy touch me because I was so ashamed of my body hair. Now I'm twenty-four and married and have a wonderful husband, but we have had no luck conceiving. I remember that once a doctor told me that a lot of male hormone in my body made me hairy. I wonder if the male hormone and the hairness are connected to infertility.
—W.E., Sumter, South Carolina

Hirsutism, or excessive hair growth, on a woman's body can be hereditary. Certain Mediterranean groups are hairy. Nordic groups are practically hairless. So much depends on ancestry. A woman who once consulted me felt, as the writer of this letter did, that she was some sort of social aberration because she had facial and body hair. She was afraid of dating, but she did make a brave effort to overcome her fear and she found out that a lot of men are "turned on" rather than "turned off" by hair. If a man is attracted to a woman, her body hair will not diminish his attraction.

However, a woman who has hair on her chin and around her nipples, and pubic hairs that grow in a triangular fashion upward toward her navel, might be living with another aspect of PCOS. This condition was pinpointed decades ago by two Chicago-based physicians who diagnosed women with excessive hair growth, irregular periods, and enlarged polycystic ovaries, such as those described in the previous section, as sufferers of the disease. The doctors also analyzed hormones.

Every woman produces estrogen, progesterone, and testosterone, and if her ovaries enlarge, they will generate more of each hormone. Sometimes, when hormonal balance is off, there is a high amount of male hormone, testosterone, secreted. The increased male hormone can cause extra hairiness, which signals the syndrome. A woman with PCOS will also have irregular bleeding, and she might be overweight due to her increased hormonal production.

Ms. E. mentions that a doctor told her that she had too much male hormone, testosterone. If she also has an irregular menstrual pattern, she might have the syndrome, which might, indeed, be the cause of her infertility.

A blood test will confirm the condition and then a woman can be given Clomid fertility tablets to help her ovulate regularly. Not every woman with polycystic ovaries is infertile, but if a woman with the condition wants to become pregnant, Clomid will help her to pinpoint her ovulation and time her intercourse.

In the past, a surgical procedure called a wedge resection of the ovaries, in which a portion of each ovary was removed to make each ovary smaller, was undertaken as treatment. Today, the newest surgical approach is a technique called ovarian drilling, in which laser or electrocautery is used to puncture ovarian tissue and stimulate ovulation. More traditionally, doctors treat PCOS with oral contraceptives *alone* to regulate menstruation and lower androgens, or in *combination* with the drug sprionolactone, which offers added blockage of androgens and suppression of hair growth. Depilatories and electrolysis to remove facial hair, and waxing and shaving for the elimination of body hair, are still the best ways to overcome hirsutism.

A woman who has excessive hair growth and irregular periods should ask her doctor to test her for PCOS because her increased hormone production, especially the influx of estrogen caused by the disease, could put her at a higher-than-average risk of developing cancer of the endometrium—the uterine lining—or breast cancer. Early detection of the disease is important so that the situation can be corrected with medication. A woman with polycystic ovaries should also be diligent about monthly breast self-examination (see chapter 16, pages 586 to 589).

I Have No Menstrual Periods; Does That Mean I'm Not Ovulating?

Four years ago, when I was twenty, I had an abortion. I had irregular periods before my abortion, but after my abortion, I had no periods at all. The loss of my menstruation didn't worry me until this year. I have met a man I plan to marry soon and we want to start a family. When I first lost my period I went to a doctor who did a battery of tests and could not find a real reason for my amenorrhea. He wanted to give me hormones, but I didn't want to take them. At the time I didn't feel the need to have a period. Now I know I have to ovulate in order to become pregnant, but can a woman be ovulating without having periods? If I'm not ovulating, what can I do to change the situation?
—C.A., Sarasota, Florida

A woman could ovulate and become pregnant without having a menstrual period, but she would be a rare person indeed. Ms. A. is probably like the majority of amenorrheic women who are not menstruating and not ovulating. The answer to why she has no ovulation is difficult to determine. Perhaps she has a malfunction of the pituary gland and the brain hormones LH and FSH, which initiate the menstrual cycle, are not being released. She might also have polycystic ovarian syndrome, as described in the previous section, which goes unnoticed by many doctors. Any number of emotional situations could be causing her amenorrhea and the absence of ovulation. The fact that she did conceive a child in her past is a positive sign that her female organs are intact and that her problem probably does not come from structural, physical abnormalities.

This woman's cervix is probably closed all the time and her vagina is no doubt dry. As a first step, menstrual bleeding might be induced by treatment with progesterone tablets or by progesterone injections, which, if there is enough estrogen present, will instigate a menstrual cycle. On the fifth day of her menstruation, this woman, if she wants to become pregnant, might be given clomiphene citrate (CC) in the form of Clomid or Serophene to assure her ovulation. If after having taken five days of CC she does not conceive, and she repeats this regimen for three menstrual cycles without conception, she might be a candidate for additional fertility drugs.

From the time she begins taking clomiphene citrate, a woman is superovulating, which means that she is producing more eggs of higher quality. Health insurance companies can demand that CC be used for at least three months before other, more expensive, fertility drugs are considered. The next step is usually to combine CC with a fertility drug containing human menopausal gonadotropin (hMG), which contains luteinizing hormone (LH), and follicle-stimulating hormone (FSH), normally released by the brain's pituitary gland to stimulate the eggs within the ovaries. Very often, after hMG is introduced, a woman conceives.

FERTILITY DRUGS THAT STRENGTHEN SUPEROVULATION

A physician might recommend one or a mix of the following fertility drugs to support superovulation:

- Pergonal, a time-honored, natural human menopausal gonadotropin, better known as hMG (a combination of LH and FSH), originally derived from the purified urine of postmenopausal Italian nuns

- Repronex or Humegon, synthetic hMG
- Metrodin, a pure FSH
- Follistim or Fertinex or Gonal-F, synthetic FSH

A woman's doctor, who should be a qualified fertility specialist, monitors her hormonal levels through blood tests. By evaluating the results of the blood tests in relation to a woman's age and her response to the drugs, a doctor might suggest different injectable drugs, or might adjust or alter the mix of drugs she is already taking. Metrodin was the first available pure FSH. That was followed by synthetic FSH drugs such as Fertinex, Follistim, and Gonal-F. The latter two drugs are now the ones most frequently used in combination with Repronex and Humegon.

NOTE: *These are expensive, powerful drugs.* Close monitoring is a must, since these later stage fertility drugs might lead to hyperstimulation of the ovaries and the release of more eggs than needed to conceive.

Fertility drugs also increase estrogen, and when blood tests show that estrogen has risen to a certain point, a woman is about to ovulate. A doctor might administer an injection of human chorionic gonadotropin (hCG), a synthetic drug similar to the brain hormone LH, to prompt the expulsion of eggs.

When all goes well, only one or two eggs are released from an ovary, thirty-six to forty-eight hours after hCG is injected. An ultrasound examination can sometimes give a doctor a definitive look at ovulation. An ovulation predictor kit, which is normally a valuable tool for determining ovulation, is not useful when a woman is taking fertility drugs. The kit measures the level of LH in a woman's body, and that level is affected by fertility drugs. On the other hand, at this time a basal body temperature reading (see pages 216 and 217), is useful for determining ovulation.

A recent study in the *New England Journal of Medicine* showed that if a woman's Fallopian tubes are healthy, fertility drug injections in combination with sperm washing and intrauterine insemination (IUI)—artificial insemination into the uterus—has a high rate of success.

Could a Thyroid Problem Be Causing My Infertility?

Three years ago I gave birth to a daughter by cesarean section. Two years ago I had an operation in which a benign tumor and part of my thyroid gland were removed. Lately my husband and I have been trying to have another baby but I haven't been able to conceive. Also, I don't feel 100 percent healthy. Since the thyroid operation my throat has felt very tight and I have dizziness and diarrhea. My doctor says that my thyroid might be a little sluggish but that I'm OK. He says I don't need medication. I don't know what to do. I'm depressed because I don't feel well and I'm depressed because I can't get pregnant. Somehow I feel that the thyroid problem and this new infertility problem might be related.
                                         —H.D., Naugatuck, Connecticut

Perhaps during surgery too much of this woman's thyroid gland was removed and now she is not producing enough thyroid hormone for her body. An underactive thyroid gland would make her feel dizzy, depressed, and drained. Her doctor says she is fine, and her blood values might indeed be adequate, but she is not feeling well. He is not looking at the clinical symptoms. This fatigued, dizzy woman who cannot become pregnant might need a small amount of thyroid medication to return her body to normal. A small dosage of Synthyroid—for example, 100 micrograms daily—might stimulate her metabolism and aid her in conception. If she becomes pregnant, she should continue taking the drug until the time when she is not at high risk for miscarriage, usually after her first trimester.

It might be wise for her to consult another physician, a doctor who would consider her blood values and her clinical symptoms together. She does not mention any pelvic problems, and since she was pregnant once before, a small amount of thyroid medication might be all she needs. I have personally seen infertile women conceive very shortly after they began taking thyroid medication. Their previous doctors had told them that they were okay, but they were borderline underactive thyroid cases. A sluggish thyroid is a minor problem easily corrected.

Can I Get Pregnant During Menstruation?

My husband and I have been trying to get pregnant for months. We have sex all the time, before, during, and after my menstruation. Nothing has happened. What could be the problem?
—P.T., San Antonio, Texas

There are a great many misconceptions about the possibility of conception during menstruation. We all know that when animals are bleeding they are "in heat," ready to be impregnated. Female animals, however, do not have menstrual flows—they bleed when they ovulate. Their endometriums—uterine linings—are reabsorbed by their bodies.

A human female sheds her uterine lining in the form of menstrual blood after her ovulation is over and her monthly egg can no longer be fertilized. A woman can never become pregnant while she menstruating.

Sometimes a woman will say that she conceived during her period but what has happened is that she might have had sexual intercourse during a time when her ovulation caused spotting. She might have mistaken ovulation bleeding for menstrual blood. There are times when the hormones surrounding the egg that bursts forth from the ovary stimulate bleeding for a day or two. A woman might think that she is having her period, but she is not.

Usually ovulation bleeding is brief, but a patient of mind was once admitted to the hospital because she was flowing profusely. She thought she was miscarrying or having an exceptionally heavy period, but actually she was pregnant. Conception had occurred in her Fallopian tube and had caused her to bleed in mid-cycle. This heavy ovulation bleeding is rare, but it can happen. If a woman conceived due to intercourse timed with a flow, she became pregnant during ovulation bleeding, not during menstruation.

To determine her ovulation, the woman who wrote this letter might purchase an over-the-counter ovulation predictor kit, or chart her basal body temperature, as explained on pages 216 and 217, or she might check her cervical mucus for signs of ovulation, as described on pages 61 to 63. The best time for conception is a day or two before, and during, ovulation. If a woman is unable to conceive during this fertility peak, she should consult an infertility specialist for an infertility workup, as explained earlier in this chapter.

When Endometriosis Causes Infertility

I have been trying to have a baby for five years, but I have endometriosis. I have taken Clomid, had two laparoscopies, two D & Cs, two X rays of my uterus and tubes after dye injections, and nothing has helped. My doctor wants to put me on Danocrine, but I'd like to know the effectiveness of the drug. Will Danocrine help my fertility or am I walking down another dead-end road?
                                        —F.H., Chicago, Illinois

After having tried for almost a year to conceive I went to an infertility specialist who performed a laparoscopy and told me that I have endometriosis. The doctor gave me a choice of danazol therapy or major surgery and I chose to take the danazol. After six months I stopped the medication and my husband and I tried again, but nothing happened. My doctor did hydrotubation therapy twice and still no pregnancy followed. He performed an edometrial biopsy and then put me on Clomid along with injections of HCG. No results yet. I think he should have performed a second laparoscopy after I finished the danazol to check on the state of my endometriosis. Shouldn't he be attacking the endometriosis to help me get rid of my infertility?
                                        —S.V., New York, New York

These alert, knowledgeable women are typical endometriosis patients. Endometriosis makes them infertile because wayward endometrial tissue that implants itself on pelvic organs can block, narrow, or damage the Fallopian tubes and cause adhesions that bind down the uterus and ovaries.

When a woman has been either clinically or surgically diagnosed as having endometriosis, she should immediately be placed on Danocrine, Lupron, or Synarel to melt away the diseased tissue. The woman who wrote the first letter might have been better off with Danocrine tablets, Lupron injections, or Synarel nasal spray for six months—or longer, depending on the extent of her disease.

At the completion of therapy a woman should have a hysterosalpingogram, an X ray of her uterus, to assure the free passage of dye from the uterus to the ovaries. If a woman's organs look good and there are no signs of adhesions, she might begin taking her basal body temperature (see pages 216 and 217) to determine her ovulation, the best time for conception. She has probably already undergone an infertility workup, but she should also have a thyroid test, and if her thyroid hormone production is low, a medication like Synthyroid, 100 micrograms daily, might correct her deficiency and help her to conceive. Extra vitamin B_6 might also be included in a woman's daily vitamins to enhance fertility.

The hysterosalpingogram after medication for endometriosis flushes out the tubes and sometimes, in the process, cleans out any small obstructions that have resulted from endometriosis. Many women find that pregnancy is easier after medication, but sometimes women who have taken a drug such as Danocrine have continued for an additional six months and conceived afterward. The woman who wrote the second letter might benefit from six months to a year more on Danocrine, but before taking the drug, a laparoscopy, as she mentioned, might be called for to be sure that her infertility is not caused by pelvic adhesions.

Danocrine gradually melts away diseased endometrial tissue, and as it shrinks growths around the ovaries, the drug especially enhances fertility. If a woman has extensive endometriosis that requires surgery,

Danocrine should be administered for three months to reduce the advanced stages of the disease before an operation is undertaken. Surgery might be necessary to eliminate the adhesions between the tubes and ovaries. Such a delicate, difficult procedure should be performed only by a skilled microsurgeon who has experience in handling the modern, fine microsurgical instruments and knows how to avoid bleeding problems.

During surgery the fimbriated ends of the Fallopian tubes must also be freed so that they can reach down and grasp an egg that is ejected by an ovary. If endometrial growths and adhesions have tilted a uterus, the womb can be repositioned during the operation. As mentioned in chapter 7, there's a good chance that a woman will conceive after Danocrine treatment alone. After Danocrine and microsurgery it is also hoped that a woman will have suppressed her endometriosis sufficiently to restore her fertility.

Could Just a Little Bit of Endometriosis Cause Infertility?

I have been going to the doctor for two years to find out why I can't have a baby. I had one tubal pregnancy and three D & Cs. The doctor did a laparoscopy and found adhesions between my uterus and tubes and a slight case of endometriosis. He said he didn't know if the endometriosis was causing my infertility. What do you think? I want a child very badly and I would like to know what's wrong with me before something terrible happens and I'm never able to have children.
—N.Y., Richmond, Virginia

I am twenty-seven years old and I have been trying to become pregnant for four years. During a recent laparoscopy my doctor discovered a small amount of endometriosis. He did not think such a minor case could cause infertility and he didn't treat it for several months. When I still failed to conceive he decided to put me on danazol medication, which I am taking now. Please help me. Could this little bit of endometriosis be my problem?
—A.O., Minneapolis, Minnesota

Even a minimal amount of endometriosis can cause infertility. Doctors still don't know exactly why infertility results no matter what the degree of the disease; however, new studies show that ovulation often does not occur when endometriosis has attacked the ovary. This finding might explain why women with just a little bit of endometriosis have great difficulty becoming pregnant unless they are immediately treated.

It is speculated that endometriosis might cause a filmy adhesion around the ovary that prevents the egg from escaping as it should during ovulation. A past study showed that women with endometriosis also produce high levels of prostaglandins, which could result in increased tubal and uterine cramping. The tube could squeeze out an egg before conception occurs. One to two tablets daily of a prostaglandin-blocking drug such as Motrin or Anaprox, taken from ovulation to menstruation, can lower the level of prostaglandins and promote conception. If a woman becomes pregnant while she is taking a prostaglandin inhibitor, the drug should not harm the embryo.

A prostaglandin-blocking drug would only be an adjunct to the essential Danocrine, Lupron, or Synarel, which should be given for even a slight case of endometriosis. Since this disease carries with it the potential for horrendous problems, it should always be treated immediately. The mildest cases of endometriosis have melted away after women have taken medication for six months. Once such medication is stopped, a high percentage of women have become pregnant.

Could I Have Both Endometriosis and Polycystic Ovarian Syndrome?

I want so desperately to give my husband a child, but we have not been having any luck. I went to a doctor who said I had endometriosis, so I went to another doctor to confirm the first physician's opinion since I was told surgery might be involved. The second doctor said I had polycystic ovarian syndrome and he wasn't sure

about the endometriosis. I went to a third doctor who told me I had
both endometriosis and PCOS. Is this possible? Could I have both
diseases?

—R.U., Dallas, Texas

A woman certainly can have both endometriosis and polycystic ovarian syndrome or PCOS. However, the endometriosis is the more likely key to her infertility. A knowledgeable doctor might treat her with Danocrine tablets for six months, after which he would give her a hysterosalpingogram, an X ray of her uterus, to make sure that her reproductive organs are in fine working order.

A further infertility workup might follow to give the doctor an opportunity to check out other possible causes of her infertility. If a woman takes her basal body temperature every day, as explained on pages 216 and 217, she should be able to know when she is ovulating. If she is not ovulating properly, she might have polycystic ovaries, and Clomid fertility tablets or an ovulation-inducing drug of her doctor's choice might help to regulate her ovulation.

If all the above treatments are conducted and this woman still cannot become pregnant, she might need further Danocrine medication followed by microsurgery to remove adhesions caused by endometriosis. The presence of both diseases makes this woman's situation slightly more complicated than that of a woman who has only one condition. The availability of today's treatments, however, gives her a good chance for conception.

Could I Be Allergic to My Husband's Sperm?

My husband and I wanted to start a family right away so we
tried getting pregnant one month after we married. We have now
been married six years and we still don't have a child. My
husband's sperm checks out fine. I've been to seven doctors and no
one can seem to find anything wrong with me. I even underwent a
laparoscopy and was told I look good inside and have no signs of
endometriosis. My current doctor says he wants to do a test to see if

*I am allergic to my husband's sperm. I never heard of such a thing!
Could my body really be rejecting my husband's sperm? If so, what
do we do? No one, not my friends or any of the doctors I visit, can
know the determination we have to have a child. We will do
anything.*

—S.F., Blaine, Washington

This woman has seen seven doctors and she has not yet had a postcoital test. Astonishing! This test is usually done as part of a normal infertility workup. A couple has sexual intercourse during the woman's ovulation and within hours thereafter, the woman visits the doctor so that he can analyze samples of her cervical mucus. Using a microscope, the physician will be able to determine whether or not the sperm are surviving in the mucus. If a high number of the sperm en route to the uterus have died in the mucus, the odds for conception are certainly decreased. The woman's mucus and her partner's sperm are incompatible, and this might be an allergy case.

A blood sample from the woman and a semen sample from the man are sent to an immunology specialist for evaluation, and if there is an allergic reaction present, *condom therapy* is often suggested. For at least three months a man uses a condom during sexual intercourse to prevent the sperm from contact with the mucus. After the three months are over, a man should continue to use a condom on all days except his partner's fertile days, when she is ovulating. The woman, during condom therapy, can also take steroids to decrease her immunity so that when sperm and mucus finally meet, the thriving sperm will not be killed and will, with full vigor, hasten toward the egg.

A woman's sperm allergy, as bizarre as it might seem, is a possible cause of infertility that a doctor should be sure to investigate.

Do Fertility Drugs Have Side Effects?

*I took the fertility drug Clomid along with shots for three years
before I finally became pregnant. I was also on Premarin for about
a year. Before I decide to have another baby I want to know if there*

are any long-term side effects from these drugs. Am I jeopardizing
my health or the well-being of my children?
                                        —E.H., Burgettstown, Pennsylvania

In the past, women were concerned about whether fertility drugs
might affect any unborn babies they might conceive. The good news
is that the drugs have not been found to be harmful to a growing
fetus, but today the focus of concern has shifted to the women
themselves. Several studies have suggested a possible link between
fertility drugs and ovarian cancer, but a connection is hard to prove
because ovarian dysfunction and abnormality, which cause infertility, are known conditions for increasing a woman's risk of ovarian
cancer. The most popular fertility drugs, Clomid, Serophene, and
Pergonal, however, have carried warnings of a possible link to ovarian cancer since a 1992 population study was made known.

That study analyzed medical records from decades ago, when fertility drugs were in their early years of development and taken orally
for prolonged periods. Dr. Alice Whittemore of Stanford University
found that among 2,197 women who had taken fertility drugs, there
was a small group that was 2.8 times more likely to develop ovarian
cancer. Among women taking the fertility drugs in the Whittemore
study, the usual figure—1.8 to 2 women out of 100 develop ovarian
cancer—jumped to 5 to 5.6 per 100. A 1994 study headed by Dr.
Mary Anne Rossing of the Fred Hutchinson Cancer Research
Center in Seattle, reported that women on Clomid for more than
twelve menstrual cycles (which is far too long) had a sevenfold
increase in their risk of developing ovarian cancer. Clomid is not
recommended for more than six consecutive cycles, and no link has
been detected on this regimen. To put the matter in perspective,
Drs. Beth Karlan and Robert Bristow reviewed all medical literature
relating to a possible link, and in 1996 concluded that infertile
women might have a higher risk for ovarian cancer irrespective of
their use of fertility drugs.

No link has thus far been found between today's injectable fertility drugs and ovarian cancer. One theory holds that superovulation,

which causes many eggs to break out and rupture an ovary in a single month, might be wounding the ovary so much it becomes susceptible to cancer, but as mentioned before, infertility itself is a risk factor for ovarian cancer. I recommend that women on fertility drugs take daily vitamin supplements, especially supplements that include high doses of antioxidant vitamins A, C, and E, to reduce their risk of developing cancer.

However, a woman should not conceive while on Premarin or other synthetic estrogens. Some natural estrogens have been beneficial in helping women conceive, but the influx of estrogen that the synthetic hormone creates somewhat raises the chances of birth defects and increases the possibility that a daughter might face vaginal or cervical cancer during her teens or twenties.

Fertility Drugs Didn't Work

My husband and I have been trying to have children for six years. I had surgery for possible endometriosis but lab analysis of the tissue was inconclusive. I've had all kinds of tests and I've used Clomid on several occasions. Every morning I take my temperature. I've miscarried a number of times after pregnancies of less than two months. My new doctor is pushing Clomid again, but I don't think this fertility drug works for me. Do you think more Clomid is my answer?

—L.Z., Des Moines, Iowa

Sometimes fertility drugs appear to be ineffective because a woman's hormonal balance has not been properly appraised. If Clomid is given to a woman who does not need the drug, it might actually act like a birth control pill and prevent ovulation. It's important that a fertility drug help a woman to compensate for an imbalance in her system, which is why a careful hormonal evaluation by an experienced infertility specialist is essential.

This woman has miscarried several times. Perhaps genetic counseling, a chromosome analysis conducted on her and her husband, would help. Genetic problems often exist when two people, even if they are cousins several times removed, are trying to conceive. This woman and her husband are probably not related, but her many miscarriages suggest that they might share an as-yet-undiscovered genetic difficulty. One patient of mine was found to have a genetic abnormality that permitted only one out of four conceptions to develop properly. After five miscarriages she maintained a healthy pregnancy and delivered a perfect baby boy.

Genetic counseling might be the answer for Ms. Z., but it is also possible, from what she writes, that she might have endometriosis. As explained earlier, even a minimal amount of the disease can severely cripple a woman's chances of becoming pregnant. If Ms. Z. has pain before her periods, severe menstrual cramps, and if her doctor tells her that she has a tilted uterus, she might have endometriosis and she might be helped by a six-month treatment of a GnRH agonist. While she is on the medication, genetic counseling might be undertaken.

Stress and Infertility

> *The doctors all say that getting pregnant is on my mind too much, that by thinking about it I'm making myself a nervous wreck and it's harder for me to conceive because I'm "obsessed." What am I supposed to do? I've been trying for three years. About a year ago I miscarried during my first trimester and I haven't been able to get pregnant since. I'm twenty-eight and getting older all the time. Yes, I am worried. I've had all the tests. I keep hearing that everything is fine, but I still don't have a baby. Everyone says "relax." Relax, relax—easy to say but not so easy to do.*
>
> *—D.A., Fairfax, Virginia*

Without a doubt, stress plays a part in infertility, but how great a part is difficult to determine. A woman who is worried about her perceived "failure" to conceive a child could easily be creating a stressful situation that might upset her hormonal balance. Once her hormones are unbalanced a woman's ovulation might not proceed properly, and her chances for conception might not be optimum. The mind/body connection is powerful.

A woman who is stressed might have a tubal spasm—her Fallopian tube might squeeze out the fertilized egg before it implants itself in the uterus. The physical reaction in her tube can come from anxiety. If her stress were removed, she might conceive. The tales of infertile couples who become pregnant after they adopt children are endless. Sometimes a woman cannot become pregnant with her husband because there is tension in the marriage. A couple might be trying to have a baby when they should be thinking about a divorce. If a woman in this kind of marriage has an affair, she frequently conceives with her lover. Gynecologists have seen many of these conceptions.

A miscarriage, like the one this woman experienced, can sometimes be related to stress, too. A pregnant lioness, if she is trapped in a stressful position, does not carry to term. The growth of the potential cub is halted and the fetus is reabsorbed in the animal's body. If stress can physically affect a four-legged animal, it can certainly affect a human being. It is also possible that Ms. A. conceived with an imperfect sperm and her body was expelling an abnormal embryo. A physical abnormality *or stress* might have terminated her pregnancy.

There is no sure way to solve the problem of Ms. A.'s infertility when, after she has had a workup, a doctor tells her nothing is wrong. Extra vitamin B-complex might help her handle stress. If her current doctor is upsetting her, she might want to find a different physician. Sometimes couples become pregnant when they go on vacation, relax, and make love. They forget their troubles. Ms. A. and her husband might plan a romantic getaway and see what happens.

The Sun and Fertility

Both my husband and I work long hours and even though we'd like to have a baby, sometimes we're just too tired to have sex. Needless to say, I haven't conceived yet. To solve the problem, we're

thinking of taking a vacation around the time of my ovulation. I
had also heard that sunshine would make us more fertile, but when
I told my husband he laughed at me. Is it true about the sun and
fertility? I hope you know.

—G.N., Chevy Chase, Maryland

Sunlight does benefit more than the plants. Years ago researchers discovered that a hormone called melatonin is secreted by the brain's pineal gland at night. In certain animals this tiny gland, this "third eye" on their heads, sends day-and-night messages to the brain. In humans, light must pass through the eye to the optic nerve and go through a series of neural transmissions before the message gets to the pineal gland. If it's night or dark outside, the pineal produces

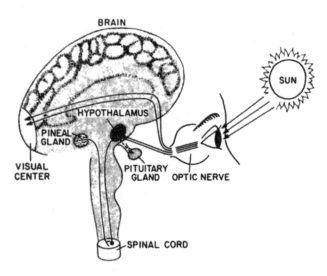

8-4   **The Effect of Sunshine on Fertility.** Light waves from the sun travel through the eye, separate, and move in two directions: (1) to the vision center of the brain, and (2) to the hypothalamus, spinal cord, and back up to the tiny pineal gland, in the brain. The production of melatonin, a hormone that comes from the pineal gland, is inhibited by the light impulses. Although scientists are still not sure how melatonin works in the body, the less melatonin, the more fertility seems to increase. Sunlight, a melatonin inhibitor, is probably the reason more conceptions occur during bright, clear, summer days.

melatonin. If it's day or bright, melatonin production slows down or stops completely.

The blockage of melatonin by natural light seems to encourage fertility. During summertime in Finland, sunlit days are twenty hours long and women become pregnant in dramatically higher numbers. Even in the United States, there are more conceptions in summer than in any other season—maybe the sun is increasing fertility, maybe the relaxing atmosphere of a vacation is balancing the hormones, or maybe both sun and relaxation are combining to make conception ideal. Whatever the reason behind the statistics, a vacation in the sun might definitely help this couple start a family.

Could an STD Be the Cause of My Infertilty?

A year ago I went to a nearby clinic to be checked for a discharge. I was trying to get pregnant. The doctor said nothing was wrong and I went home. The discharge got worse and then I got boils so I went back to the clinic. A different doctor looked up my records and told me I had gonorrhea. He wanted to know why I didn't come back for treatment, but I didn't even know I had an STD. The second doctor gave me antibiotics and the gonorrhea cleared up but I still haven't been able to have a baby. Will the gonorrhea prevent me from ever getting pregnant?

—S.S., Muncie, Indiana

Any discharge alters the vaginal milieu and kills sperm. Whether the discharge is from a yeast or a bacterial infection, or from a sexually transmitted disease, a culture should be taken and the discharge should be treated immediately.

This woman was carrying gonorrhea without knowing it and the disease spread. Gonorrhea can travel through a woman's reproductive system, obstruct and damage her Fallopian tubes, and cause infertility. Ms. S. should have a hysterosalpingogram, an X ray of her uterus, to learn whether her tubes are occluded. If the tubes are obstructed, she might need microsurgery to restore her prospects for pregnancy.

As for the STD, Ms. S. must inform her mate or any other sexual contacts that they should be checked for the disease. Since gonorrhea can damage sperm production, a man who has been exposed to the disease should be immediately evaluated through a sperm count and a culture test.

Can I Get Pregnant with Just One Ovary?

Three years ago I had my left ovary removed because a large ovarian cyst was causing pressure on my bladder and giving me great pain. Since the operation, my husband and I have been trying to have a child but so far, we haven't succeeded. Please tell me, can I become a mother with just one ovary?
—W.M., Torrington, Connecticut

When a woman has ovarian cysts, her doctor should make every effort to remove her cysts and save her ovaries. Years ago, when gynecological surgery was performed by surgeons who were not gynecologists, these doctors would remove the ovaries as a matter of routine. Today, gynecological surgeons try to preserve the ovaries when they operate on cysts. If one ovary is removed there's a chance that, if the other one becomes diseased, a woman will be sterile.

It is always a good policy to leave as many organs intact as possible, but a woman needs only one healthy tube and one healthy ovary to become pregnant. Sometimes when a woman has one Fallopian tube and two ovaries, a doctor might remove the ovary on the side without the tube to ensure ovulation on the side that is best equipped to result in conception. If a woman has one healthy ovary and one healthy tube but they are on opposite sides, she can still become pregnant, but her chances are not as good as those of the woman who has a healthy ovary and tube on the same side.

This woman should have a thorough infertility workup as described on pages 213 to 218. Her workup should include a thyroid test and a hysterosalpingogram, an X ray of her uterus, to determine whether or not her tubes are obstructed. If nothing seems to be wrong, the X ray alone might increase her chances of conception since the dye used during the X ray might flush out small tubal obstructions.

Could a D & C Cure My Infertility?

My husband and I have been married for five years and for the last two and a half years we have been trying to conceive. We've each been tested but the results have not made any difference. There doesn't seem to be anything specifically wrong. In the last six months I've started gaining weight. I think I've been overeating to compensate for my depression because I'm not a mother. Anyway, my period has become very heavy. Last month I even saw clots. A friend of mine suggested that I might need a D & C. She said a D & C might even help my fertility. Do you agree?
—J.N., New Orleans, Louisiana

When a D & C is performed on a woman who has a regular menstrual pattern, fertility will not be affected at all. Too often D & Cs are conducted unnecessarily, but in this woman's case a D & C might help.

When a woman gains weight, her added body fat produces high amounts of the female hormone estrogen. This estrogen can cause the endometrium, the uterine lining that replenishes itself monthly, to become especially thick and spongy, too rich for an egg implantation. If an egg cannot implant itself in the uterine lining, pregnancy cannot exist. The lining will shed itself as heavy, thick menstrual blood that might contain clots.

A D & C (see chapter 5 for a detailed description of the procedure) will remove the overproduced uterine lining and return the uterine cavity to its normal expansiveness, and the chance of conception will possibly increase. Then this woman must try to diet, keep her weight down, and allow her regular menstrual pattern to return.

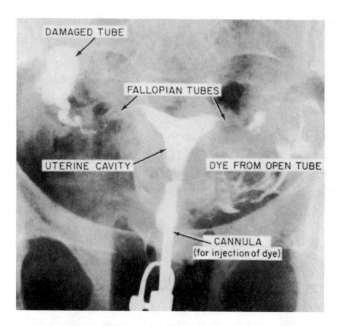

8-5 **Hysterosalpingogram.** A hysterosalpingogram is an X ray of the uterine cavity and the Fallopian tubes. The test is performed while a woman is resting on an examining table. A speculum is inserted into the vagina and the woman's cervix is visualized. The cervix is then steadied with a clamp. A cannula (a small hollow tube) for injection of the dye is placed inside the cervical canal as illustrated at the bottom of the photo. The dye, which fills the uterine cavity, can be viewed by the doctor on a fluoroscope screen and an X ray can be taken at the same time. The uterine cavity should normally be small and triangular, as seen in the picture. If any fibroids or polyps are found inside the uterine cavity, they show up on the picture as irregular spots. The dye will subsequently be pushed through the Fallopian tubes, which are connected to the top upper corners of the uterus. A normal tube is hair-thin and can often be difficult to see. In a healthy tube, the dye will be expelled and located around the ovary and bowel, as illustrated on the right side of the picture. The ovary itself cannot be seen. If a tube is damaged, as the left tube is in the picture, the dye will not escape from the tube but will be trapped inside an extended outer portion of the damaged tube. Pregnancy cannot occur through a damaged tube like the one on the left; but if a woman has one healthy tube, pregnancy can take place. If a woman has two damaged tubes, microsurgery is needed to correct her infertility.

I Have Scar Tissue in My Fallopian Tube; Must I Have Surgery?

I have a three-year-old son and for two years I have been trying to give him a brother or sister but I haven't been able to get pregnant again. I am twenty-five years old and I didn't expect to have any problems but I did go to a doctor for a complete infertility workup. I had the hysterosalpingogram, the X ray where the doctor injects blue dye into the uterus and it comes out the Fallopian tubes. This showed that my right tube was perfect but my left tube was blocked. The doctor said I have scar tissue that must be surgically removed. He said if I didn't have surgery I'll never get pregnant again. I would like to know if I have any other options besides surgery. I heard that vitamin E reduces scar tissues and I've started taking it. Is there anything else I can do?
—A.P., Bethany, Oklahoma

A Fallopian tube can become damaged and marred with scar tissue after an infection from a pelvic inflammatory disease, from gonorrhea that has traveled into the tube, from infection caused by an IUD, or from endometriosis. Sometimes an infection can go unnoticed. A woman who wears an IUD might have pain and irregular bleeding that she attributes to the IUD, and she does not realize that she has suffered a mild infection. Later on, this infection can show up as scar tissue, which might interfere with the egg's journey through the tube.

With her one good tube and one good ovary this woman should certainly be able to get pregnant. If in six months to a year's time she has not conceived, she might need a laparoscopy, an operation in which a surgically designed periscope is inserted through a small incision inside a woman's navel. A doctor can observe the woman's organs and check for abnormalities. If at this time everything seems fine, she might set aside another six months to a year to conceive.

After this second time period, if she still has not become pregnant, Ms. P. might undergo an exploratory laparotomy, an operation that allows a surgeon to investigate a woman's organs and remove adhesions that might be binding the uterus, tubes, and ovaries. When this surgery or any subsequent surgery is needed, Ms. P. should select a microsurgeon, one of the new breed of infertility specialists who know how to operate with the aid of magnification, fine instruments, and in the bloodless manner needed for successful infertility surgery. Such a doctor can usually be found at a teaching hospital or a university medical center.

Ms. P. also asked about vitamin E. Although some people claim that vitamin E removes skin scars, it does not eliminate internal scar tissue.

Do X Rays Decrease Fertility?

Last year I was involved in an auto accident and it seemed like I broke every bone in my body. I had dozens of X rays. I had been trying to get pregnant before the accident and I've continued to try since my recovery, but I haven't succeeded. My doctor thinks I might have some damage to my internal organs and he wants me to agree to a hysterosalpingogram, an X ray of my uterus and tubes. I'm worried that I'm already full of radiation and another round of X rays will overexpose me even more. Too many X rays can make you sterile, can't they? What do you think? Will this hysterosalpingogram harm my ovaries?

—R.C., Cherry Hill, New Jersey

In general, men and women should limit their exposure to X rays. The days when children were given annual lung X rays in schools and shoe stores had machines to X ray the feet of customers are over. Even dentists are much more aware of the X rays they give their patients. When a person must undergo extensive X rays, a lead apron should be worn over the genital areas.

This woman has had above-average exposure to X-ray radiation, but her doctor must consider a hysterosalpingogram necessary for diagnosis of her infertility. An X-ray examination is always weighed against an individual and her particular problem. An X ray is a diagnostic tool that is chosen when absolutely necessary.

The amount of radiation from a hysterosalpingogram is low. The X ray is taken right after a woman's menstruation when the doctor can be assured that she is not pregnant. The dye that is used during the procedure could flush out a conception if one existed, so it is especially important that the X ray be properly timed. Ms. C. might benefit from the X ray, and it is not likely to put her in any danger. The X ray is being used to help her gain her fertility, not lose it.

Can My Tubal Sterilization Be Reversed?

Whenever I see a woman with a baby I feel a longing. I am in my second marriage and I want so badly to give my husband a child. I had three healthy babies by cesarean section in my first marriage and then I had my tubes tied. I've been to a doctor who said that my surgery might be irreversible. I am planning to go to another doctor for a second opinion. I want to cry for my husband, myself, and the child who would make our lives complete. Doctor, is there any hope?

—K.B., Mobile, Alabama

Tubal sterilization should only be performed on women in their late thirties or forties who are absolutely sure that they do not want more children. This woman's story is very common. A child dies or a woman remarries and she finds herself with a change of heart. She had her tubes tied but now she would like a chance to have another child.

I am very much against tubal ligation until a woman's childbearing years are practically at an end. Today's oral contraceptives are now being prescribed to women who are over age forty, and although only 1 percent of women in their childbearing years use an IUD, it remains an option. A tubal ligation too often can lead to abnormal bleeding, pelvic pain, and a subsequent unnecessary hysterectomy.

The possibility of reversing a tubal sterilization varies with the type of surgery that was initially performed. When sterilization is done at the time of a cesarean section, a small midsection of the Fallopian tube is usually removed. If this is what happened to Ms. B., microsurgery to reanastomose—reconnect—the tubes is possible. Using the latest procedures, a microsurgeon can trim the damaged tubal ends and bring the two new healthy ends together with fine sutures.

If tubal sterilization was done during laparoscopy and the tubes were cauterized, a large portion of the tube might have been damaged by the burning process and a reversal might be extremely difficult. There must be at least two remaining inches of normal healthy Fallopian tube attached to the uterus for reanastomosis to be undertaken successfully. If the tube has been removed quite close to the uterus, a tubal implantation might be the only alternative. During a tubal implantation, a hole is made in the patient's uterus and the end of her tube placed directly into the opening, but chances of conception are only 10 to 15 percent after this type of surgery.

If a woman wants her tubal sterilization reversed, she should know that she might have to undergo extensive, expensive surgery. Before she submits to an operation her husband should have a sperm count and a physical examination to make sure that he is in good reproductive shape. The woman should be examined to confirm the fitness of her reproductive system, the functioning of her ovaries, and the position of her uterus. A hysterosalpingogram will reveal the amount of remaining tube, and a physician will suggest, depending on the condition of a woman's tube and her age, whether the surgical ordeal would be a good idea. Even after a successful reanastomosis of a tube, a woman's chances of conception might be only 50 percent. She will never have 100 percent fertility.

A woman must weigh her desire for motherhood, the projected outcome of the surgery, and the emotions she will experience if she goes through the operation and does not become pregnant, before she makes her decision to reverse her sterilization.

The Ends of My Tubes Were Crushed

I only recently learned that I had a tubal sterilization that the medical establishment considers permanent. The doctor removed the distal third of my tubes and crushed the ends. I thought he was going to tie my tubes and I felt that this type of operation could be reversed. Now I find that there is virtually no chance of reversing the way I was sterilized. I've written to the AMA and consulted several gynecologists and nobody gives me any information or hope. I can't believe there's nothing I can do.

—T.R., Manteca, California

The fimbriated (fringed) end of a Fallopian tube reaches down and catches an egg as it bursts from an ovary. The surgery this woman underwent—a fimbriaectomy—destroyed the ends of her tubes, and it is very difficult to change what happened. As mentioned in the previous section, she and her husband must be examined to make sure that their reproductive capabilities, with the exception of her tubes, are fine in every respect before surgery can be contemplated. She must have a hysterosalpingogram so that a doctor can see what portions of her tubes remain. Then she should undergo a laparoscopy to give her doctor the opportunity to see the condition of her tubes. If a repair is possible, she will need exploratory surgery using microsurgical techniques; however, the success rate of this type of surgical repair is very low. I feel that Ms. R would have a greater chance at conception, as well as avoid invasive surgery, if she considered in vitro fertilization (IVF), an assisted reproductive technology technique explained in chapter 9. IVF was created for women with blocked or damaged Fallopian tubes.

Should My Husband Take Viagra?

I am thirty-nine years old and my husband is fifty. When we got married two years ago, we agreed that we wanted to have a baby together. Lately my husband is very often impotent and we

don't know why. He does not have any medical conditions. We are
under a strain because I see my biological clock ticking. Should my
husband take Viagra?

—M.P., Katonah, New York

Viagra has been helpful for many couples trying to conceive, and
it might help you. In a survey of Massachusetts men, Dr. Irwin
Goldstein of the Boston University School of Medicine reported
that about half of the men aged forty to seventy had difficulties
obtaining or maintaining erections. Vascular problems were common among the men, and this is the key to Viagra's success. Viagra,
also called sildenafil, increases blood flow to the penis, enhancing
erections. Other drugs for erectile dysfunction (ED) require inserts
into the urethra or penile injections, and they work whether a man is
about to have sex or not. Viagra, an easy-to-take pill, is effective only
if a man is sexually aroused. However, Viagra will not change a low
sperm count, and it should not be taken by anyone using nitrate
medications. Viagra can cause a sudden drop in blood pressure that
could send a man on nitroglycerin or blood pressure medication into
shock. A man should consult his physician before he uses Viagra,
especially if he is at risk for heart disease. Other side effects such as
headaches, indigestion, blurred or bluish vision, and flushing have
not stopped men from continuing use of Viagra.

Should I Have a Sperm Count?

My wife and I have been trying to start a family. We have had
sex at different times of the day and night all throughout the
month. We have been trying for the better part of the year and she
has still not gotten pregnant. She thinks she might need a D & C,
but I'm wondering if I'm not the one who should go to a doctor.
Should I have a sperm count? I'd like to know if I am able to get
my wife pregnant. If my sperm count is low, what can I do?

—Mr. B.P., Sparks, Nevada

Approximately 40 percent of all infertility problems are caused by the male. A man might have a low sperm count or his sperm might have poor motility (movement) or abnormal morphology (structure, shape). There might also be infections among sperm if a man has had a previous bout with gonorrhea. Years ago, many Vietnam veterans were found to be infertile due to sperm infections from gonorrhea that they contracted while on duty in Southeast Asia. A man's sperm could also be infected by mycoplasma, a microorganism found in the vagina and cervix of many women. If mycoplasma is found to be the cause of infertility, a man and a woman could be treated with vibramycin tablets, 100 mg twice a day for ten to twenty days.

When a man and a woman are faced with the problem of infertility, it is very important that the man have a sperm count before his wife undergoes many painful, expensive tests. Quite often men have low counts due to malformations in the genitals, stress, excessive drinking or smoking, jogging in tight nylon shorts, or soaking in hot tubs, and these are just a few of many reasons.

Usually a man must abstain from sex for two to four days before he ejaculates for a sperm count. He should collect his semen in a wide-mouth jar because if any of the specimen is lost, he will have to discard it and use the semen from another ejaculation or after intercourse and withdrawal. Sometimes a man ejaculates in the bathroom in the doctor's office or in a private area in a laboratory. A sperm count is a medical analysis, and a man who goes to a doctor's office will not find an erotic room with a lab assistant to aid him in his ejaculation. His surroundings will be quite clinical.

Men can sometimes have misconceptions about a semen analysis. They think that the test might diminish their manhood, and they can become awkward and fearful. A sperm count is an important part of an infertility workup; it is not a measure of masculinity. The semen should be collected in the morning and delivered to the lab within the hour. The sperm is examined immediately and two, and then four, hours later.

A man usually releases 3 to 5 cubic centimeters (cc) of semen with a pH ranging from 7.05 to 7.80. The normal sperm count is routinely greater than 40 million per cc. In the 1930s, 1940s, and even in the 1950s, it was assumed that 100 million sperm per cc was average. By 1974 a median sperm count had dropped to an average of 65 million. In a study of 150 students at Florida State University in 1975, the average sperm count was 60 million per cc with 23 percent of the men having fewer than 20 million. The 60 million figure is now considered the overall average and 20 million is thought to be the lowest amount possible for conception. This greatly reduced sperm count is attributed to modern-day stress, infections, environmental pollutants, and physical conditions such as varicocele, the bulging of the veins near the testicles, a condition that inhibits sperm motility.

Vitamin B-complex seems to enhance a state of well-being in people, and it might work to increase a man's sperm count. A man might also avoid excessive exercise, overeating, heavy drinking, and smoking. He should try to keep himself fit, well-rested, and as stress-free as possible. If his low sperm count is not due to a physical problem, and he keeps himself in good shape, his sperm count should increase.

Can I Have My Vasectomy Reversed?

I was married with three children when my wife developed a terrible infection from her IUD. I didn't think it was fair for the burden of contraception to be placed on her when she was suffering. I got a vasectomy. This story would have had a happy ending if it stopped here, but we had our problems and eventually got divorced. I remarried two years ago and I would very much like to have a child with my current wife. She's a wonderful person and I know she would be so happy to be a mother. What are the chances that I will be able to be a father again?

—V.L., Hoxie, Kansas

A vasectomy can be reversed by delicate, intricate surgery that should be performed only by a skilled microsurgeon. This man should contact the heads of both the urology and infertility departments at the teaching hospital closest to him. The chief physicians of these departments would be able to advise him about *vasovasotomy*, the surgical reversal of a vasectomy. Selection of a surgeon is crucial if the reversal is to succeed, and Mr. L. should choose a doctor who has performed this type of surgery in the past. One of the two top doctors with whom he consults is likely to be a practiced microsurgeon who can help him.

An experienced microsurgeon will reanastomose—join together—the severed ends of a man's vas deferens, his sperm-carrying duct. The vas is only about 2 millimeters in diameter, so the surgery is particularly precise. The doctor cuts the damaged ends and connects them with very fine sutures. He operates under magnification with special microsurgical instruments. The operation is bloodless.

The better the microsurgeon, the greater the chance of a successful reversal, but even with the best of everything there might be no more than a 20 to 40 percent chance that a man will be able to impregnate his partner. Scar tissue can block the passage of sperm or a man can manufacture antibiotics that attack the sperm he is trying to produce. This time around, Mr. L. will need a great deal of patience to become a father.

INFERTILITY AND AWARENESS

Years before a man and a woman actually want to start a family they should monitor their fertility. There's a chance that some of the problems causing infertility can be averted if they are noticed when people are young.

A man might have periodic sperm counts to gauge the level of his potency, while a woman might keep a basal body temperature chart to mark the regularity of her monthly ovulations. If a woman has had an IUD, an infection from the contraceptive can damage the Fallopian tubes. She should be diagnosed and treated immediately. It is also important that endometriosis be caught in its early stages (see chapter 7) and treated with a Danocrine or GnRH agonist medication before it severely cripples the female organs. A woman who is concerned about the workings of her reproductive system might have a hysterosalpingogram to assure herself that her tubes and ovaries are normal.

At the first question of infertility, men and women might contact the following organizations for information and advice:

RESOLVE, the National Infertility Association
1310 Broadway
Somerville, MA 02144-1731
HelpLine: 617-623-0744
Fax: 617-623-0252
E-mail: resolveinc@aol.com
Web site: http://www.resolve.org

American Society for Reproductive Medicine
11209 Montgomery Highway
Birmingham, AL 35216-2809
Telephone: 205-978-5000
Fax: 205-978-5005
E-mail: asrm@asrm.org
Web site: http://www.asrm.org

9.

Assisted Reproductive Technology (ART)— Modern Answers for the Infertile Couple

Science has shifted some solutions to the problem of infertility. In the past, after years of trying unsuccessfully to conceive, infertile couples who wanted to raise children turned to adoption. Today the adoption alternative has become the more difficult one. Improved techniques for contraception and abortion have decreased the number of babies born, and the supply of infants is not great enough to fulfill the never-ending requests from potential adoptive parents. Where does an infertile couple turn? To other possibilities. Science, it seems, might be counterbalancing the loss of adoptable newborns by providing new ways for infertile couples themselves to have babies.

With modern methods of conception, a husband and a wife who have not conceived a child through sexual intercourse might still be able to have a baby who embodies their genes, or at least the genes from one of them. Depending on the cause of their infertility, a couple might choose to have a child through artificial insemination, in vitro fertilization (IVF), gamete intrafallopian tube transfer (GIFT), zygote intrafallopian tube transfer (ZIFT), intracytoplasmic sperm injection (ICSI), egg donation, or surrogate motherhood.

These revolutionary methods of babymaking are so new that the legal and ethical questions surrounding them have not yet been answered and cannot be explored at length here. In this chapter, innovations in conception will be explained medically, and answers to questions from couples who are contemplating these daring ways of conception can clarify the latest options for all infertile partners.

THERE IS NOTHING ARTIFICIAL ABOUT ARTIFICIAL INSEMINATION

A one-year-old boy smiled up at me from the stroller that his mother had wheeled into my office. As she adjusted the strap that held her child, the young mother spoke. "My son is beautiful," she said, "and you know that he was conceived through artificial insemination." Then she paused, and after a thoughtful moment continued. "That's such a terrible term—artificial insemination. Those words make the process seem so unreal. This child is my flesh and blood. There is nothing artificial about him. Really, you must change the term." I agreed.

Artificial insemination is referred to as either TDI (for therapeutic donor insemination), AID (artificial insemination with donor sperm), or AIH (artificial insemination with husband sperm). If doctors called the procedure "*aided* conception with donor sperm" or "*aided* conception with husband sperm," we might be offering a more inviting alternative to childlessness. Often the words *artificial insemination* give a science fiction quality to the method.

Artificial insemination describes the placement of semen inside the vagina, cervix, or uterus at a time appropriate to conception. (Intrauterine insemination [IUI] can only be performed by a doctor who does sperm washing, as on page 256.) After both partners have undergone infertility workups, as described in chapter 8, and they have learned that the woman is completely fertile but that her husband has an uncorrectable infertility problem, only then would they investigate this very helpful and painless procedure, which I prefer to call "aided conception."

As pointed out in chapter 8, there are many reasons a man might have impaired sperm production. A mature sperm, or *spermatozoon*

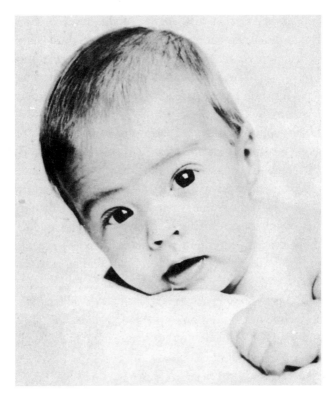

9-1 **"I am not artificial, no matter how I was conceived."** Photo of baby boy conceived through "aided conception." He is beautiful, he is real, and he is loved. *Photo:* © *Sheldon Moskowitz/Contact Press Images*

has three sections—head, midpiece, and tail—within approximately 55 micrometers. The head, which is 5 micrometers long and 3 micrometers wide, contains all the vital chromosomes with genes that transmit inherited characteristics. In fertile men, about 20 percent of the sperm that appear to be normal might be abnormal when scrutinized under a microscope. In infertile men, this percentage is even higher. Sperm might be damaged by bacteria that stem from an infected prostate gland or some other inflammation. A percentage of sperm might be immature and unable to fertilize a woman's egg.

A woman might be rejecting her husband's sperm in a rare immune response. A husband's sperm might be completely absent, a condition called *azoospermia,* or he might have *oligozoospermia,* which is a minimal presence of sperm. A man might have had neurological disorders that make ejaculation impossible. He might have undergone a vasectomy at some time or had an accident or an infection that affected his testes. Also, prostatic surgery might have damaged sperm production.

Depending on the husband's sperm count and quality, a physician might suggest artificial insemination with his (the husband's) fresh sperm. A recent study has shown that when a woman takes fertility drugs and is inseminated within her uterus—intrauterine insemination, or IUI—she is three times more likely to conceive than if she had cervical insemination, and twice as likely when compared to having IUI without drugs. Conception rates are as high as those of in vitro fertilization, IVF (see pages 275 to 278). This finding is significant.

NOTE: If a man's sperm are very weak, he can still father a child through a technique called *intracytoplasmic sperm injection,* or ICSI (explained on page 273), which must be used in combination with IVF.

How Sperm Are Handled

If a woman is being inseminated with her husband's sperm, the man is advised to abstain from sex for forty-eight hours before he ejaculates to keep his sperm count at a peak. No more than two hours before the insemination, the husband should masturbate and ejaculate into a wide-mouth jar. The woman keeps the semen warm and alive by placing the container under her armpit or near her breast when she takes it to the doctor's office. The semen must remain at body temperature.

Fresh sperm do not need to be washed for vaginal or cervical insemination, but sperm washing is necessary for intrauterine insemination (IUI). The ejaculated sperm sit in a container for about a half hour in order to liquefy. Then sperm and seminal fluid are separated in a centrifuge. The concentrated pellet of sperm that is produced after an approximate ten-minute wash is used for insemination.

Some doctors inject fresh sperm into a woman's vagina or cervix, but most fertility specialists, who know the technique and are equipped to do sperm washing, prefer IUI. With or without fertility drugs for superovulation, IUI is the most successful technique for conception. When a partner's sperm is available, the fresh kind is used for insemination.

On the other hand, sometimes a woman might be inseminated with frozen donor sperm for a variety of reasons. For example, her husband's/partner's sperm might be too weak or damaged to impregnate an egg, or he might carry a genetic disorder, or there might be an incompatibility of blood types. Conception with high-potency donor sperm can be quite successful for healthy women.

Frozen sperm thaw within a woman's body after insemination. The finally freed, live, healthy sperm begin their swim to the Fallopian tube, but unfortunately, they're not going to be as energetic as their fresh counterparts. During the freezing and thawing process, sperm lose a certain amount of motility, and this fact leads many physicians to prefer insemination with fresh sperm.

Donor sperm are frozen for at least six months before use, in order to allow a waiting period for a second round of testing to make sure no viruses have developed. Sperm are screened and tested for, among other things, hepatitis C and several forms of HIV, the AIDS virus. Immersed in vats of liquid nitrogen, test tubes of frozen sperm can stay alive indefinitely.

Doctors try to find donor semen that will carry the characteristics of the man who will become the child's only known father. Sperm banks claim that they can easily match characteristic traits from the sperm provided by a great number of semen donors. They also argue that they keep an ample sperm supply from each donor so that if a man and a woman want to give a sibling to the child who was conceived through artificial insemination, they can request the same donor semen for a true brother or sister.

A couple must use their intuition when they select an infertility specialist and quiz him about his semen supply source. Commercial sperm banks are known to profit from frozen semen analysis. Which sperm bank is your doctor using? Is it reputable? Is your doctor affiliated with a well-known teaching hospital or university medical center? Your knowledge and your trust in your doctor (see chapter 2) are often essential for a successful conception.

However, the need for donor sperm has dramatically dropped in recent years. Hormone treatments and improved surgical techniques that open the epididymis, the coiled tubes atop each testicle where sperm mature, have restored fertility to many men who would have remained infertile. Also, using the ICSI technique, today's doctors can take ejaculated sperm or remove sperm from the testicles and inject a single sperm cell into a single egg for fertilization.

How Artificial Insemination Is Performed

After a woman has had an infertility workup and has been found to be a fertile female with a healthy uterus and Fallopian tubes, she might be a candidate for artificial insemination. Of course, her husband's infertility should be clearly determined, and the couple, as a unit, should wholeheartedly agree to the procedure.

Artificial insemination can be performed by a doctor in two ways: (1) by monitoring a woman's *natural menstrual cycle* to gauge ovulation and the optimum time for insemination, or (2) by administering *fertility drugs* to stimulate superovulation of eggs, and performing an intrauterine insemination (IUI).

The Natural Cycle Method. A woman should begin keeping a basal body temperature chart, or BBT (see pages 216 and 217) for two to three months, if she has not done so as part of her infertility workup. BBT is based on morning temperature readings. At ovulation, her temperature either drops slightly or remains the same, and a day or two after ovulation, her temperature jumps a degree and remains at this new, higher level until menstruation. An over-the-counter ovulation predictor kit is also recommended to gauge the time of ovulation.

A doctor studies a woman's ovulation pattern through BBT and/or through an ovulation predictor test, and also checks her cervical mucus for changes that signal a favorable insemination. A "fern" pattern usually appears in the mucus a day or two before ovulation or during ovulation. Channels shaped like the fronds of a fern are visible under a microscope after the mucus dries and crystallizes. These channels are pathways that give the sperm clear sailing into the uterus. Another prelude to ovulation is the stretchability of the mucus, the spinnbarkeit phenomenon that permits a woman to thread her cervical mucus between her fingers (see figure 3-2 on page 61).

The Fertility Drug Method. BBT and ovulation predictor kits cannot pinpoint ovulation when fertility drugs are used because the drugs affect the rise of LH, the hormone that signals a natural ovulation. When a woman is on fertility drugs, a doctor determines her ovulation through ultrasound.

There is some controversy over the exact lifetime of a sperm that enters a woman's body. It is known that sperm cannot survive longer than six hours in the vagina, and only the hardiest sperm move out of the vagina into the uterus before time runs out. Once in the uterus and hastening toward the Fallopian tube, healthy sperm, it is generally assumed, can exist for seventy-two hours, but here a dispute arises. Some sperm move so rapidly that they travel through the tubes, right out the fimbriated ends, and into the abdomen, where they might disintegrate within a day or two. Other, less healthy sperm might not live the full seventy-two hours even within the tube. Due to this uncertainty about the life span of a sperm, some doctors feel that they achieve a higher rate of conception if they artificially inseminate a woman before the time of her ovulation. Usually a woman is inseminated every other day beginning two or three days prior to ovulation, continuing through the day of ovulation. Generally, a woman is inseminated two or three times during each menstrual cycle in which she is trying to conceive.

At the start of the artificial insemination procedure, a woman is supine on the examining table. Her legs are parted and the heels of her feet are resting in the stirrups. Her physician elevates the lower end of the table so that her buttocks are tilted upward, angled slightly higher than her head. Then the doctor inserts a speculum into her vagina.

Fresh semen should be procured no more than two hours before the insemination. When donor semen is used, sometimes for psychological reasons a couple chooses to mix the husband's sperm with the donor semen. Theoretically, if conception should occur, it might have resulted from one of the husband's sperm. However, some doctors do not like to mix semens because they're afraid that the combination might result in an immune reaction between the sperm of the two men, and thus, chances of conception might decrease. Nevertheless, a couple who prefer to have the husband's sperm included should always discuss the possibility with the doctor.

ARTIFICIAL INSEMINATION

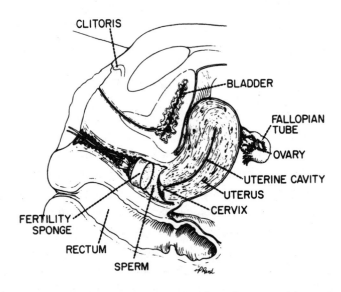

9-2 **Artificial Insemination.** After semen is injected into the uterus and the area surrounding the cervix, a fertility sponge (a plastic sponge) is inserted into the vagina to hold the sperm close to the mouth of the womb.

A fertility specialist performing artificial insemination usually chooses to do sperm washing followed by an intrauterine insemination (IUI). The doctors who lack experience in sperm washing are the ones who lean toward vaginal or cervical inseminations. When *fresh semen* is used for an *IUI,* the sperm is washed (see page 256) to remove seminal fluid, because within the fluid are hormonelike prostaglandins that can cause undesired uterine cramps. The sperm washing results in concentrated sperm that are passed through a fine plastic tube inserted into the uterine cavity. IUI brings sperm much closer to Fallopian tubes and eggs, and as mentioned before, if fertility drugs are used in combination with IUI, the rate of conception increases.

When *fresh semen* is used for *vaginal or cervical inseminations,* the sperm is aspirated into a syringe that has a soft plastic tip. The syringe is inserted into a woman's vagina and the sperm is injected around the cervix when it is open.

After any kind of insemination, to prevent leakage and keep sperm high in the vagina, a doctor often places a plastic-covered fertility sponge into the vagina, in front of the cervix. From start to finish, inseminations take only a few minutes and are often said to be as painless as a Pap smear. The woman remains on the elevated examining table with the sponge blocking a backslide of the sperm for at least thirty minutes to give the sperm time to travel into her uterus. Wearing the sponge is like wearing a tampon. A woman can carry out her normal activities and remove the sponge six to eight hours later.

Using another method, a doctor might fit a small cap over a woman's cervix with the aide of long forceps. A slim plastic tube attached to the cervical cap leads out the vagina. A doctor who uses this technique slowly injects the semen into the tube and the fluid runs down to the cervical area enclosed by the cap. There is no spillage with this method since a small plastic ball is immediately pushed into the tube to act as a stopper. Again, the woman must remain on the examining table for at least thirty minutes after insemination. The tube folds into her vagina when she stands, so she

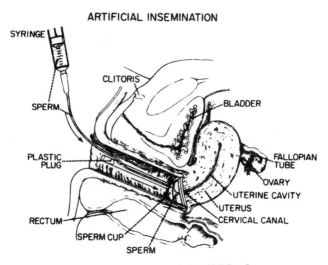

ARTIFICIAL INSEMINATION

SYRINGE

CLITORIS

SPERM

BLADDER

PLASTIC PLUG

FALLOPIAN TUBE

OVARY

UTERINE CAVITY

UTERUS

CERVICAL CANAL

RECTUM

SPERM CUP

SPERM

FIBROID TUMORS OF UTERUS

9-3 **Artificial Insemination.** This drawing illustrates an alternate technique for artificial insemination. A sperm cup is, on direct vision by a physician, placed on a cervix. The cup is attached to a long, hollow, plastic tube with a small opening on the side. As illustrated, the sperm is injected into the area around the cervix with the aid of a syringe. After the syringe is removed, a small plastic plug is pushed down to the sperm cup to prevent any leakage of the semen.

can carry out her normal activities, and like the sponge, the cap can be pulled from the vagina ten to twelve hours after insemination.

Frozen sperm is stored in small tubes or in straws. Before use, sperm are usually thawed and examined under a microscope to confirm that they are still alive. Sperm must be washed before IUI, but are sometimes also washed before vaginal or cervical inseminations. Once again, the woman must remain on the examining table for at least thirty minutes after the insemination, and the sponge can be removed six to eight hours later.

Studies have shown that under their own power, sperm can move from the cervix to the Fallopian tubes within ten minutes. By the time a woman who has been resting on the examining table for thirty minutes rises, the sperm already might have reached the egg.

How Many Times Must a Woman Be Inseminated Before She Conceives?

A woman often needs to be inseminated two or three times per cycle for three to six menstrual cycles before she conceives; however, these are average numbers. Some women conceive immediately, while others must undergo artificial inseminations for many months. It's amazing that sometimes a woman might have sexual intercourse with one man only once and she will become pregnant, while during artificial insemination, when all the conditions for conception are ideal, pregnancy eludes her.

Sometimes a woman's nervousness about the procedure constricts her tubes and inhibits conception, so it is always wise for a woman who has chosen artificial insemination to take stress-reducing B vitamins and to try to relax as much as possible. I personally have artificially inseminated women for up to fifteen months before we hit the pregnancy jackpot.

Conception is a highly individualized event, and couples should not burden themselves with deadlines and fret over inseminations that did not "take." If a couple trust their own physician, then nature must be allowed to work on its own timetable. However, a couple might visit another doctor or infertility specialist if they feel that a fresh relationship with a different physician might enhance their chances of conception.

What Does Artificial Insemination Cost?

The cost of each insemination varies with the physician's fee and the price of the semen. For donor sperm the average price runs from $200 to $250 per insemination, and two are usually needed. Donor sperm is tested extensively at the time of donation, frozen for six months, and then retested to make sure it remains negative for HIV, hepatitis, and other viruses. Sometimes donor sperm is prewashed, but sometimes it needs a washing, and that will affect cost.

Depending upon a woman's health plan, some of the cost might be absorbed by medical insurance. Money spent on these medical procedures is also tax deductible. And if a couple compares the cost of artificial insemination to the fees involved in adopting a child, they might see that, in comparison, artificial insemination is not high-priced.

However, judging from the letters I have received, women are not as concerned about the cost of artificial insemination as they are about the emotional impact the procedure might have on them and on the children they hope to bear.

QUESTIONS ABOUT ARTIFICIAL INSEMINATION

How Long Can I Continue Being Artificially Inseminated?

A year ago, after my husband and I decided that we had infertility problems, we both went for checkups at a well-known hospital, which is quite a long drive from where we live. After the doctor did my husband's sperm count and a bunch of other tests, he said that my husband was born without a vas deferens, the duct that leads the sperm from the testicles. That's why my husband has no sperm count. We had to face this sad abnormal condition and learn that the only way we would ever have a child would be through adoption or artificial insemination. I am a perfectly healthy thirty-one-year-old woman, and since artificial insemination would mean that the child would be half mine and I would be able to experience pregnancy and childbirth, I wanted to be inseminated. My husband agreed and three months ago I began the long monthly drives to the hospital. I'm still not pregnant and I wonder how long I can go on. I'm beginning to feel that this monthly ordeal might be hurting my marriage more than it's helping. I think maybe my husband went along with the inseminations because I wanted them so badly. Now I don't know if they're worth the trouble. I become so depressed each month when my period comes,

*and emotionally, I'm torn. Am I really doing the right thing by
being artificially inseminated? Should I continue the inseminations
or stop them?*

—S.N., Millens, West Virginia

An important study has shown that the fertility drug method of
insemination using IUI results in higher rates of conception than the
natural method (see page 259 to 262) without fertility drugs. I suggest the fertility drug method for Ms. N.

Also, Mr. N. should be seen by a urologist specializing in male
infertility because he might be producing sperm in his testicles. If so,
Ms. N. might be able to bear her husband's child following in vitro
fertilization (IVF), in combination with intracytoplasmic sperm
injection (ICSI) (see page 273).

If she must use donor sperm, I often suggest that a husband and a
wife have sexual intercourse on the night of the day that she has
been artificially inseminated. When a couple has sex at this particular time, the man is really showing the woman that he accepts and
wants this child. Psychologically, it is almost as if he is giving her a
baby. She needs his support during the entire insemination process.
If they cannot talk to each other about the artificial insemination,
they might ask their physician to refer them to a psychological counselor who has experience advising couples participating in this
method of conception.

Sometimes, due to the money and frustration involved, a woman
decides to stop the inseminations. Eventually, she might want to
investigate adoption. While the adoption procedures are going on, a
woman might become pregnant with her husband. I have seen these
conceptions happen too many times for them all to be coincidences.
In Ms. N.'s case, of course, an unexpected pregnancy could not happen because her husband's infertility problem eliminates a sperm
count. I would suggest that she continue her inseminations for several more months if she can feel secure in her husband's support. If
she does decide to end her inseminations and look into adoption,
she might at some point in the course of the adoption try artificial

insemination again. She might feel less pressured the second time around, and she might conceive.

Will My Baby Look Like Me and My Husband?

My husband and I were high school sweethearts who got married and bought a house in the same town where we grew up. Most of the people here have known us all our lives and practically from the day of our wedding they started asking us when we were going to have a baby. We tried, but when I never conceived we traveled to a famous infertility doctor in the closest city. We found out that a case of the mumps has left my husband sterile, and that artificial insemination with the sperm of an anonymous donor was our best way to have a child outside of adoption. We did a lot of reading and talked to a number of infertility experts who assured us that the sperm would come from a man who had the same qualities as my husband. We haven't told anyone that we're doing this because everybody around here gossips so much, but I started my inseminations this month. I want this child, but I can't seem to shake the nagging question in the back of my brain: What if the baby doesn't look like either one of us? People will think I had an affair! Can I really trust the doctors when they say the baby will resemble me and my husband?

—L.P., (name of town withheld)

A doctor who is going to perform an artificial insemination has a great responsibility to select exactly the right donor semen for his patient. A physician tries to match blood type, IQ, height, skin, color of hair and eyes, and anything else a couple has told him is important to them. He is searching for a facsimile of an existing husband and his judgment and sensitivity are crucial. Children sometimes search for their biological fathers. In the past the identities of sperm donors were kept secret, but today some laboratories and sperm banks reveal the donors.

If Ms. P.'s doctor is an accredited physician who is affiliated with a reputable teaching hospital, he probably is a person of sound judgment. And the donors who provided the frozen semen supply have most assuredly been screened for their health, fertility, and absence of HIV and genetic disorders. So, judgment on both sides is needed. A couple's reasons for choosing a doctor are just as important as the doctor's reasons for selecting a particular donor semen.

Naturally, every profession has its horror stories. I can remember hearing about one prominent physician who mixed up semen specimens he was using for artificial inseminations. He gave a white woman the semen from a black man and a black woman the semen from a white man. Without a doubt, the doctor who performs a couple's artificial insemination is a pivotal person in their lives. You want a well-organized physician with a solid reputation.

In my own practice I have seen many beautiful children born as a result of artificial insemination. These children are loved and treasured, and I have never heard any husband express disappointment or concern over his child's appearance. Some of my patients have told family members that they conceived through artificial inseminations; some patients have told no one. It's not uncommon to deliver a child from an aided conception and hear the family say, "The baby looks just like his father." And naturally, as the child grows up, she or he will adopt the father's mannerisms just as his own child, conceived through sexual intercourse, would.

Since Ms. P. and her husband have decided to keep their artificial insemination a secret, they might want to ask their physician to refer them to a psychological counselor who might be a sounding board for their doubts and fears. There are counselors who specialize in the problems of infertile couples.

No one can predict how any child, conceived in any way, will look, but couples who choose caring physicians have good starts at bearing beautiful babies.

I'm a Single Woman; Can I Have Artificial Insemination?

I'm a thirty-eight-year-old, single television producer. I was married for a few years in my twenties, but I was totally involved in building a career at the time and I did not want a child. Now I don't have too many fertile years left. I have no prospects of marriage, and I would like to have a baby before time takes away my chance to be a mother. I did become pregnant once when I was thirty and I had an abortion, so I know I am capable of conceiving. I'm ambitious, self-sufficient, and financially well-off. I could give a child a wonderful home and a lot of love, but I'm writing to you to find out if I will be able to find a doctor to inseminate me. Will I have to face medical opposition and legal hassles? Also, since I don't have a husband whose traits I'd like to match, can I pick whatever I want? Personally, I like tall, black-haired, blue-eyed Latin men.
—C.J., Studio City, California

In our free society, each person should have the right to control her or his own body. A man can choose to be vasectomized without his wife's consent. A single woman should be able to elect artificial insemination, but physician-aided conception of an unwed mother is an issue that is not without controversy.

In the past, fertility clinics were sued for making marital status a factor in the eligibility of patients for artificial inseminations. These suits were dropped or settled out of court, so there is no law either for or against the artificial insemination of a single woman. The decision to proceed with this method of conception must be made between a single woman and her doctor, and in the medical community there are many fine physicians who would agree to perform an artificial insemination with an unmarried woman. These doctors are usually at metropolitan teaching hospitals and large university medical centers, rather than in small towns.

In fact, today artificial insemination is a popular option for single women who want to become mothers before their childbearing years end. This woman obviously does not want use a man for breeding purposes, and she prefers not to have the emotional burden of knowing the father of her child. In Los Angeles, the area in which Ms. J. lives, there should be a number of physicians who would agree with her point of view. Ms. J. is presenting herself honestly. Sometimes single women who want to be artificially inseminated tell their doctors that they are married to avoid any adverse reactions.

When Ms. J. meets a doctor who will artificially inseminate her, she might ask him to match whatever traits she prefers her imaginary mate to have. Doctors consider no request unusual; after all, didn't Nobel Prize winner Dr. William Shockley want his sperm preserved only to breed with geniuses? It might be difficult for a doctor to find semen from a tall, black-haired, blue-eyed Latin donor, but it might not be impossible. In my practice a patient once wanted the donor to be a tall, red-haired orthopedic surgeon. It took a long time to meet her request, but we did succeed.

How Can My Husband Increase His Sperm Count?

I have one child, a son, from my first marriage and no children with my second husband. Recently we learned that his sperm count is very low. The doctor said that if we really want to raise a child from infancy, we could try the ICSI technique, but if we declined that, or it did not work, our best hope would be artificial insemination with donor sperm. Is there any way that my husband might increase his sperm count? What are the chances that I would conceive if I insist upon artificial insemination with his sperm only?
—B.R., Wichita, Kansas

A man's sperm count can vary with his habits. Excessive drinking, smoking, and even marathon-type jogging might lower a sperm count (see chapter 8). Stress might also reduce sperm production. Vitamin C also plays an important role in promoting healthy sperm. As little as 250 mg of vitamin C a day can make a difference to sperm quality. I recommend daily vitamin C, 500 mg twice a day; zinc, 50 mg two to three times a day; vitamin B-complex; E; and five servings of fruits and vegetables. Antioxidants from food will fight possible sperm damage from drinking, smoking, radiation, and pollution. If he has not already, Mr. R. should be examined for varicocele, a mass of varicose veins in the scrotum that warm the scrotum and interfere with sperm production. Varicocele can be surgically repaired. He might also request a thyroid test, because often a slightly sluggish thyroid, which can be corrected with medication, is at the root of a man's sperm problem.

Now that Ms. R.'s husband knows his sperm count is low, there are natural techniques he can use to try to impregnate his wife. He should only have intercourse every forty-eight hours in order to give sperm sufficient time to accumulate. Immediately after orgasm, he should withdraw, because if his penis remains in his wife's vagina it might allow for the escape of the sperm that is deposited in front of the cervix.

There are really no reliable statistics on the success rate of artificial insemination with husband semen. Remember, it takes a series of inseminations for an average of at least three to six menstrual cycles before a woman conceives with fertile donor semen. Using semen that is not as potent, conception is likely to take even longer, perhaps from six to nine menstrual cycle inseminations.

If this couple decides to try artificial insemination with husband semen, they should commit themselves to the necessary time and be extremely patient. They should also learn about ICSI (see page 273).

I'm Afraid That My Daughter Will Marry Her Own Brother

My fourteen-year-old daughter was conceived through artificial insemination. Now she is dating a young man who has her same coloring and is a similar body type. He doesn't look much like his parents and I'm worried that he might have been conceived through artificial insemination too. This is a small town. What if the same donor was used for this young man and my daughter? Could my

daughter be dating her brother? What if they want to get married
someday? How am I going to handle this?
—E.B., (name of town withheld)

There's an old saying, "Thieves think all men steal." Since this
woman underwent artificial insemination and apparently has not discussed it with anyone, she might imagine that every other woman
might have done the same. Although this method of conception is
becoming more popular, it is still not in widespread use. It is highly
unlikely that two children living in the same community would
have been conceived by artificial insemination, and even more unlikely
that they would have been conceived by semen from the same donor.
Statistical studies in Switzerland, where there are about 70,000
total births a year, have shown that the probability of a marriage of
half siblings conceived by the same donor would be one marriage in
twenty years, which is below the marriage rate of blood relatives in
normal populations. If donors were frequently varied within a population, that figure would drop even lower. So there is less than a
remote possibility that in a small community two teenagers would
have the same donor/father. Ms. B. need not worry. Besides, it's a
myth that in love "opposites attract." A person usually is attracted to
someone who looks like she or he does, or someone who resembles
one of her or his parents. It sounds like your daughter followed her
natural instincts when she chose her boyfriend.

I Would Like My Child to Be a Boy

My husband is infertile. I am keeping temperature charts
and planning to start artificial insemination this year. Since it
is such an emotional, time-consuming procedure, I will probably
go through artificial insemination only once in my life. If I do
conceive, I would like my child to be a boy. Can the doctor do
anything to increase my chances of having a son?
—W.S., Wheaton, Maryland

In spite of ethical debates, people have been attempting methods of sex selection since ancient Greek civilization. Some methods not requiring artificial insemination are described on pages 301 to 304. As for sex selection with artificial insemination, two known techniques are the Ericsson method and Microsort.

The Ericsson method has been scientifically questioned, but is still offered in sixty-five "sperm centers" and claims to be more than 70 percent effective in conceiving a boy. Fast-swimming sperm are isolated in a glass column that is filled with serum albumin, which is known to slow sperm speed. Since the smaller male sperm swim faster than the female sperm, the males race through the albumin and reach the lower end of the column quicker than the females. At the "finish," fluid at the bottom of the glass contains a high concentration of male sperm, which can be separated out by centrifuge and artificially inseminated into a woman when she ovulates. For a girl, a doctor induces ovulation and inseminates a woman with sperm identified as high in the female-producing X chromosome. Ericsson costs $600 to $800 above a doctor's fee.

Microsort, a method developed at Genetics & IVF Institute in Virginia, is sex selection based on the fact that sperm carrying the female X chromosome have 2.8 percent more genetic material than sperm carrying the male Y chromosome. First, researchers expose sperm cells to a temporary, nontoxic, fluorescent chemical. Then they shine a laser light on the sperm, and cells with the greatest amount of genetic material—the female-producing cells—glow more brightly. Separated according to their reflected light intensity, selected sperm are then used for artificial insemination. Microsort, which has a reported 65 to 90 percent success rate, is expensive at $2,500 per insemination, and usually takes a few tries before conception occurs. Although no studies are available for artificial insemination with the less costly SELNAS natural sex selection method (see page 303), a couple might look into it.

INTRACYTOPLASMIC SPERM INJECTION (ICSI):
HOW TODAY'S MEN WITH LOW SPERM COUNTS
CAN FATHER THEIR OWN CHILDREN

With intracytoplasmic sperm injection, called ICSI ("Ick-see"), the majority of today's infertile men can now father children with their own sperm. Now, any man who produces sperm at all, whether he ejaculates or not, and even if his sperm do not mature in his testes, can become a father. Doctors can use ejaculated sperm or, through needle or surgical biopsy, remove sperm from the epididymis (the coiled tubes atop the testes) or from the testes themselves. When a couple needs ICSI, the procedure must be performed along with a woman's involvement in assisted reproductive technology (see pages 256 to 262), usually in vitro fertilization, IVF; GIFT; or ZIFT.

A woman is given injections of fertility drugs to stimulate her ovaries to produce multiple eggs, or follicles. Eggs are retrieved during an ultrasound-guided needle aspiration. Next, an embryologist examines the sperm, finds the healthiest-looking one, and using designated micromanipulation devices and microscopes, injects a single sperm into the nucleus of a single egg. When all goes well, the sperm fertilizes the egg after injection, and the resulting embryo is then transferred into the woman's uterus, where it implants and develops into a normal pregnancy.

During standard IVF, a sperm placed in a laboratory dish with an egg naturally passes through the egg's outer membrane and heads for the nucleus. During ICSI/IVF, an embryologist changes the way the sperm's genetic material is introduced into the egg by performing the intracytoplasmic injection. Thousands of healthy babies have been delivered through ICSI, but there is some concern that a chromosomal abnormality might result from the maneuver. More research is under way. In the meantime, prenatal testing can determine whether the fetus of an ICSI conception has normal chromosomes. When facing male infertility, couples should ask their fertility specialists about the latest reports on ICSI.

ART: HOW ASSISTED REPRODUCTIVE
TECHNOLOGY SOLVES INFERTILITY
PROBLEMS

Baby Louise Brown, known as the world's first test tube baby, was conceived in a shallow glass Petri dish, the kind you might find in any high school chemistry lab. An egg that had been extracted from her mother, Lesley Brown, was fertilized in the dish by sperm from Lesley's husband. About two days later, after the fertilized egg had divided into several cell stages, it was carefully implanted within Mrs. Brown's womb. Like any mother-to-be, Lesley Brown lived through a normal, nine-month pregnancy and on July 25, 1978, Baby Louise was the first baby born through in vitro fertilization (IVF). We had arrived at the dawn of assisted reproductive technology (ART).

The pioneering British physicians Drs. Patrick C. Steptoe and Robert G. Edwards used *in vitro* (which means "in glass") *fertilization* for Mrs. Brown because her badly scarred tubes prevented natural conception. Without the help of her doctors, she would never have borne her own child.

Normally, at ovulation a woman's monthly egg is "caught" by the fimbriated end of her Fallopian tube. Shortly after entering the tube, if the egg is penetrated by a sperm, conception occurs (see chapter 10). As the fertilized egg makes its way through the Fallopian tube to the uterus, it begins to divide into two, four, eight cells and more until, by the time it reaches the womb, it is a thirty-two-cell blastocyst, a developing embryo. Like a fallen tree blocking a roadway, scar tissue from a previous infection, endometriosis, or some other disease or abnormality can obstruct the open tube and impede the journey of the egg as it travels from the ovary to the uterus.

With the various assisted reproductive technologies, the course of conception is no longer thwarted. ART has especially helped women over thirty-five who want to become mothers. During my years as an infertility specialist, I have gained much pleasure in seeing the beautiful babies that would not have been born without

ART. In 1996, the most recent year for available USA figures, more than 64,000 attempts at assisted reproduction were made and over 20,000 babies were born. Women using their own eggs (babies can be conceived with donor eggs as well as donor sperm) succeeded at a rate of 23 percent, or about one out of four attempts at conception.

In my book *Getting Pregnant*, published by Fireside/Simon & Schuster, I describe the different assisted reproductive technology techniques in detail and share insights gathered from my work in infertility. In this chapter, I will help you find the procedure that matches your needs. The costs are still high, with a single IVF attempt ranging from $7,000 to $10,000. (Some health insurance companies do not cover IVF, but some cover two or three attempts.) There are ethical issues that have not been resolved, such as ART-related multiple conceptions followed by reduction, and the question of maternal age limitations. That said, here's how far we have come and how many options we have created to assist conception since Louise Brown was born.

In Vitro Fertilization (IVF)

IVF was originally developed for women who had blocked or damaged Fallopian tubes, which prevented them from becoming pregnant. When tubes are blocked, sperm and egg are denied access to their natural meeting place. Over time, IVF evolved to help women who had postponed pregnancy and faced infertility due to aging ovaries and eggs of poor quality. Today, IVF continues to be an option for women who have blocked or damaged Fallopian tubes, but it is also sought by women who have ovulation disorders, anti-sperm antibodies, cervical or uterine damage, unexplained infertility, or partners with male factor infertility, such as a very low sperm count.

Every woman who attempts an IVF pregnancy is treated with injectable fertility drugs to stimulate the ovaries into superovulation—the ripening of more than one egg in a menstrual month—to enable doctors to perform egg retrieval. The eggs are captured through either laparoscopy, when a thin, probe is slid through a tiny incision made in the navel, or with a needle-guided vaginal ultrasound probe used during a minor surgical procedure that allows eggs to be retrieved through the vagina.

An embryologist carefully examines the eggs, and if they are of good quality he combines them with an appropriate amount of sperm in a laboratory Petri dish. The eggs and sperm are left to fertilize in their dish in an incubator. If the sperm quality is poor, or if only a few eggs are retrieved, the embryologist might decide to perform an ICSI procedure for fertilization (see page 273). On average, six or eight eggs are retrieved, and three or four are ripe enough to be fertilized. Sometimes immature eggs are allowed to mature in the laboratory for twenty-four hours before fertilization is attempted.

After sperm fertilize the eggs, resulting embryos are transferred into a woman's body using one of two different techniques. In the first, if a woman's tubes are blocked, the embryo transfer (ET) is made directly into her uterus about three days after egg retrieval. For ET, a woman retains a full bladder and reclines supine on a gynecological examining table with her heels in the stirrups. A speculum is inserted into her vagina and her doctor locates and cleanses her cervix. Using ultrasound guidance, the doctor locates her uterus, visualizes the uterine lining, and glides the tip of a narrow embryo transfer tube to the top of the uterine cavity. The embryologist then places an embryo in the transfer tube and slowly injects it into the uterus. The transfer tube is slowly removed, and the woman remains resting from thirty minutes to three hours.

After she returns home, she is advised to rest for three days. If all goes well, at least one of the eggs will implant within two weeks and develop for the next nine months. If a woman is healthy and her eggs easily develop into the embryo stage, there is no limit to the number of times IVF can be attempted. However, if she does not conceive after several attempts, her doctor should suggest another form of ART, such as ZIFT or GIFT (see below).

The second technique is blastocyst transfer. When an embryo is about five days old, it becomes a blastocyst of eight or more cells, and a new technique being used in association with IVF is a blastocyst transfer to a woman's womb. A problem with this method is that many embryos die before they reach the blastocyst stage due either to embryo quality or laboratory conditions. In cases where the embryos survive, however, the success rate of blastocyst transfer compares with that of standard IVF. In 1996, 45,462 attempts at IVF were made in the United States, at a 25.9 percent success rate. The younger you are when you attempt IVF, the more likely you are to succeed.

IVF with Intracytoplasmic Sperm Injection (ICSI)

The IVF with ICSI procedure (see page 273) is a major breakthrough in helping men with low sperm counts become biological fathers. In previous years, a woman had little hopes of conceiving a child with a partner who faced this fertility problem. ICSI has changed all that. When ICSI fits your needs, you follow the standard IVF procedure, whether you have blocked Fallopian tubes or not. During standard IVF, sperm are mingled with retrieved eggs in a laboratory dish (see IVF section above), allowing natural fertilization to occur. With ICSI, natural fertilization is bypassed. Sperm are actually injected into the inner cores of the eggs. Normally, a sperm sheds proteins as it enters an egg, but with ICSI that does not happen. A large microscope-type of equipment is used. The egg is held with a probe as a fine needle injects a healthy-appearing sperm into its center. Researchers have been studying whether veering from the natural process will cause genetic problems or chromosomal defects in the developing fetus. Many babies born through IVF/ICSI appear to be fine, but a woman could ask her fertility doctor what the latest information is.

Once ICSI fertilizes eggs and they develop into embryos, they are transferred into a woman's uterus either in standard IVF fashion or using the ZIFT (see below) procedure. The hope is that they will implant and result in pregnancy. About 15,000 attempts at IVF with ICSI were made in 1996, and 27.8 percent of those attempts were successful.

Gamete Intrafallopian Tube Transfer (GIFT)

A woman must have at least one healthy Fallopian tube, and be producing healthy eggs, to be able to choose GIFT. This procedure helps women who have endometriosis, lack of ovulation, cervical mucus abnormalities, unexplained infertility, male factor infertility, damaged fimbria (the fingerlike projections at the ends of the Fallopian tubes), antisperm antibodies, a history of ectopic pregnancy, and one healthy Fallopian tube/one healthy ovary but on opposite sides of their bodies.

The procedure for GIFT is the same as for IVF until the point of egg retrieval. Most often, eggs are retrieved during laparoscopy, which gives the doctor a chance to visualize the ovaries and aspirate eggs. He then delivers the eggs to an embryologist, who prepares them and mixes mature eggs with the appropriate amount of sperm in a transfer tube: egg, then sperm; egg, then sperm. During the same laparoscopy, the transfer tube is carefully guided to a Fallopian tube and the mix is ejected into the outer portion of the tube, where the egg can be fertilized naturally. A fertilized egg develops into an embryo during the next five to seven days and moves through the Fallopian tube to the uterus. There is no technological embryo transfer to a woman's uterus, as with IVF. Sperm and egg fertilize in the Fallopian tube, the way they do during a natural conception. Of 2,892 GIFT attempts in 1996, 28.7 percent were successful. GIFT has a more successful rate of childbirth than standard IVF; perhaps that's because fertilization takes place in nature's meeting ground, the Fallopian tube, and implantation in the uterus is done at the most optimum time, or perhaps the women who choose GIFT start out with fewer problems and do not have the tubal damage shared by most women who attempt standard IVF.

Zygote Intrafallopian Tube Transfer (ZIFT)

Any woman who has one healthy Fallopian tube, but who also has any of the fertility problems mentioned above in connection with GIFT, might choose ZIFT. Superovulation, egg monitoring, and vaginal egg retrieval are the same with ZIFT as with standard IVF. The ZIFT procedure deviates from standard IVF when it comes to transferring the embryos, or zygotes, to a woman's body. With ZIFT, sperm fertilize eggs in a laboratory dish, but rather than transfer the resulting embryos directly to a woman's uterus, the ZIFT transfer is made into a woman's Fallopian tube during a laparoscopy about two days after egg retrieval. Of 1,225 attempts at ZIFT in 1996, 30.3 percent succeeded. Although ZIFT is the least performed ART technique, it has the highest rate of sucess.

MONITORING MULTIPLE CONCEPTIONS

All of the ART procedures require a woman to be injected with fertility drugs that bring on "superovulation," the ripening of a number of eggs for retrieval. Today, if many eggs are retrieved from a woman, she can choose to donate extra eggs to another woman for that woman's use. During IVF, several retrieved eggs are fertilized by sperm in a laboratory dish, and the resulting embryos are then transferred to a woman's womb. In general, no more than four healthy, high-quality embryos are transferred. Whether a woman is attempting conception naturally or through ART, if she is taking fertility drugs, the chance that she will have a multiple birth increases by 25 percent. The result is usually twins, but there is still the outside chance of a higher number of babies being born. We have all heard the news of six, seven, or eight babies being born to one mother during a single childbirth session.

If a multiple pregnancy occurs, a woman must be cared for by a high-risk obstetrician, a perinatologist. She also must be very careful to eat properly, take extra prenatal vitamins, and rest more than other pregnant women. A cervical cerclace (a type of suture) may be placed on her cervix to prevent it from dilating. She usually will be treated with medications that control premature labor and will be involved in home uterine activity monitoring (HUAM). Available through a national service such as Matria, HUAM requires an expectant mother to have telephone checks of signals emitted from a computerized abdominal belt that she wears. It is my experience that if a woman is treated in this high-risk fashion, she has a healthy multiple childbirth.

There are physicians who recommend the so-called fetal reduction technique of eliminating a number of fetuses so that only one or two babies will be born. I do not believe in this practice; instead, I feel that multiple gestation can be successfully managed if a woman starts her high-risk care early in pregnancy.

PREGNANT WITH A DONOR EGG OR EMBRYO

Women who cannot produce healthy eggs, even if the reason they cannot produce good eggs is that menopause has stopped their reproductive capacity, can still become pregnant. The oldest known ART pregnancy is a sixty-three-year-old woman who used donor eggs, IVF, and the transfer of a frozen embryo, but most clinics limit maternal age to fifty-five. Ethical questions swirl around the issue of egg donation. Most women who become egg donors are paid from $2,000 to $3,000. In 1999 a couple offered an absurd amount—$50,000, and advertised in the newspapers of Ivy League colleges and other top academic institutions for a 5'10" athletic egg donor who had scored at least 1400 on her SATs. This is unusual, unnecessary, and totally unrealistic for most couples.

Being an egg donor is more complicated than being a sperm donor. A woman must take fertility drugs to induce superovulation, have her egg development ultrasound-monitored by a doctor, and her eggs retrieved during a minor procedure using a vaginal ultrasound probe. The donor egg is then fertilized in a laboratory dish with sperm from the male of the recipient couple, or with donor sperm.

While all this is going on, the woman who will be the recipient is treated with a series of hormone injections and oral medications to bring her womb into a condition where it is primed for acceptance of a fertilized egg, or embryo, two or three days after the eggs have been retrieved. Twists of fate that result from this procedure are that aunts can give birth to their nieces and nephews, and grandmothers to their own grandchildren. In South Africa in 1987, a woman gave birth to her daughter's triplets. In the United States in 1991, eggs retrieved from a woman who had ovaries but no uterus were fertilized and transferred into the womb of the woman's mother. That grandmother became pregnant with twins, and was delighted to give her daughter and son-in-law the babies they so desperately wanted, her own grandchildren. Embryos not transferred during a cycle are usually frozen and can be used at a later date. Fertility specialists also are able to offer fresh or frozen embryos to women when both partners are facing fertility problems.

Other options for women who cannot produce healthy eggs are also on the horizon. *Cytoplasmic transfer* technique is one. Although as of this writing no embryos have been produced, scientists have been able to remove the nucleus from a younger woman's egg and replace it with the nucleus of an older woman's egg. The surrounding cytoplasm of the younger eggs help the newly created egg's development. This means that once this new egg is fertilized, an embryo, a potential baby, should be able to grow with the older woman's chromosomes intact.

Although fertilized eggs, embryos, are preserved through a freezing process called cryopreservation for future use, unfertilized eggs have been too fragile to preserve. With new technology, scientists are very close to creating ways to freeze and preserve unfertilized eggs for the future. This would allow women who are older to use their own, younger, stored eggs when they want to become mothers, and have the option that men who preserve their sperm have.

THE FIRST OVARIAN TISSUE TRANSPLANT

In 1999 the first ovarian tissue transplant was performed on a thirty-year-old woman whose ovaries had been surgically removed due to cysts and other noncancerous problems. The woman's first ovary was removed when she was seventeen, and her second at age twenty-eight, when some of her ovarian tissue was preserved through freezing. Two years after her second surgery, in 1999, Dr. Kutluk Oktay of New York Methodist Hospital in Brooklyn, New York, surgically re-implanted her ovarian tissue. Four months later, the woman received fertility drugs to stimulate ovulation, and they worked. She menstruated like any other fertile woman. To become pregnant, the woman will have to take fertility drugs again to stimulate her ovarian tissue, and then she will require IVF. This first ovarian tissue transplant, however, holds a promising avenue of fertility for women who are at risk of losing both ovaries.

ART DIMINISHES THE NEED FOR SURROGATE MOTHERS

In the 1980s and 1990s about 4,000 American women entered into arrangements to be surrogate mothers. Usually, they were paid $10,000 to be inseminated with sperm from men whose wives were infertile. Although the experience worked well for some couples, the aftermath of surrogacy sometimes generated legal battles and emotional pain for everyone involved. Surrogates gave birth to their own babies, albeit conceived with the sperm of strangers, and on occasion fought to keep their rights as mothers. Today, as assisted reproductive technology has advanced, the surrogacy of the 1980s has faded. These days, surrogate mothers are more likely to be sought by gay male couples.

In 1998, Dr. Nancy Reame, a researcher in reproductive science at the University of Michigan, surveyed the emotional impact of surrogacy on ten surrogate mothers who had given birth eleven to fifteen years before the study. Four of the ten women were quite satisfied, with two of the four remaining close with the families they had helped. Among the other six women, a few reported anger or bitterness, but others had separated from the families in a healthy way. Generally, most of the women felt good about the past. That said, Dr. Reame also reported that surrogate mothers fantasize that someday, when their children are over eighteen, they will come to find them.

ADOPTION, MORE OPEN THAN EVER

Although this chapter focuses on the latest options a woman has to become a mother biologically, there are many avenues a couple might follow that will lead them to parenthood. Whether through agency or independent adoptions, whether from newspaper ads or the Internet, birth mothers and infertile couples have been finding each other in droves. For older partners, foreign adoption is a good choice, because the age limitations for adoptions are more flexible in foreign countries. Perhaps this is why adoptions from foreign countries have doubled. Many beautiful boys and girls around the world need, and will thrive in, stable, loving homes and families. A woman who has not become pregnant after attempts at assisted reproductive technology might consider the adoption option.

Patience is key. For couples who want to adopt a newborn baby, a match with a birth mother takes time, and then after that, there is the wait for childbirth. Couples who are open to an older child, a preschooler rather than a newborn, or a child of special need, might find a son or daughter faster. No matter how long it takes, though, your child will return the love you have waited to give, a hundredfold.

10.

How You Know You Are Pregnant

CONCEPTION—A DAILY MIRACLE

Since every day women become pregnant, conception might be regarded as "nothing special," but conception is a daily miracle. No computer could invent a reproductive system as complete and as fascinating as the one that belongs to a woman. When a woman is involved in conception, even if she has just had an unplanned pregnancy confirmed and she feels less than marvelous, she is a miracle worker. Wondrous events within a woman's body lead to the conception of a child.

A woman's reproductive organs are always busy. The uterus, which is shaped like a lightbulb, is three inches long and the largest organ. Its outer wall is strong and muscular. The interior of the organ is a cavity, the womb in which the fetus will grow. As explained in chapter 3, during a woman's monthly menstrual cycle the endometrium, the uterine lining that will nourish the fetus, becomes thick and spongy and cushions the inner wall of the uterus. The endometrium develops into the perfect bed for a fertilized egg. A monthly egg that is traveling from an ovary through a Fallopian tube, if fertilized by a sperm, will implant itself in the endometrium. If the egg-of-the-month is not fertilized, the endometrium will shed itself. The vascular uterine lining will move down to the lower, narrow end of the uterus, progress through the cervix, and flow out the vagina. The portal of the uterus, the cervix is the opening at the juncture of the uterus and the vagina. The endometrium *exits* through the cervix in the form of menstrual blood. During intercourse, the sperm *enter* through the cervix.

Opposite the cervix, at the full upper end of the uterus, the two Fallopian tubes extend from either side. The tubes, which are the pathways between the uterus and the ovaries, are about four inches long and, at the most, a quarter of an inch in their diameters. They are comprised of sections.

The *isthmus* of the tube is the narrow part connected to the uterus. The *ampulla* is the midsection, the mating ground for sperm and egg. The tubes terminate at their fingery *fimbriated ends,* which

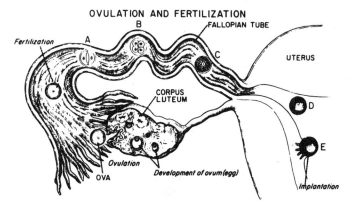

10-1 **Ovulation and Fertilization.** This illustration depicts several phases of ovulation and fertilization. The ovary, the Fallopian tube, and the uterus are greatly enlarged to portray the miracle of conception. A cross-section of an ovary, which contains an egg in developing stages, is shown. As ovulation occurs, the ovum (egg) is expelled from the ovary. Note how the fimbriated (fringed) end of the Fallopian tube reaches down toward the ovary to catch the ovum and assure its entry into the tube. The egg will now be beginning its seven-day journey through the tube; however, if it is not fertilized, the egg will die in twenty-four hours. The egg is seen surrounded by sperm, and fertilization occurs as one sperm enters the ovum. Cell division begins as the fertilized egg (A, B, and C) begins its trip through the tube. Soon after the egg enters the uterine cavity (D), it implants itself into the endometrium (E). The fertilized egg has at this time evolved into the blastocyst stage. Note how the ovarian tissue from which the ovum has been expelled transforms into the corpus luteum, which produces the progesterone needed to maintain pregnancy.

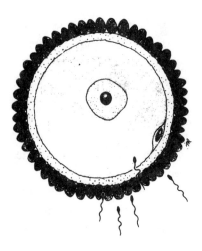

10-2 **Conception.** Conception occurs when a sperm breaks through the cell membrane of
an egg (ovum) and enters into its nucleus, as shown in the illustration. As soon as one
sperm has moved into the ovum, chemical changes occur that inhibit the entry of other
healthy sperm, which are pictured surrounding the egg.

reach down like tentacles and grasp the eggs that escape from the
ovaries.

Like two pearls, the ovaries are pinkish gray ovals situated at the
fimbriated ends of the Fallopian tubes. Each ovary is only about one
and a half inches long, one inch wide, and about one half inch thick.
The ovaries contain the entire supply of ova, all the follicles—also
called eggs—that a woman will use for reproduction during her lifetime. As many as 500,000 eggs might be locked within the ovaries
when a female is born. Needless to say, hundreds of thousands of
eggs will not be expelled for fertilization, and these will disintegrate
during menopause.

When ovulation occurs and an egg is released from an ovary, the
organ turns its ovulation side toward the fimbriated end of the
Fallopian tube. The fimbria, the tentaclelike extensions, reach down
and catch the freed egg, which at this stage is a nucleus surrounded
by nourishing cytoplasm or egg white. Once trapped in the tube, the
egg is moved toward the uterus by the cilia, microscopic hairs that

flutter like thousands of tiny eyelashes lining the Fallopian channel. The egg is now embarking on its seven-day journey through the tube. The egg will only live for twenty-four hours if it is not fertilized, but if intercourse has coincided with ovulation, a multitude of healthy sperm might have reached the Fallopian tube at just the right time to make fertilization possible.

Electrical charges enable the sperm to attach themselves to the egg cell. Under a microscope, the sperm actually look like missiles bombarding the egg. When one sperm breaks through the cell membrane and enters into the nucleus of the egg, *conception* occurs, and in most cases the egg chemically alters to prevent the entry of another sperm. On those rare occasions when two eggs are released during ovulation, if both are fertilized by sperm, fraternal twins might be born.

Conception usually occurs in the farthest portion of the tube, near the fimbriated end. The cilia then move the fertilized egg toward the uterus. When the egg reaches a point approximately one third away from the womb, it rests for two days while cell division begins. The egg divides in two, then four, then eight, then sixteen, and starts its move into the uterus. By the time the egg completes the seven-day trip and implants itself in the endometrium, it has divided at least thirty-two times and has evolved into the *blastocyst* stage, an early phase of embryonic life.

If the Fallopian tube is abnormal or obstructed in some way, the fertilized egg might not reach the uterus. It might implant itself where it is in the tube and an ectopic pregnancy might result. Sometimes the conception disintegrates in the tube or is expelled due to tension. Many snags can deter pregnancy. A fibroid tumor in the uterus, scar tissue from an IUD infection, unidentified growths, polyps—so many things can sabotage an otherwise potentially perfect pregnancy.

Nevertheless, if all goes well, a woman will conceive, the developing embryo will implant itself in the rich vascular uterine lining, and a woman will notice that she has missed her monthly period.

SIGNS OF PREGNANCY

A woman ovulates thirteen or fourteen days before the onset of her menstrual flow. Once ovulation occurs and an egg leaves an ovary, a woman is fertile, but her fragile egg will only live for twenty-four hours unless a conception occurs. It is generally believed that sperm that have entered the uterus and the Fallopian tubes can survive up to seventy-two hours (the sperm that remain trapped in the vagina die after six hours), so intercourse that takes place up to three days before ovulation might produce a healthy sperm that impregnates an egg. Since a woman will be fertile for a day after ovulation, any sex within about a four-day interval—three days prior to ovulation to one day after ovulation—might lead to conception.

Usually once a woman is pregnant she cannot become "more pregnant" because she can conceive only once a month with one man. There is one historic case in Germany, however, where a woman had sex with two different men during her fertile days and gave birth to twins—one fathered by a black man, one sired by a white man. So unique is this incident that the story is constantly retold in gynecological circles.

The more common occurrence is the single conception, the one-baby pregnancy that a woman discovers when she skips a period. Then her body begins to change. Her breasts become larger, with noticeable veins, and the brown areolar/nipple areas darken. Fatigue can overtake her due to an increased progesterone level, and sometimes she can feel bloated, too. Morning sickness, of course, is not to be forgotten.

If she takes her basal body temperature, as explained in chapter 8, and it does not drop below 98.5 degrees, she is pregnant without a doubt. During a pelvic examination a doctor will see a blueness in the cervix and the organ will be softer and more pliable than usual. This cervical change is known as Hegar's sign of pregnancy. Several tests to confirm pregnancy will be described in this chapter's questions and answers, but the physical signs can let a woman know her condition well before she receives an official confirmation.

HOW FAST DID THE SPERM TRAVEL
TO MEET THE EGG?

Just before ovulation the estrogen level in a woman's body increases and causes the cervical mucus to become thin and stretchy. A woman can reach inside her vagina, feel the wetness at her cervix, and thread out the mucus in a phenomenon known as spinnbarkeit, which is explained in chapter 3. As mentioned in chapter 9, when seen under a microscope, this preovulatory mucus contains *fern-patterned channels,* tracks to facilitate the self-propelled sperm.

Studies conducted during general anesthesia and artificial insemination have shown that, without the aid of orgasm or any extrauterine contractions, sperm can move from the vagina, to the cervix, to the uterus, and into the Fallopian tube *within ten minutes.* It was initially thought that if a woman had intense orgasms she would be pulling in sperm fast and efficiently, but now we know that if the time is right, sperm swim with speed and they don't need orgasm. (This rapid movement of sperm tells us that douching is a completely ineffective form of contraception. By the time a woman organizes her douche equipment, she could already be fertilized.)

Only the fastest and healthiest sperm will reach the Fallopian tube within ten minutes. The male sperm, which is smaller than the female sperm, usually get to the Fallopian tube first. The best sperm enter into the uterus immediately after sex, and the sperm that remain in the vagina die after six hours.

After having sexual intercourse, a woman who wants to conceive should remain supine, with a pillow elevating her hips, for at least thirty minutes to hold the sperm within her body. Her position will help the sperm's journey and will aid conception. If a woman rises right after intercourse, the semen containing sperm might drip from her vagina, and this decreases her chances of conception.

QUESTIONS ABOUT PREGNANCY
AND CONCEPTION

Questions about pregnancy and when conception occurs trouble many women, whether or not they are trying to conceive. Happy notes have come from women who have accurately predicted their own pregnancies, but women with irregular menstrual patterns, and women who have relationships with more than one man at the same time, have written searching letters.

Since every woman should know what is happening within her body at all times, no questions about conception and pregnancy should go unanswered. Conception and pregnancy are miracles, not mysteries, of life.

If I Had Sex During Menstruation How Could I Be Pregnant?

I had my period and then two weeks later, while my husband and I were having intercourse, I began to bleed. My abdominal pain was so severe my husband took me to the hospital. I was bleeding in clots by the time we arrived at the emergency room. I was given intravenous fluid and admitted to the hospital for two days' observation. The pain subsided and I was sent home. Eventually I became worried because my period never came again. After more than a month of waiting, I went to the doctor. He examined me and conducted a urine test and told me I was pregnant. When did I become pregnant? When I was bleeding during intercourse I thought I was having my period. Could I have become pregnant then? I'm concerned because I had an affair a week before I was admitted to the hospital. I want this baby to be my husband's. Please tell me. When could I have conceived?
—S.L., Buffalo, New York

A woman can only become pregnant for approximately four or five days during the middle of her menstrual cycle, or more precisely, exactly two weeks before the onset of her flow. A woman might bleed during her ovulation and suspect that her period has started, which is what Ms. L. did. She ovulated and the hormones that triggered her ovulation initiated the bleeding, which coincided with sexual intercourse. The bleeding might have been more intensified because sperm contain prostaglandins, which can cause cramping. She also might have been experiencing *mittelschmerz*, the pain in mid-cycle caused by irritating ovulation fluid that has spilled into the abdomen.

After two days, she felt better because the ovulation fluid began to be reabsorbed in her body, and the ovulation pain and bleeding stopped. Meanwhile, her newly ovulated egg, which was most likely fertilized by her husband's sperm just before ovulation bleeding, was still safely following its course in the Fallopian tube.

Right after menstruation, when Ms. L. had her affair, she could not have become pregnant because her cervical mucus would have formed a natural diaphragm to prevent the entry of sperm. It bears repeating that *a woman can only become pregnant during a four-or-five-day span two weeks before the first day of her period.* These four or five days, which cover her ovulation, are the only times conception can occur. Conception only occurs during ovulation, not during menstruation.

Is There Any Way to Know If I've Ever Been Pregnant?

I've had surgery twice for endometriosis and I've tried very hard to become pregnant. My husband and I desperately want a child to make us a family. Three times during the last year and a half I've had late periods that were very heavy and full of clots when they came. I think I might have had three miscarriages. Is there any way to know if my late periods were pregnancies? Also, if I am miscarrying, how can I prevent it?

—J.Q., Tustin, California

If a woman is a few days late with her period, she is not necessarily pregnant. The menstrual cycle responds to the brain hormones, and the secretions of the brain hormones can be affected by stress. Pressure and anxiety, therefore, can delay a period. Stress can sometimes be so great that it tenses and contracts the Fallopian tube, which might, in turn, eject a newly ovulated, unfertilized egg.

A woman who wants a baby so much that her body cries for it can exhibit the signs of pregnancy without ever having conceived. She might experience a false pregnancy, have a late period accompanied by breast growth and morning sickness, but she might never have conceived. Such is the power of the psyche.

If Ms. Q. finds herself with a late period again, she might want, after ovulation but before a period is missed, a radioimmunoassay (RIA) blood test performed by a doctor. Cost ranges from $30 to $50. A less expensive home pregnancy test is most accurate ten days after ovulation, still giving results before a missed period.

As far as past pregnancies are concerned, there is no way to determine whether Ms. Q. has ever been pregnant. It is possible that Ms. Q., since she seems worried about conception, might be experiencing stress-induced uterine contractions after ovulation. These contractions might be preventing conception. A woman with endometriosis is typically subject to cramping contractions. Ms. Q. might possibly be helped by prostaglandin-blocking drugs such as Motrin or Nuprin. Studies have shown that women with endometriosis have high prostaglandin levels. If Ms. Q.'s prostaglandins were blocked, her contractions and risk of miscarriage might diminish.

I Always Know the Moment I'm Pregnant

I've been pregnant twice and each time I've known the day after conception. My whole body felt different. I told my close friends I was pregnant and they said I couldn't possibly be so sure so soon. Two of them had not even believed they were pregnant after their tests had confirmed it. Nobody has to tell me I'm pregnant. Am I some kind of weirdo because I know my pregnancy before the doctor does?

—C.H., Wilmington, Delaware

A woman who is attuned to her body usually knows when she ovulates, and it is very possible that she would recognize some internal changes after conception. Her increased progesterone level, due to pregnancy, would elevate her temperature and she might feel a little warmer all the time. Her uterus, which usually contracts to shed the unused endometrium as menstrual flow, would be calm. A woman who is aware of her body would notice these subtle changes even before the differences in her breasts became obvious.

Ms. H.'s friends might not have reactions to internal activities. They might be used to missing their periods now and then, and they might dismiss any bodily fluctuations as "normal." Sometimes people do not focus on their physical changes because they're worried that they might discover something is wrong with them. This fear keeps them ignorant and often results in lengthy illnesses that could have been avoided if they had been discovered early. A woman who listens to her body, senses her pregnancy, and is proven right time and again, can only be applauded for an awareness that will probably give her a long and healthy life.

How Can I Be Pregnant and Still Have My Period?

I was getting fat for no reason. I had my period each month but I couldn't fit into my clothes. I went to the doctor because I thought I had a problem with my metabolism. I knew I wasn't eating a lot. He told me that I was four months pregnant. How could that have happened? He never really explained how I could be pregnant and still have periods. Now I'm really worried that the baby will be harmed because I've bled during pregnancy.
—L.D., Washington, Missouri

Spotting can occur when a fertilized egg implants itself within the uterus. As the egg settles into the uterine lining, there might be a slight bleeding from the implantation site. A woman might notice bloodstains, not as dark and thick as her regular menstrual blood, but pink and thin. Sometimes this implantation bleeding might be considered a menstrual flow. A woman will think she is having a period when she is actually pregnant.

During the second month, progesterone, the hormone that is initially produced by the corpus luteum after ovulation, begins to be manufactured by the placenta. A tricky kind of timing is involved here. Before the placental production of progesterone reaches its optimum level, the corpus luteum's generation of the hormone goes down. At this moment, the low progesterone level might not be strong enough to prevent a slight cramping in the uterus, and another spotting might occur. This bleeding might again be interpreted as a period. So it could seem to a woman who has bled in her first and second months of pregnancy that she is not pregnant at all, but menstruating normally.

A woman might also stain or even flow during the third and fourth months, and the reasons for these episodes, which tend to occur when a period is expected, are not known. A fetus will not be harmed by any of the bleeding I've described. However, if a woman's uterus begins to cramp painfully, it might then be cutting off the oxygen supply to the baby and a miscarriage or fetal damage might ensue.

A woman who has had spotting and wants to take no chances with her baby's survival should stay in bed and avoid physical activity during the times of the month when she normally had a menstrual period. It is also wise to avoid sexual intercourse on those days. Such a woman is at high risk for miscarriage, and these preventive measures are designed to help make her a mother.

I Only Had Anal Sex; Is It Possible That I Could Be Pregnant?

I normally use a diaphragm for contraception since I am not married and I don't have a regular boyfriend. Recently, a man I've known for some time invited me to his house for dinner. We drank wine and smoked grass and pretty soon we were in bed together, except I didn't have my diaphragm with me. I'm so afraid of getting pregnant that I didn't let him come inside me. We did a lot

*of heavy necking and had anal sex, which I didn't think would
make me pregnant. Now my period is late and I'm really worried.
Could I be pregnant? How is it possible? I swear he didn't come
inside me.*

—M.Y., Atlanta, Georgia

Conception is amazing. Even when a woman is artificially inseminated with thousands of sperm planted in the right place at the
right time, conception might not occur. Yet, pregnancy takes only
one sperm to fertilize one egg, and some people don't seem to need
perfect timing to make this happen.

If this woman only had anal sex, and absolutely no sperm was
spilled into her vagina, she could not possibly be pregnant. After
anal intercourse, however, some sperm, inadvertently spilled in her
perineal area, might have entered her vagina. Couples who use
coitus interruptus as a form of birth control often conceive a child
due to this same principle. If sperm are spilled around or near a
woman's vulva, they might, through their own movement, enter her
vagina and proceed toward the ovulated egg. It is also possible that
during sex play after ejaculation sperm might be spread through the
touching and fondling of a woman's external organs.

A woman can have a blood test for pregnancy as early as a week
after a missed period, and Ms. Y. might be wise to find out as soon
as possible whether she is pregnant. She might want to decide
whether to continue or to interrupt the pregnancy. Since Ms. Y. was
"high" at the time of her lovemaking, she might not have been fully
aware of everything that happened to her and she might have
become pregnant.

Can a Man Have a Baby?

*I saw a newspaper headline that said men can have babies. I
can't believe it! Is is true?*

—E.A., Campbell, Ohio

Researchers in England implanted an embryo in the testes of a male mouse in a highly successful experiment. In New Zealand a woman gave birth to a baby girl eight months after she had her uterus removed in a hysterectomy. (A fertilized egg had been moving through her Fallopian tube at the time of her surgery and the developing embryo implanted itself on her bowel.) The fetus created a placenta, an umbilical cord, and generated its own means of survival.

Years ago, these findings led Australian scientists who were studying forms of in vitro fertilization to theorize that if a fertilized egg were implanted into a man's abdominal cavity, the embryo would be able to nourish itself and be delivered by cesarean section. An abdominal pregnancy, wherein the fetus matures outside a woman's uterus and arrives in the world by cesarean section, is well known in medicine.

The fetus, scientists are discovering, is self-sustaining. Hormonal fluctuations, breast development, and most side effects of pregnancy are caused by the fetus's influencing the mother and not by the mother's controlling the fetus. Therefore, it seems to follow that if a man became an incubator for a fetus, the developing baby would give him weight gain, morning sickness, lactating breasts, and anything else a woman experiences. The man would also face a risky delivery after carrying the baby for nine months.

The cesarean section that removes an abdominal pregnancy can cause tremendous bleeding. The placenta from this type of pregnancy does not easily shed itself at the time of birth. Women who have undergone cesarean sections for abdominal pregnancies have been known to bleed to death. Men having these operations would be subject to the same, possibly fatal, bleeding complication. In one such case, a woman with an abdominal pregnancy was successfully delivered by cesarean section, the placenta was removed, and she seemed recovered. On the seventh day after her surgery she was discharged from the hospital but she never made it home. She died on the steps of the hospital due to a blood clot that had been produced by the abnormal placenta vessel in her abdomen.

The delivery problem, I think, would reduce the possibility of men carrying babies, but these findings and theories certainly bring the sexes closer together. Men and women might not be as different as they think they are.

Beyond the Rabbit: The Latest Pregnancy Tests

Is a rabbit killed each time a woman is tested for pregnancy? Is this really how pregnancy tests are done today?

—P.L., Jacksonville, Arkansas

Only in the movies. "The rabbit test" is historically interesting, but it is not used any longer. Pregnancy testing dates back to the Egyptians, who, in those days before modern plumbing, noticed that the urine of pregnant women caused certain flowers to bloom. The urine contained biotropic substances. In 1927, the first "modern" pregnancy test was developed—a bioassay based on the studies of Drs. Aschheim and Zondek, two physicians who discovered that specific hormones developed during pregnancy. Their test changed forever the way women would know they were pregnant.

Ironically, the first bioassay pregnancy test was performed on a mouse. A woman's urine was injected into a mouse that had not yet begun to ovulate. Five days after being injected, the mouse was killed and its ovaries were examined by a lab technician. If the urine was from a pregnant woman, it would contain hormones that would have caused the mouse ovaries to mature rapidly and develop blood spots. If the urine was from a woman who was not pregnant, the mouse ovaries would still be small and immature. Depending on the state of the mouse ovaries, a woman would be told whether or not she was pregnant. This method was used from 1927 to 1929.

In 1929, an improved pregnancy bioassay, which took only two days, was developed using immature rabbits instead of mice, and henceforth the bioassay was known as the rabbit test. But all the wives who told their husbands they were pregnant by using the

HOW YOU KNOW YOU ARE PREGNANT

expression "The rabbit died" were saying something that didn't apply. In the rabbit test, *all* the rabbits died, not because they were injected with a pregnant woman's urine—they were killed by the doctors who were examining their ovaries. Fortunately, with the advances in pregnancy testing today, no rabbits are dying because no one is doing bioassays.

The urine test is not one of the innovative testing methods, but it is still frequently used. Two weeks after a woman misses her period, her urine might be tested for the presence of HCG (human chorionic gonadotropin), a hormone that pregnancy causes to rise. Physicians often perform convenient urine slide tests in their offices by putting a drop of a woman's urine on a slide and adding a test solution and HCG antibodies. Within two minutes, if the test is positive, the mixture turns a milky-white but remains smooth. When the result is negative, the mixture stays clear and gets a lumpy sour milk consistency.

If a doctor prefers not to conduct a slide test in his office, he might send the urine to a lab for analysis. The laboratory test of a woman's morning urine is based on the same principle as the slide test. The urine is mixed in a test tube with a test solution and HCG antibodies. After two hours, if a red ring appears at the bottom of the test tube, the test result is positive. A woman learns she is pregnant, but she has to wait two weeks beyond a missed period before she knows. The new pregnancy tests eliminate the wait.

A radioimmunoassay (RIA) blood test for the beta-subunit HCG, the placenta-produced hormone that increases with pregnancy, can determine a pregnancy within a week after conception, even before a missed period. It is probably the most popular pregnancy blood test today. The RIA is extremely sensitive, and if it is carefully conducted in a reputable laboratory, it is virtually free from error. A woman can also use an over-the-counter home pregnancy test, which is most accurate ten days after conception (see page 299). A home test should still be followed by a blood test so her doctor can determine the exact level of her HCG.

How Good Is a Home Pregnancy Test?

I found out I was pregnant by using a home pregnancy test, but my doctor said he didn't trust the result. He insisted on testing me himself. After my blood test proved positive, I realized that I had to pay a second time to learn what I already knew. Why didn't he believe me the first time? Are home pregnancy tests ever wrong? I have some of the kit left over but I don't want anyone else to use it if the results are going to cause confusion.

—T.N., Brownsville, Texas

Manufacturers of home pregnancy test kits claim that their products are 97 to 99 percent accurate. However, Duke University researchers compiled data from five studies that evaluated sixteen different kits. When volunteers tested the kits on urine samples collected by investigators, test sensitivity averaged 91 percent. That sensitivity dropped to 75 percent when women followed kit instructions on their own.

The kits are designed to determine pregnancy based on an increased level of HCG in a woman's urine. Most home pregnancy testing picks up levels of 50 mIU/ml, whereas a blood test can detect levels of HCG as low as 5 mIU/ml. A blood test is far more sensitive. Although some test kits advertise that they can be used within one week after fertilization, it is best to wait ten days while HCG rapidly rises, and then follow the directions carefully. It is always wise to follow home pregnancy testing with a visit to a doctor, clinic, or nurse practitioner for confirmation.

Why Didn't the Doctor Know If I Was Pregnant?

I was in such terrible pain I couldn't walk when I arrived at my doctor's office. He examined me, felt a mass on my ovary, and admitted me to the hospital immediately. He ordered a urine test for pregnancy and a day later, when my pain had started to

*subside, he told me the test was positive and that I had an ectopic
pregnancy. I was wearing an IUD but I knew that there was a
chance that with an IUD I could have an ectopic pregnancy. The
doctor scheduled a laparoscopy and the next day I was in the
operating room. While I was under anesthesia, he looked at my
organs. He found nothing unhealthy. I had ovulated but I
definitely was not pregnant. A blood test for pregnancy proved
negative. The surgery had been unnecessary. Why didn't the doctor
have his facts straight? Why didn't he know if I was pregnant? Is
there any way I can help other woman avoid such an ordeal?*
                              —D.M., Seattle, Washington

Ms. M. was obviously suffering from middle-of-the-month ovulation pain. She might have even had a cyst that had broken and disintegrated, but she definitely did not have an ectopic pregnancy. If she had had such a pregnancy she might also have had bleeding from her vagina and pain that would have increased rather than lessened as the days progressed. It is true that with an IUD there is a higher incidence of ectopic pregnancy, but if her doctor had carefully observed her clinical symptoms he would have known that she was not a pregnant woman.

It is recognized that sometimes a urine test can give inaccurate results, whereas an RIA blood test is totally reliable and fast. If her doctor had ordered a blood test, Ms. M. would have known the negative outcome within a day and she could have avoided surgery. Her ovulation pain was disappearing as her unnecessary surgery was being scheduled. Even though a laparoscopy is only exploratory, it is still an operation usually performed under general anesthesia, and it entails a risk. Ms. M. might have benefited from a second opinion. She was beginning to feel better before the operation and she might have listened to her body and postponed her laparoscopy.

If she had known her menstrual cycle, Ms. M. might have realized that she was ovulating when she was in pain. A woman should try to be as alert as possible to her bodily changes.

Can I Choose the Sex of My Child?

My husband and I want to have a baby but there is hemophilia in my family. I vaguely remember reading something about being able to choose the sex of your child by timing intercourse. When would be the right time to conceive a female child? Anything you could tell me would be helpful.

—H.B., Red Bank, New Jersey

Hemophilia is an inherited disease that affects only male offspring. This woman definitely could benefit from conceiving a baby girl—who might carry, but would never have, hemophilia.

There are no fail-safe methods for determining the sex of your child, but the timed-intercourse technique to which Ms. B. refers is probably the one developed by Dr. Landrum B. Shettles and described in his book *Your Baby's Sex: Now You Can Choose.*[1] Dr. Shettles discovered that smaller, round-headed male sperm move much faster than larger, oval female sperm. His research also showed that female sperm like an acidic milieu, while male sperm survive better in an alkaline environment.

Considering the speed and survival capacities of the two kinds of sperm, Dr. Shettles created a natural method of sex selection for his patients. He combined a timing technique with before-sex douching to make the vagina either acidic or alkaline. Physicians have debated and often disparaged the Shettles technique, but many couples swear that it has worked for them. Dr. Shettles himself has reported an 85 percent rate of success with his method.

Here, in summary, are Dr. Shettles's instructions for having girls and boys:

HOW TO HAVE A GIRL

1. A couple might have intercourse any time except two or three days before, and the day of, ovulation. No sex on those days. (A woman can determine her ovulation by using the BBT chart on pages 216 and 217, mucus checks described on pages 61 to 63, and ovulation predictor kits.)

2. In order to encourage the acidic environment that inhibits male sperm and gives female sperm a definite edge on survival, a woman should precede each intercourse with an acidic douche of two table-spoons of white vinegar added to one quart of lukewarm water.

3. Since orgasm makes the vaginal environment more alkaline and better for male sperm, a woman who wants a girl should make every effort to prevent herself from climaxing. (This might require a force of will for some women, but thoughts of a baby girl might add to determination.)

4. The classic, man-on-top, missionary position should be used during intercourse, and male penetration should be shallow. The missionary pose will lessen the chances that sperm will be deposited directly at the mouth of the cervix, and a shallow penetration will give sperm time to experience the acidic vagina.

HOW TO HAVE A BOY

1. Timing is crucial for boy babies. Intercourse should coincide exactly with a woman's ovulation, and in order to insure a high sperm count, intercourse during ovulation should be the only sex a couple has all month.

2. To promote an alkaline environment favorable to male sperm, a woman should precede each intercourse with an alkaline douche of two tablespoons of baking soda mixed with one quart of lukewarm water. To allow the baking soda to dissolve, the douche mixture should stand for about fifteen minutes before it's used.

3. A woman should have an orgasm either before or at the same time as her partner.

4. Whatever position a couple favors that allows a man to enter a woman's vagina from behind should be used, and male penetration should be deep.

The *new French natural sex selection method, SELNAS (in French, Sélection Naturelle du Sexe)*, is based on the polarity cycle of the ovum. French cellular biologist Patrick Shoun discovered that at certain times during a month, the human egg changes its electrical charge. Some days the ovum is positively charged to attract the X, or girl, sperm, but on other days it is negatively charged to attract the Y, or boy, sperm. Through a questionnaire, and with information given by the woman, the SELNAS method determines her polarity cycle and creates a personal calendar of favorable days for intercourse for conceiving either a boy or a girl. There is a fee of $399 for having your twelve-month calendar created, but the technique is totally natural. No drugs are used. You are instructed to have unprotected sex on lab-indicated days.

The method, which is popular abroad, has an international success rate of 95 percent for having a child of the desired sex. Critics of the SELNAS method say the research is not conclusive, but Laboratories PROKIAD in France, distributors of the method, offer a money-back guarantee if you fail to have a baby of the sex you desired. PROKIAD is making the method available in the United States under the name SELNAS-USA; a woman can call toll-free: 1-877-NUBIRTH (1-877-682-4784), or visit the Web site: www.SelnasUSA.com for information.

The *French Diet Technique* was discovered by Drs. J. Stolkowski and J. Choukroun of Puteaux Hospital, France, after studying the outcomes of forty-seven births. They found that a diet high in potassium and sodium predisposes a woman to conceive a boy, whereas a diet high in magnesium and calcium increases the chances for a girl.

For methods of preselection involving the separation of male and female sperm followed by artificial insemination, see chapter 9, page 272.

The Drano Test

Like a juicy bit of gossip, word of the Drano test has spread among women in the United States and Canada. It has been said that if the morning urine of a woman who is more than six months pregnant is added to liquid Drano, the Drano will change color. The growing legend is that the mixture turns green for boys and golden brown for girls.

Although there is no scientific proof that the Drano test works, a Canadian physician has found it to be accurate in twelve out of fourteen cases. The Drackett Company, manufacturers of Drano, are trying to stop the story, and they have announced that the latest Drano is made with new ingredients that make the test impossible.

WARNING: If you try the Drano test, run out of the room after you've added the urine. The Drano smokes, smells foul, and could be harmful to your eyes if you're standing too close. Check your results after the solution has calmed down.

Is There a Difference Between Firstborn and Secondborn Children?

I am considering having another baby and I had heard that there are differences between firstborns and secondborns. My firstborn is a boy. Does the sex of the secondborn matter?
—G.T., West Allis, Wisconsin

Studies have shown that firstborns of either sex are different from later-born children. Firstborns are highly motivated to achieve. In general, they are more serious, self-controlled, ambitious, and creative than siblings of lower birth orders. Yet, while firstborns are likely to become educated and prominent, they might also be anxious because they want to be all things to all people and they fear that they might fail. Firstborns are described as having what are stereotypically called "masculine" traits.

Secondborns are usually outgoing, charming, more at ease in social situations than firstborns, unafraid to ask for help, practical, and somewhat nervous. They embody the stereotyped "feminine" characteristics.

In sex preference studies, 80 percent of those questioned chose male firstborn/female secondborn as the most desirable combination. If sex selection of offspring became a reality, it could lead to a great disparity of the sexes. We can be thankful that nature cannot be totally controlled and hope that in the future female firstborns might be first choice, too.

11.

Miscarriage, Ectopic Pregnancy, and Abortion— Do They Harm Your Body?

The time after either a miscarriage or an abortion can be a trying one in which a woman feels hopelessly depressed. Especially in the case of a miscarriage, she might blame herself for what happened. Rarely can an early miscarriage be prevented, but the powerful force of guilt feelings can generate waves of self-doubt. In the aftermath of a miscarriage or an abortion, a woman might be understandably shaky. She might see only joylessness around her, but she can eliminate some heartache if she realizes that these events do have a positive side. Miscarriage and abortion show a woman that she is fertile, and if pregnancy can occur once, it can happen again.

An ectopic pregnancy is potentially much more harmful than a miscarriage or an abortion, because if it is not discovered early, an ectopic pregnancy might seriously damage a woman's organs. In an ectopic pregnancy, a fetus develops outside a woman's uterus, usually in her tube. This type of pregnancy is painful for every woman, and it can be extremely upsetting to a would-be mother who strongly wants the child. If an ectopic pregnancy is not noticed in its early stages, a woman's tube might burst and she might have internal bleeding, but if recognized shortly after conception, an ectopic pregnancy can be arrested through microsurgery and reproductive organs can be saved. Although it is not a happy occurrence, an ectopic pregnancy is definitely a sign of a couple's fertility, and it alerts a woman and her doctor to a pregnancy problem that they can hope to overcome when she wants to conceive again.

As the answers to this chapter's questions will show, miscarriage, ectopic pregnancy, and abortion, if they happen, will hinder childbirth and might bring on sadness, but they also provide women with information about their bodies. A woman might experience an internal mourning, but she also might grow wiser and more determined because of these events.

MISCARRIAGE—WHEN NATURE ENDS A PREGNANCY

A miscarriage is a loss, but it is nature's way of stopping an abnormal pregnancy as soon as possible. Healthy pregnancies can remain intact after hours of horseback riding, jogging, and even after self-abortion attempts. It is certainly not a pregnant woman's fault if she miscarries—the American College of Obstetricians and Gynecologists once estimated that 50 percent of *all* conceptions result in rejection and miscarriage. A prospective mother might feel upset and depressed, but eventually she should be pleased that her organs functioned properly, that she became pregnant.

Naturally, it is understandable that a woman who has just experienced a miscarriage might not find her fertility comforting, but she should know that she does have a childbearing future that many infertile women would be happy to exchange for their own. A miscarriage, known medically as a "spontaneous abortion," might possibly be viewed as a beginning rather than an ending.

People think of a miscarriage as the early birth of a baby, the passing of an embryo before its time. A miscarriage is called a spontaneous abortion because the body unexpectedly terminates a pregnancy on its own. (Naturally occurring miscarriage should not be confused with planned, therapeutic abortion.) Actually, this sudden end to gestation provides an opportunity to create a possibly better life, because it is likely that had the miscarried conception been borne to term, it might have resulted in a baby with birth defects.

A woman might miscarry soon after conception because the sperm and the egg, for some reason, do not develop in the right way. Nine out of ten miscarriages occur during the early months of pregnancy, due, in large degree, to chromosomal abnormalities. During that first trimester, nothing can be done to change the course of a miscarriage when a body decides to cleanse itself of an abnormal fetus.

In the second trimester, a miscarriage might be provoked by an infection, an illness contracted by a mother-to-be, or an incompetent cervix—one that opens as the growing fetus stretches the uterus. In these cases there will be various signs preceding the miscarriage. High fever, viral or urinary tract infection, vaginal pressure, or bleeding should send a woman to her doctor immediately. He might be able to treat the symptoms and prevent the miscarriage from occurring, if a woman listens to her body and responds.

How to Know Whether You're Having a Miscarriage

About 25 percent of all expectant mothers have some bleeding during pregnancy. Spotting might occur when an embryo implants itself in the uterine lining during the first month of pregnancy. A woman might also notice staining in the second month, before the progesterone level in her body has increased enough to support the pregnancy. Neither of these episodes signals miscarriage, but a woman should always consult her doctor when she notices bleeding. She might need bedrest to calm a sensitive uterus.

Anywhere from a few hours to several weeks might pass from the time a pregnant woman notices some bleeding to what might become a miscarriage. At the first sign of spotting, she should go to bed, avoid any physical activity, and contact her doctor. Her staining might be a "threatened abortion" that will subside with rest, but if the bleeding is accompanied by mounting abdominal pain, miscarriage might be imminent.

Miscarriage does not occur unless bleeding is paired with intensifying pain. When a woman has both pain and bleeding, her doctor will probably want to see her in the hospital. When the uterus begins a steady cramping, the blood supply to the fetus diminishes, the cervix stretches and opens, and the miscarriage—bright red or brown blood—flows heavily from the vagina. If a woman is in a hospital bed, she most likely will be given intravenous fluid and medication to help control the blood loss, which, at times, can be health-threatening. Uncontrollable bleeding during a miscarriage means that blood is being lost from a woman's own circulatory system, beyond her reproductive organs, and she might need a transfusion. This severe blood loss happens only occasionally.

It is worth repeating that a miscarried pregnancy is one that might very well have led to a malformed child. The law of natural selection is at work here, not a woman's habits or her diet. A couple should try as well as they can to understand the event and to eliminate any guilt they might feel. *They are blameless.*

How Is Miscarriage Treated?

A doctor who learns that his patient is bleeding might examine her with the aid of ultrasonography, the method by which sound waves produce a moving picture of the fetus on a television-type screen.

If the ultrasonography reveals a living fetus with an intact fetal sac, the prospective mother will be advised to have strict bedrest either in the hospital or at home. The hope is that by lying supine with her feet elevated, she will stop bleeding and ward off miscarriage.

If an "empty sac" without an embryo appears on the ultrasound screen, a woman might have a *blighted ovum,* a failed conception that has not grown normally. This type of pregnancy is often referred to as a "missed abortion," because the fetus has disintegrated and been reabsorbed by the body. The physician might admit the woman to the hospital to remove the remaining placental tissue with a D & C or by the suction method.

Most obstetricians have access to ultrasonography equipment and can monitor the condition of an unborn by ultrasound and by measuring the level of HCG in a pregnant woman's blood. If HCG counts taken two weeks in a row show that the hormone level is dropping, the fetus is not likely to be developing normally. The doctor might perform a D & C or use the suction procedure to remove the remaining tissue from the uterus. Since the woman has been bleeding and expelling tissue, he will merely be completing an "incomplete abortion."

In the beginning of pregnancy the placenta and the uterus are integrated, so when a miscarriage occurs during the first trimester, there's a good chance that the placental tissue will not completely shed itself. If there is tissue left behind, the cervix will remain open, the uterus will continue cramping, and bacteria could be sucked into the womb. A "septic abortion" might result, and this must be treated with potent antibiotics to prevent a woman from becoming sterile. To avoid such a tragic outcome, immediate medical help is needed for treatment and, possibly, a D & C.

Even if a woman has miscarried in her second trimester, her uterus might not have expelled all the placenta and she might still need a curettage. No matter what stage of pregnancy a woman is in, if she has a miscarriage anywhere but within a hospital, she should collect the passed tissue in a jar and bring it to her doctor. After tissue analysis, he will be able to tell her if a D & C is needed.

As previously mentioned, the two basic surgical methods for uterine cleansing are D & C (see figure 5-5, page 133) and suction curettage. Many doctors today prefer to use suction followed by exploration with a curette (shown in figure 5-5). This way, the tissue can be removed from the uterine cavity with less possibility that the womb will be damaged in the process. The cleansing is very gentle with suction, but with a D & C a lot depends on a doctor's individual technique. If a physician scrapes just a little too much uterine lining, he might create areas of scar tissue, intrauterine adhesions that might grow and cause future infertility.

A woman who has learned that she needs a postmiscarriage curettage might ask her doctor if he plans to use the suction method. If he tells her that he prefers to do a D & C, she might diplomatically remind him that she would like children in the future and that he should scrape as little as possible. Some women, of course, will not have to worry about a D & C or suction procedure because their miscarriages are complete when they occur—the embryo and placenta both exit the body and no leftover tissue remains.

Whether or not a woman needs a surgical cleansing, a few months after miscarriage her body will be in fine shape if she wants to conceive again. A miscarriage represents a great loss to a woman and a man who longed for a child, but as the responses to the following letters show, hope and future childbirth exist to make miscarriage merely a memory.

QUESTIONS ABOUT MISCARRIAGE

When Can I Get Pregnant After Miscarriage?

I am twenty-five years old and the mother of a three-year-old son. I was hoping to give my little boy a brother or sister but just as I was getting into my fourth month of pregnancy, I miscarried. The doctor could not tell me why it happened. My previous pregnancy was normal except that the delivery was by cesarean section because I was so small. Anyway, I do want our family to grow, and I want to have another baby. My miscarriage happened two months ago. I've been very depressed about it, but I think getting pregnant again would be the best thing for me. How long should I wait before I try to get pregnant?

—C.O., Taunton, Massachusetts

After a miscarriage, a woman's uterus usually needs six to eight weeks to heal, so generally, a woman should be able to conceive again after two or three menstrual cycles. She should at that time feel physically and emotionally strong.

The prenatal vitamins a woman might have been taking before her miscarriage, in addition to iron, will help to strengthen her blood count and rebuild her body. The uterine muscle must regain its lost power, and rest and proper nutrition will aid in quick recovery. It is also believed that a woman who takes special care of herself with increased rest and adequate vitamins, and eliminates drinking, smoking, and drugs during the first three months of pregnancy, reduces her chance of miscarriage.

I also suggest that pregnant women drink either bottled water or filtered tap water, especially during the first trimester. An EPA study in California found a *possible link* between the trihalomethanes (TTHMs) in chlorinated water and a higher risk of miscarriage.

Ms. O. miscarried after the critical three-month period. She had passed the time when the future of the fetus is somewhat uncertain, and perhaps she miscarried at this late date because she has uterine scar tissue from her cesarean section. The embryo might have implanted itself in the scar tissue, from which it could not receive its needed blood supply. If Ms. O. experienced a combination of bleeding and pain, the miscarriage was probably due to a thwarted blood supply.

It is also possible that she was carrying a malformed child that her body rejected. If her next conception contains no chromosomal abnormality, she should be able to carry to term without any difficulties; however, considering her previous miscarriage and the cesarean section, her uterus might be somewhat weakened. She will need to take it easy and reduce her physical activity during her next pregnancy.

Ms. O. and her husband might look upon her miscarriage as a sign, at least, that they are still able to make a baby together. One miscarriage is not uncommon for a woman who is expanding her role as a mother. Ms. O. seems to have a mature attitude about her past and future pregnancies, and with luck, her next pregnancy will be just as smooth as her first, although a repeated miscarriage is always a possibility.

Did My Past Abortion Make Me Miscarry?

*The first time I got pregnant I was eighteen years old and a
freshman in college. There was no way I could have raised a child
at that point in my life and I had an abortion. Now I'm twenty-
four, and I've been married for six months. I've had to relocate with
my husband and find a new job, and we've both been anxious
about the changes in our lives. We were using a diaphragm during
intercourse when I became pregnant. Of course, I didn't want
another abortion, so we adjusted ourselves to thinking of having
our family sooner than we had expected. Then, two months into the
pregnancy, I miscarried. I'm still very sad about the whole thing,
and I feel guilty. I think it's my fault because I had an abortion.
My husband says the abortion has nothing to do with the
miscarriage, but I seem to be inconsolable. What can you tell me?
Could the abortion I had years ago have made me miscarry our
child? What are my chances of having a normal pregnancy?*
—R.E., Los Angeles, California

If this woman underwent a legal abortion under careful, sterile
conditions in a reputable medical center, she should have no problem with subsequent pregnancies. Before therapeutic abortions were
legalized in 1973, the rate of first-trimester miscarriage for a woman
who had had an abortion was more than three times greater than
usual. Today, Ms. E.'s one abortion should have no bearing on her
ability to carry a child to term.

Recent studies, however, do show that when a woman conceives
while using contraceptive jelly, the sperm-killing agent in the jelly
might alter the impregnating sperm and cause a malformed embryo.
The result might be the miscarriage of a potentially birth-
defective child. This might have happened to Ms. E., since she was
wearing a diaphragm with jelly when she conceived. Also, since she
and her husband have been living with stress, they both might have
been smoking more, if they are smokers. Smoking and drinking,
common stress relievers, can harm an egg and a sperm before and

during conception, and the resultant embryo might be expelled by the uterus.

Several variables might have caused Ms. E. to miscarry, but as I've mentioned before, one miscarriage is very common. With the hundreds of thousands of eggs a woman holds within her body, there might be a few imperfect ones, and even a completely healthy woman might conceive with one of her defective ova. Once a woman has healed after miscarriage, there is no reason whatever to think that she will not bear a robust baby the next time she conceives.

For the first three months of her next pregnancy, her doctor might advise increased rest for her during the days when she would normally have a menstrual flow, and he might ask her to decrease or refrain from intercourse until the crucial trimester has passed. With the right kind of awareness and care, a woman who fears a repeated miscarriage can reduce her worry.

Does the Pill Cause Miscarriage?

After five years of marriage and five years on the pill, I decided to become pregnant. My husband and I jog, ski, and sail together and we're in such good shape that we never thought we would have any problems with pregnancy. I thought it was perfectly normal for me to get pregnant right after I stopped the pill, but one night when I was about seven weeks into the pregnancy, I woke up with such severe cramps I was crying. The pain increased and I began to bleed. My husband and I got scared, called the hospital, and an ambulance rushed me into emergency, where I was admitted for a D & C. It never occurred to us that anything could go wrong when we planned to have our baby. I never had any concern about miscarriage. What happened? Did the pill do something to my body to make me miscarry? Could I lose another baby this way?

—P.V., San Diego, California

Ms. V.'s miscarriage could quite possibly be related to the pill. According to recent studies, a woman who stops taking birth control pills and conceives immediately doubles her chances of having a miscarriage. It could be that the miscarriage rate is greater because the pill keeps a woman's uterine lining at minimal development each month. The endometrium, the home for a fertilized egg, does not become as thick as it normally would, and even after a woman goes off the pill it might take several cycles for her lining to become as lush as it used to be.

A fertilized egg needs a rich uterine lining for nourishment, and if it implants itself into an underdeveloped endometrium, it might not be able to maintain its hold. An embryo might miscarry. However, waiting to conceive overcomes this situation.

Recent studies in the United States and Great Britain have shown that if a woman waits three months after she stops the pill before trying to conceive, her chances of miscarriage will not increase. The pill will not affect a woman or her baby as long as the waiting period is observed. After three menstrual cycles have passed, the endometrium should be at its thick, rich, vascular best—the perfect site for the implantation of a fertilized egg.

Ms. V. should also know that if she was exercising or jogging excessively, she could have diminished the blood supply to the developing fetus and triggered bleeding and miscarriage. As soon as a woman becomes pregnant she should immediately begin to slow down by decreasing her exercise in order to give the baby the best chance for proper intrauterine development.

Ms. V., and every woman who has been on the pill and wants a child, should add folic acid and vitamin B_6 to her daily vitamin intake, and wait those three months before conceiving. If a woman wants to continue exercising after conception, swimming and bicycling are much safer for the baby than jogging, which might result in a bouncing of the uterus.

I've Had Three Miscarriages: What Can I Do?

I had one normal pregnancy and, using Lamaze, I gave birth to my daughter, who is now four. I've been trying to have another

child for the past few years but each time I become pregnant I
miscarry, and I don't know why. My first miscarriage was at four
weeks, the second was a six-month-old fetus that had to be
surgically removed, the third was during my fifth month. I was
really careful with this last pregnancy. I rested a lot and didn't do
anything strenuous. My doctor said my placenta tore loose, but why
would it do that? Will I ever be able to have another child?

—M.J., Butler, Pennsylvania

A woman who suffers repeated miscarriages should be evaluated by her doctor for hormone imbalances that might be corrected with progesterone or other hormones. A basal body temperature record (see pages 216 and 217) will help a doctor judge the hormonal fluctuations within a woman. She should also have a hysterosalpingogram, a uterine X ray, to see if there is any problem in her womb. Since Ms. J. underwent surgery for the removal of a fetus, she might have scar tissue from the operation, or if she had a D & C after miscarriage, the scraping might have caused the formation of scar tissue inside the womb. If Ms. J. does have scar tissue, her placenta might not be able to grow normally, and it might become detached, as her doctor said it did.

A current theory is that multiple miscarriages might be caused by problems in a woman's immune system, which marks a fetus as "foreign" and causes her body to reject the conception. Some doctors have had success treating women with immunoglobulin, a blood product that tempers action in the immune system's killer cells. Ms. J. might ask her doctor about immune therapy. Daily or biweekly injections of heparin, paired with a progesterone suppository, and daily baby aspirin (80 to 100 mg), might also help reduce her chance of miscarriage.

Ms. J.'s daughter is living proof that she is able to bear a child. I sense a high probability that she will do so again.

Ms. J. does not mention whether the fetal tissue from her miscarriages was analyzed. A large number of couples who live through the anguish of repeated miscarriages are known to have greater-than-average likelihood of carrying genes with chromosomal abnormalities. Ms. J. and her husband each have forty-six pairs of chromosomes that join together to create their child. Among these essential forty-six, there might be certain chromosomes that do not complement each other, and only one out of four pregnancies might work.

How Can I Prevent a Miscarriage?

I'm twenty-five years old and I have battled with endometriosis ever since I was a teenager. I thought I might never be able to get pregnant, but I did. I actually conceived a child and I was devastated when I miscarried in my second month. I know miscarriages aren't unusual, but I don't want this to happen to me again. My husband is very optimistic about trying to have another baby right away, but first I want to know everything about preventing miscarriages. What can I do to have a healthy child?
—F.E., Vernon, Connecticut

As mentioned before, an early miscarriage is often the result of a chromosomal abnormality in a fetus; the body cleanses itself of an imperfect conception. The recent news; however, is that *defects in chromosomes might more often be attributed to sperm, not egg, problems.*

Sperm abnormality increases with a man's age. Heavy drinkers and smokers often have damaged sperm, as do men who have had numerous sex partners and more chance of exposure to infections. A man's sperm should be examined for bacteria cultures. Mycoplasma, a microorganism that attacks a man's sperm, might have caused the development of a defective conceptus that led to miscarriage. If a man has mycoplasma, he can be treated with antibiotics such as vibramycin or erythromycin, taken daily for at least twenty days. Extra vitamin B and a reduction in smoking and drinking will also improve a man's sperm quality.

While a man tries to upgrade his sperm, a woman might also keep herself fit with prenatal vitamins and exercise to maintain an optimum body weight. Ms. E. might take extra precautions because women with endometriosis are at higher-than-average risk of having a miscarriage. Prostaglandins, which increase with endometriosis, cause uterine contractions that might squeeze out a newly implanted egg. A woman like Ms. E. might deactivate her prostaglandins and calm her uterus if she takes a prostaglandin-blocking drug such as Motrin (see chapter 3). Also, it is known that after at least a six-month treatment with Danocrine or a GnRH agonist (see chapter 7), a woman who suffers from endometriosis has a much better chance of conceiving and bearing a healthy child.

Before Ms. E. experiences another miscarriage she might also want to have her thyroid checked. If she has a low/normal reading, thyroid medication might help to prevent a second miscarriage. When a woman lives through miscarriage after miscarriage, her doctor should check, in addition to her thyroid, her progesterone level. If her progesterone is low, she might benefit from natural progesterone treatment. There are reports that women getting synthetic progesterone for miscarriage have a slightly increased possibility of bearing children with birth defects such as cardiovascular malformations and shortened limbs. On the other hand, there have also been reports that the offspring of mothers who have taken synthetic or natural progesterone during pregnancy have increased intelligence, self-confidence, and ambition. Findings related to the effects of progesterone during pregnancy, however, are still under debate.

It is certain, though, that a woman who fears miscarriage must lead a fairly sedentary life during her first trimester, just in case physical exertion could dislodge the embryo. A woman is advised to slow down her physical activity, decrease her jogging, and limit or refrain from sexual intercourse until the critical three months have passed.

Does an IUD Cause Miscarriage?

I was pregnant once with an IUD and my doctor gave me an abortion. At the time I didn't question him but now I'm wondering whether the IUD would have caused a miscarriage or could I have carried the baby to term?

—J.K., Pleasanton, California

A woman who is wearing an IUD can conceive if the contraceptive has slipped down to the lower part of her uterus or if a fibroid tumor or some other condition has caused the upper portion of her womb to expand so that the IUD cannot cover the area in which a fertilized egg implants itself. The IUD does not generally cause miscarriage because the misplaced device is not situated near the embryo. Thus, when women who do not want to conceive find themselves pregnant with an IUD, they should not wait and hope for a miscarriage.

Pregnancies with IUDs have been known to have been carried to term. However, years ago the Dalkon Shield IUD caused a crisis. Doctors felt that if a pregnant woman wore a Dalkon Shield and broke her water, the Shield was responsible for ensuing severe infections that led to hospitalization and even death in some cases.

After the Dalkon tragedy, doctors were inclined to give women abortions if they became pregnant with IUDs, to avoid the possibility of infection. Today, attitudes are changing. Some doctors who are worried about infection still say that abortion is a must when an IUD is involved, but a growing number of physicians have come to believe that since an IUD is usually situated in an area of the uterus away from the developing embryo, it can be removed without harming mother or baby. A woman must be informed that there is a possibility of miscarriage after IUD removal, but to give herself the best chance for a healthy pregnancy, she must permit the device to be taken out.

If a doctor cannot remove the IUD without harming the embryo, then he will have to perform an abortion in conjunction with IUD withdrawal. There might be a problem if the tail of the IUD has traveled up into the uterus because the device then becomes more difficult to extract.

Once a doctor has removed an IUD and a woman has no bleeding or cramping for a few days, the pregnancy should continue without interruption. Of course, a woman who becomes pregnant with an IUD has every right to choose a legal abortion since she was attempting to prevent pregnancy in wearing the IUD, but no woman should let her doctor insist that abortion is the only way to handle a pregnancy conceived with an IUD. *The IUD alone must be removed.*

NOTE: If a woman has unprotected intercourse and is fearful that she is pregnant, she might have heard that the insertion of an IUD is an effective morning-after method. The hope is that the IUD might bring on a miscarriage, but the device must be inserted within seventy-two hours after the intercourse and a woman might find herself in great pain afterward. For current information on emergency contraception, check pages 354 to 355.

Could a Fibroid Tumor Bring on Miscarriage?

I'm a twenty-eight-year-old black woman with fibroid tumors. I've miscarried twice in the last two years and now my doctor is saying that the miscarriages could be due to the fibroids. Does this mean I'll never be able to have a baby? Will I need a hysterectomy?
—A.H., Washington, D.C.

Fibroid tumors are predominant in black and Eastern European women. Fibroids that have grown outside the uterus or within the uterine wall generally do not prevent conception or lead to miscarriage, but a submucous fibroid penetrates the lining of the uterus, breaks into the uterine cavity, and intrudes upon a healthy pregnancy (see chapter 15). The uterine area taken up by a submucous fibroid disrupts the blood supply to the developing fetus. Cramping and miscarriage might follow.

Mrs. H. needs to have a D & C to give her doctor an opportunity to look for a submucous fibroid inside her womb. If she does have such a fibroid, she can have it removed during a myomectomy, a major operation designed to eliminate tumors while leaving a woman's organs intact. Some doctors do not like to perform myomectomies, which they find are a bit more complicated than hysterectomies, but a woman should know that she has this choice. She should seek out a doctor who is capable and willing to perform the myomectomy procedure and allow her to hold on to her uterus and conceive again.

If Ms. H. does not have submucous fibroids, which her doctor should have discovered during her second miscarriage anyway, then she should be given a hysterosalpingogram, an X ray of her uterus, to see where her fibroids are positioned. If no other abnormalities appear on the X ray, she might try to conceive once more, but if she miscarries a third time, she and her husband will need further evaluation and genetic counseling.

Why Don't Doctors Pay More Attention to Miscarriages?

I gave birth to my son two years ago and recently became pregnant again. I was about six weeks into my pregnancy when one day at work I began to have severe cramps. I went to the ladies' room and blood was flowing out between my legs. My boss, who fortunately is a woman, came in to see how I was and when she realized that I was slipping into a fainting spell, she drove me to the nearest hospital emergency room. We sat and waited while doctors milled around us. I was still bleeding but no one seemed to care. It was only after I passed out that a doctor took charge. I had to be given a blood transfusion and a D & C because I had lost so much blood. The doctors did not seem to think that a miscarriage was a serious condition. They practically ignored me. Why don't doctors pay more attention to miscarriages? Don't they know that a miscarriage is traumatic?

—D.Y., Terre Haute, Indiana

The chance of miscarriage increases after a woman has already had a child, so Ms. Y. was more susceptible to miscarriage during her second pregnancy. Her personal obstetrician should be doing his best to find the cause of her miscarriage by following it up with X rays, a thyroid test, and other evaluations. He should carefully guide her through her next pregnancy to avoid the possibility of another miscarriage.

As for her emergency room experience, Ms. Y. is undoubtedly right about the doctors not paying enough attention to her. Perhaps this attitude is a carryover from the days when women arrived in emergency rooms suffering from self-induced abortions. Many of these women were damaged for life, and the young doctors could not cope with the emotional trauma of watching them. Remember, the majority of doctors in emergency rooms are not gynecologists. They are surgeons, interns, and residents in training. Many of them are not yet educated about the severity of miscarriage. This woman might have bled to death. If she had been properly treated with intravenous fluid and medication, her bleeding might have been controlled without the need for a transfusion.

Not only gynecologists, but all physicians must be alerted to the serious effects of miscarriage. The American College of Obstetricians and Gynecologists is encouraging more physicians to educate and counsel their patients in the area of women's health. If couples were more informed about miscarriage, its causes and treatments, women might possibly prevent themselves from suffering as Ms. Y. did.

Once a woman has been tested for the cause of a spontaneous abortion, she can take better care of herself in a subsequent pregnancy. She can restrict her physical and sexual activities and visit her doctor frequently. Her cautious program should allay her anxiety and generally increase her chances for successful childbearing.

Could Sex Cause a Miscarriage?

My husband and I were having sexual intercourse one night when I got stabbing pains across my abdomen. I couldn't move and he had to call an ambulance. I was rushed to a hospital immediately.

I had had a miscarriage and had been hemorrhaging internally
when I was admitted. I didn't even know I was pregnant and I
wonder: Could sex have caused my miscarriage? How can I avoid
miscarriage again?

—M.T., Margate, New Jersey

A miscarriage will not occur easily if a pregnancy is healthy. Women who have not wanted their pregnancies have tried everything from jumping off tables to having hours of sexual activity, and nothing has dislodged their conceptions. Ms. T. probably did not have a normal pregnancy. Perhaps she had an ectopic pregnancy that happened to burst during intercourse. It's also possible that the fertilized egg had not implanted properly in her womb and that sex moved the egg into her abdomen and caused her internal bleeding.

In general, sex will not disturb a healthy, well-nourished embryo, but a woman who knows she is at high risk for miscarriage, as Ms. T.'s experience tells her she now is, should refrain from sex when she thinks she might have conceived. After a pregnancy is confirmed, it is wise to avoid sex and orgasm until a few months after conception, when the egg has achieved a strong hold inside the uterus. There will then be less chance of miscarriage.

How Does an Incompetent Cervix Cause Repeated Miscarriages?

Last year I had two miscarriages, one at nineteen weeks and
another at twenty-two weeks, and both were healthy babies. My
doctor says my cervix isn't strong enough. He called my cervix
"incompetent," but he never really explained what that meant.
How does an incompetent cervix cause repeated miscarriages?

—W.N., Boca Raton, Florida

An incompetent cervix has a weak muscular tissue that cannot withstand the pressure of the expanding uterus. Usually, in the second trimester, during about the twentieth week of gestation, the cervix painlessly opens and the woman loses the pregnancy. Incompetent cervixes are common in women who have had their cervixes forcefully opened during repeated therapeutic abortions.

Ms. N. should have a hysterosalpingogram to make sure that she has no abnormality aside from the incompetent cervix. The X ray will also show the width and depth of her cervix. If she miscarries a third time, she will be considered a person who suffers from "habitual abortion," so on her next conception measures should be taken to strengthen her weakened cervix.

Her doctor has two choices. As soon as this woman completes the first three months of her next pregnancy, he should admit her to a hospital or clinic for a Shirodkar procedure or a McDonald suture. In both procedures a drawstring type of suture is placed around the cervix to prevent the pregnancy from escaping. Using the Shirodkar method, a doctor buries a suture underneath the cervical skin tissue, not irritating the vagina but closing the relaxed cervix. A McDonald suture is placed around the cervix, and the stitches are exposed. In both cases, when a woman reaches term the doctor will cut the suture and remove it. This removal is painless because the nerves around the suture are usually numbed. If the suture is really well-placed, and a woman intends to become pregnant again, a doctor might perform a cesarean section and leave the suture behind so that it does not have to be replaced during the next pregnancy.

Any woman who has endured at least two miscarriages in the second trimester might be suffering from an incompetent cervix. She should consult a perinatologist, a doctor who specializes in high-risk pregnancies; he will be highly skilled at saving her next baby with the possible aid of a Shirodkar or a McDonald suture. Then, to assure the success of the treatment, after she has her cervix stitched, a woman should still decrease her physical and sexual activities and take it easy throughout the pregnancy.

What Is the Difference Between an Incompetent Cervix and Premature Labor?

I lost my first baby due to a blighted ovum, but two months after the miscarriage I become pregnant again. The pregnancy was fine until the twenty-fifth week, when I had "strange twinges." I went to the doctor and he said my cervix was starting to expand and I should go home and stay in bed for the rest of the pregnancy. My cervix was incompetent, he told me, and I could lose my second baby if I didn't lie down. After thirty-six weeks I was allowed to get out of bed and two weeks later I gave birth to an eight-pound, six-ounce baby girl. Now my baby's pediatrician says that he doesn't think I had an incompetent cervix but a threatened premature delivery. What's the difference? And will I be able to have another child someday without spending the whole pregnancy in bed?

—B.Z., El Paso, Texas

A woman miscarries due to a blighted ovum because a chromosomal or genetic abnormality has caused the embryo to disintegrate and leave behind a little sac of amniotic fluid. There's no particular reason why a woman gets a blighted ovum. It could happen to anyone, and it has no effect on future pregnancies. However, since she might be problem-prone, a woman who has had a miscarriage as a result of a blighted ovum deserves special attention from her doctor during the months that she is bearing a child. Ms. Z.'s doctor should have been carefully following her second pregnancy.

Regarding her second pregnancy, her pediatrician is right. When a cervix is incompetent, it opens painlessly. A woman often feels only pressure and maybe a slight staining. the fact that Ms. Z. felt "twinges" could indicate that she was beginning premature labor. Her bedrest probably saved her baby's life, but it is impossible to make an absolute judgment based on her letter. Her symptoms could be diagnosed as one of three conditions: incompetent cervix, threatened premature labor, or false labor.

If Ms. Z. does become pregnant again, she should visit her obstetrician frequently during her nine months of expectancy to give him opportunities to inspect her cervix. A woman's cervix should remain closed during pregnancy. If any cervical changes occur without labor, she might have an incompetent cervix, which could be corrected with the Shirodkar or McDonald suture, as explained in the response to the previous letter. If premature labor begins, she could be treated with one of a group of drugs called beta-mimetics, medications that stimulate the womb's beta cells to relax uterine muscles.

A newer approach to miscarriage prevention comes from a regimen of folic acid, heparin, baby aspirin, erythromycin, and a progesterone suppository. The *folic acid* helps prevent birth defects that might lead to miscarriage. The drug *heparin* and the *baby aspirin* are blood thinners that prevent possible microcoagulations to the fetus. The antibiotic *erythromycin* helps to prevent infections in the developing embryo. A *progesterone suppository* relaxes the uterus, slows contractions, and aids in the implantation of an embryo.

What Is a Molar Pregnancy, and Why Did It Cause My Miscarriage?

I'm a twenty-three-year-old woman of Chinese descent. Six weeks into my pregnancy I miscarried and my doctor said it was because I had a molar pregnancy. He mentioned something about Asian women being more inclined to have this type of pregnancy but he never said anything more. What is a molar pregnancy, and why did it cause my miscarriage?
—C.C., New York, New York

A molar pregnancy, also know as a hydatiform mole, occurs when the placenta, possibly for some genetic or immunological reason, is overtaken by small molar cysts that look like clusters of grapes. The cysts multiply and replace the entire placenta; their very presence cuts off fetal oxygen and nourishment and results in fetal death.

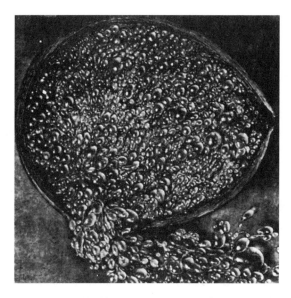

11-1 **Hydatiform Mole.** This picture shows a molar pregnancy in which the fetus and placenta have been completely replaced by small molar cysts that look like clusters of grapes. The molar tissue is surrounded by the uterine wall. At the bottom of the picture one can see the molar tissue being expelled from the uterus through a partially dilated (opened) cervix. *Reproduced by permission from* Textbook of Obstetrics, *by Henricas J. Stander, 1945, D. Appleton-Century Co., New York.*

Whenever a woman notices slight or heavy bleeding during her pregnancy, she should visit her doctor for an examination. A woman with a rapidly growing hydatiform mole usually has a uterus that is larger than expected, considering her delivery date. A doctor who suspects a molar pregnancy from his patient's symptoms can confirm his suspicions with the aid of ultrasonography. A higher-than-normal beta-subunit HCG level, which can be determined by a blood test, is also a sign of a hydatiform mole.

As soon as the condition is diagnosed, the molar pregnancy must be removed by a D & C or the suction method because, although the mole is usually benign, it can become cancerous. If a woman miscarries before her doctor has been able to remove the mole surgically, she should collect the discharged tissue in a jar and bring it to the doctor for a pathological analysis. Since the tissue is potentially cancerous, it must be tested immediately, and a woman will want a D & C to make sure that all of the hydatiform mole is eradicated.

After a physician has carefully cleaned the uterine wall and removed all the harmful cysts and tissue, a woman's HCG should be monitored to assure all concerned that the molar pregnancy is definitely over. Since a mole can become cancerous, some physicians used to recommend preventive chemotherapy after the pregnancy was terminated, but this course of action is no longer favored. The recurrence of molar tissue can be monitored with regular checks of the beta-subunit HCG. Actually, any sensitive blood test that is normally used to determine pregnancy can provide readings that will indicate whether the molar cysts are encroaching.

For at least a year after she has experienced a molar pregnancy, a woman should visit her obstetrician or an oncologist frequently. There is a chance that the mole could spontaneously return within a year, but if her beta-subunit HCG remains low, another molar invasion is not likely to happen. During the year that she is being observed and guarded, a woman should be sure to use contraception to avoid pregnancy. Birth control pills are especially recommended at this time because they keep the body's HCG level naturally low. This is important since an increase in HCG could mean that the disease has recurred.

A woman will be at less risk for cancer if her hydatiform mole developed late in her pregnancy and she miscarried molar tissue along with a coexistent fetus. With this type of molar miscarriage, the fetus is usually female, and the choriocarcinoma, the deadly cancer that a molar pregnancy might generate, rarely occurs. However, this late-in-the-pregnancy mole growth is not the norm. Most of the time a molar pregnancy starts during the first months of gestation, and after it is terminated a woman must be carefully monitored for at least a year.

If, after a year, a woman has been declared free of any metastatic cancer from the mole, she is not likely to have a recurrence of the disease. She might try to conceive again, and if she does become pregnant, she should be carefully monitored throughout her nine months. Her labor and delivery should be no different from any healthy woman's, and her baby will not be affected by the previous molar pregnancy.

ECTOPIC PREGNANCY—
AN INCREASING DANGER

Unlike a miscarriage, which is often provoked by an abnormality in the union of sperm and egg, an ectopic pregnancy results from a normal conception that grows in an inappropriate place. When a fertilized egg does not move into a woman's womb, but instead implants itself in her tube, on an ovary, or somewhere within her abdominal cavity, it creates an ectopic pregnancy. The tube is the most common site that a conceptus chooses for its gestation outside the uterus. That's why the term "tubal pregnancy" might be more familiar than "ovarian pregnancy" or "abdominal pregnancy," although all are ectopic, troublesome, and biologically remarkable.

Potentially life-threatening ectopic pregnancies are on the rise, occurring in about one in every sixty pregnancies. Tubal pregnancies alone increased 400 percent from 1970 to 1989. Yet, with improvements in early detection, the mortality rate from ectopic pregnancy has dropped to 5 in 10,000. So the numbers are climbing, but the survival rate is improving.

Only human beings—no other animals—have ectopic pregnancies. In a tubal pregnancy the egg, which is normally only fertilized in a Fallopian tube and then moved into the uterus by the cilia, for some reason stops before it reaches the womb. An egg that is impeded in the tubal passage should not be able to grow, but, logic aside, it often does. Changes in the tubal environment apparently can make the channel more conducive to implantation, and these changes are obviously occurring in more and more women.

It seems that an increased frequency of tubal infection is turning the Fallopian tubes of fertile women into grounds, though unsafe, for implantation. The chance of infection increases as the number of sex partners grows. A woman who has been sexually active with a variety of men might have picked up a sexually transmitted disease or an infection that did not render symptoms when it occurred. No matter where it comes from, an infection that invades a Fallopian tube can cause scar tissue that destroys the unbroken movement of the cilia and thereby disrupts the journey of the fertilized egg.

Some women are at increased risk for ectopic pregnancy if they smoke or they have had tubal sterilization. On average, a woman who smokes before conception is almost twice as likely to have an ectopic pregnancy than a nonsmoker. And for every 1,000 tubal sterilizations, about seven ectopic pregnancies occur within ten years. If it is not terminated, an ectopic pregnancy can lead to internal bleeding and eventually death. Only early detection can change this potentially devastating situation into a manageable event.

How to Know Whether Your Pregnancy Is Ectopic

When a pregnancy is ectopic, certain signs will alert a woman to the fact that something is wrong. Most ectopic pregnancies occur in the Fallopian tube (tubal pregnancy). At first a woman might assume that she has a normal pregnancy because she has no out-of-the-ordinary symptoms. The fetus grows as it would in the uterus. However, the tube is not made for expansion, and between the sixth and eighth week of pregnancy a woman might begin to feel pain as the tube stretches. Often, she might also notice vaginal bleeding. If her bleeding continues, she might pass a clot that she could interpret as a miscarriage because the blood is in layers and looks different than her usual menstrual flow.

A woman in the throes of a miscarriage has severe uterine cramps before she miscarries, but her pain ends as soon as the fetal tissue is expelled. During an ectopic pregnancy a woman bleeds, passes clots, but continues to have abdominal pain, so a woman whose pain does not stop with bleeding should strongly suspect that her pregnancy is ectopic.

The signals of a *tubal pregnancy* are clear: pain—either diffuse abdominal pain or specific pain on the right or left side—and possible vaginal bleeding. Sometimes pain is present without bleeding. When a woman who knows or suspects she is pregnant recognizes the symptoms of a tubal pregnancy, she must phone her doctor immediately so that he can assess her condition.

Only a minimal number of ectopic pregnancies implant themselves on the ovaries or in the abdomen. An ectopic pregnancy on the ovary will never be carried to term, but will result in rupture and intraabdominal expulsion of the fetus. No fetal tissue passes through the vagina as it does during miscarriage. Symptoms of an *ovarian pregnancy* are somewhat similar to those of a tubal pregnancy, but the pain can be less intense or completely absent. The condition is often diagnosed only after the pregnancy ruptures and internal bleeding begins. Before a woman becomes seriously ill, an immediate laparotomy is needed to stop the bleeding. If surgery is not performed, an ovarian pregnancy might lead to more extensive internal bleeding, shock, and even death.

Abdominal pregnancies are very rare. An abdominal pregnancy will usually disintegrate, but can occasionally progress all the way to term. Should this happen, a baby will be delivered by cesarean section. After the delivery of a child carried in the abdomen, a woman might have dangerous internal bleeding because the placenta might not be shed as it would after normal childbirth. In the saddest cases, women have died from internal bleeding after abdominal pregnancies. The seriousness of an abdominal pregnancy cannot be overemphasized.

How Is Tubal Pregnancy Treated?

The progesterone that is normally produced by the placenta during a healthy pregnancy is not secreted in a high enough quantity to maintain the uterine lining during an ectopic pregnancy. This progesterone deficiency might lead to mild uterine cramping and sometimes, but not always, vaginal bleeding. The abdominal pain, often rhythmic in nature, comes and goes like the pain during labor. Rather than take painkillers, a woman who is suffering all the signs of a tubal pregnancy should contact her doctor. If he is not available, she should go to the emergency room of the nearest hospital. After pain and possible bleeding begin, only one or two days might elapse before a tube bursts. Sometimes a tube breaks very soon after a woman feels the pain. As soon as the symptoms of a tubal pregnancy appear, a woman should seek immediate medical attention.

An ectopic pregnancy is a life-threatening situation. A doctor must perform a thorough pelvic examination. If he discovers a painful cyst or mass in the area of the tubes, whether or not vaginal bleeding is present, he must verify his finding by administering blood hormone tests to check levels of progesterone and beta human chorionic gonadotropin, known as beta HCG. The levels of progesterone are useful in diagnosing women who are unsure of the date of their last menstruation. Depending on progesterone levels, a doctor might continue to suspect, or completely rule out, ectopic pregnancy, or he might turn his attention to a viable pregnancy. In a normal pregnancy, beta HCG doubles every two days. In a suspected ectopic pregnancy, beta HCG will rise abnormally and have a longer doubling time.

When there are abnormal hormone patterns, a doctor should use a transvaginal ultrasound probe to visualize the possible ectopic pregnancy. This type of ultrasound can provide a doctor with the size and condition of an ectopic mass. If the mass is unruptured, a laparoscopy can be performed to remove it, and at the same time an attempt can be made to save a woman's tube. (Sometimes a pregnancy damages the tube beyond salvation.) If a mass is large or inaccessible to laparoscopy, a woman might be treated with the drug methotrexate, as explained in the "How Your Fertility Can Be Saved" section.

After an ultrasound shows that there is no pregnancy in a woman's uterus, a doctor might perform a dilatation and curettage (D & C) to obtain samples from the uterine lining that will prove beyond a doubt the absence of pregnancy.

When an ultrasound cannot verify the presence or absence of pregnancy, either within or outside the uterus, a doctor will assess the results of the blood hormone tests and might then decide to proceed with a D & C or a possible laparoscopy. An ultrasound might not show whether an ectopic pregnancy has ruptured, so a blood pressure check should be done to help the doctor take appropriate measures.

A *culdecentesis,* the insertion of a needle through the vagina into the abdomen, is a slightly painful procedure, but it is an essential test. If blood can be aspirated into the needle, internal abdominal bleeding is occurring, and if the doctor sees that the aspirated blood is not coagulating, he knows the tube has burst and he must immediately perform a laparotomy in order to control the internal bleeding.

When a tube breaks, blood instantly begins pumping into a woman's abdomen and the sudden internal hemmorhage can lead to shock and even death. During the laparotomy, a doctor might have to remove the damaged portion of the Fallopian tube, which would diminish a woman's ability to conceive again. Blood transfusions would probably be needed, too. After recovery, a woman can consider herself a survivor of a catastrophe, but she will be less fertile. Before her operation, if she thinks she would like to bear a child in the future, she should ask the doctor to save as much of her tube as possible because a microsurgeon later on might be able to repair her tube and restore her fertility.

If no blood is aspirated during the culdecentesis, but a woman is still suffering intolerable pain, a physician must perform a laparoscopy to find out whether she has an ectopic pregnancy, as he suspects she does. If an unruptured tubal pregnancy is found, the tube and the woman's fertility can be saved either through laparoscopic surgery or with the drug methotrexate.

How Your Fertility Can Be Saved. The best way a doctor has for examining an ectopic pregnancy is through *laparoscopy.* A small incision is made within a woman's navel, and fine microsurgical viewing instruments are passed through the opening. If a doctor sees an unruptured tubal pregnancy, he might remove the mass during the laparoscopic surgery using laser removal or cauterization to try to save the tube. If a mass is 4 centimeters or smaller, he might elect to treat it with *methotrexate*, a drug that kills the developing cells of the placenta and leads to a miscarriage of an ectopic pregnancy. Methotrexate is becoming popular as a single 50-mg intramuscular injection. This medical treatment of ectopic pregnancy keeps a woman's internal organs intact. However, some doctors prefer to perform a laparoscopy to treat a tubal pregnancy regardless of its size. In the best situation, a small incision is made in a Fallopian tube, the ectopic pregnancy is removed, and the tube stays intact.

When Your Fertility Might Be Lost. If a woman has complications such as blood in her abdomen, or a large amount of pelvic scar tissue, she might have to undergo a more invasive and less desired operation, a *laparotomy*. A surgeon will perform a bikini cut, a transverse incision below a woman's pubic hair line, and in this case, a Fallopian tube, an ovary, and possibly the uterus might be removed.

QUESTIONS ABOUT ECTOPIC PREGNANCY

What Are the Chances of a Second Ectopic Pregnancy?

When I was twenty-six I had an ectopic pregnancy and I had to have an immediate operation. My right tube was removed along with an ovarian cyst the size of a grapefruit. The doctor said it had all matter of hair, bone, etc., in it. After this major surgery I had all sorts of fears about having another ectopic pregnancy. I want to have a child and my husband and I are trying to listen to our new doctor, who tells us to have sex at least three times a week for six months, and then he will do a laparoscopy. Now I'm thirty-one,

I've had painful periods since I was fifteen, and I wonder if they could have anything to do with my problems getting pregnant. Also, does the ovarian cyst have any bearing on my infertility? My husband's sperm checks out fine. Still, in the back of my mind, I have a nagging, haunting fear that it will all repeat again, that I will have another ectopic and lose my only remaining tube. What are the chances that that will happen?

—R.J., Marathon, New York

The chance of having an ectopic pregnancy is, as mentioned before, about 1 percent for all women, although women who have had infections, endometriosis, or other abnormalities are at greater risk. Only 50 percent of the women who have had an ectopic pregnancy will be able to conceive again, and then, the chance of a second ectopic pregnancy is about 25 percent—a percentage that increases if a woman's tube was seriously damaged after her first tubal pregnancy. These figures are particularly tragic for a woman who has no disease or abnormality. Sympathetic doctors are making strong efforts to change the odds by encouraging the use of microsurgery. If an ectopic pregnancy is diagnosed early, a microsurgeon can make a fine incision in the tube, remove the pregnancy, and save the tube and a woman's fertility.

Ms. J. lost her tube after her first ectopic pregnancy and her fertility is now diminished. The ovarian cyst that was removed during her surgery sounds, from the letter, like a dermoid cyst, one that contains hair and glands but is not cancerous (see chapter 15). This long-gone cyst should have no influence on her ability to conceive again if, indeed, it was a dermoid cyst. Ms. J. writes that she has painful periods, so perhaps the cyst was an endometrial growth. If so, she might have infertility problems due to endometriosis (see chapters 7 and 8).

Ms. J. might benefit from a hysterosalpingogram, which would flush out her remaining tube with dye used for the X-ray process. If the X ray does not show any abnormalities and her tube is cleansed, she might continue her attempt to become pregnant. If after six months no conception occurs, further investigation is needed. At that time her doctor would be right to suggest a laparoscopy and possible microsurgery for removal of adhesions.

If Ms. J. does become pregnant, she and her doctor must monitor her pregnancy closely in case it should be ectopic. Any extraordinary pain, either with or without vaginal bleeding, must be considered a strong warning sign. If Ms. J. does conceive ectopically again, conservative microsurgery can remove the pregnancy before her tube ruptures, and she can recover as a fertile woman. By understanding that she will not lose her tube if she listens to her body, Ms. J.'s fear might be lessened and she might be in a better frame of mind to conceive.

I Had Two Ectopic Pregnancies; Will I Ever Have a Baby?

When I was twenty-three I had a tubal pregnancy that required immediate surgery and my tube was removed. I was told that I only had a fifty-fifty chance of getting pregnant again but I did not give up hope. A little over a year later I got pregnant again. I was happy until I learned that I had another tubal pregnancy. Once more, I was back in the hospital having surgery. This time the surgeon placed a plastic inserter into my tube and it stayed there for two months to keep the tube open. Afterward the doctor said that I had too much scar tissue to ever conceive naturally. Is IVF my only chance for having a baby now?

—D.R., Norfolk, Virginia

As mentioned in the response to the previous letter, there is a 25 percent chance of a second ectopic pregnancy. This woman should have had a hysterosalpingogram after her first ectopic pregnancy to make sure that she had no damage in her remaining tube. Then, when she became pregnant a second time, she and her doctor should have been monitoring her case, trying to catch a possible ectopic pregnancy early. Obviously, Ms. R. did not know her chances of having a second ectopic pregnancy or she would have been watching her symptoms.

If she felt she had an ectopic pregnancy and had consulted a microsurgeon at a teaching hospital or a large university medical center early enough, he might have removed the conceptus without causing scar tissue to form in her tube. Rather than place a plastic inserter into her tube, he probably would have used fine microsurgical instruments to repair her tube after he had ended the pregnancy.

Ms. J. had bad luck twice, but perhaps all is not lost for her. A skilled infertility specialist/microsurgeon who would be willing to treat her might be found at a large teaching hospital or university medical center. Such a physician might examine her with X rays and, possibly, a laparoscopy in order to decide whether he would be able to perform surgery to heighten her fertility. If only a portion of her remaining tube is damaged, he can remove the troublesome part and reanastomose (join together) the healthy sections. This reanastomosis is the same procedure used to reverse tubal sterilization. As long as the fimbriated end of her tube is whole and infection has not altered a major area of the tube, her fertility might be increased as much as 30 or 40 percent.

In vitro fertilization (IVF) one of the assisted reproductive technology techniques available today (see pages 274 to 279), was developed to help women with blocked or damaged Fallopian tubes, and it is certainly an option for Ms. R. I suggest that before she undergoes further surgery, she consult an infertility specialist about her chances of conception with IVF.

Ms. J.'s experience illustrates the importance of early and proper treatment of ectopic pregnancy. It might not have been necessary to remove her entire tube. Perhaps only a portion could have been taken out so that reanastomosis could have been performed by a microsurgeon at a later date. A woman who discovers that she has an ectopic pregnancy must remind her doctor before surgery, please, to save as much of her tube as possible. When her fertility is at stake, a woman must become an activist on her own behalf.

I Have Used an IUD; What Are My Chances of Having an Ectopic Pregnancy?

I used an IUD when I was in college but I developed such a severe infection that the doctors in the infirmary put me in the local hospital for treatment. My IUD was removed and I received intravenous fluid with antibiotics. The doctors at the hospital told me that I should not use an IUD if I wanted to have children later on in life. I went on the pill for a few years. Now I'm married and ready to go off contraceptives and start a family. Friends tell me they have heard that if you ever used an IUD you might be infertile or be susceptible to an ectopic pregnancy. Do you think I could be infertile? I did have that infection. What are my chances of having an ectopic pregnancy? Every now and then I have a pain on my left side and, of course, I think my tube is hurting and damaged. I need an expert opinion.

—M.C., Rogers, Arkansas

Studies have shown that there is a higher incidence of ectopic pregnancy when a woman has used an IUD in the past. Older IUDs sometimes caused tubal infections, which could be either silent or marked, like Ms. C.'s. Ms. C. might be better off than the woman whose infection goes unnoticed because in the first case, the inflammation might remain untreated and cause tubal scarring that inhibits conception. Ms. C. was appropriately treated with high doses of antibiotics and her infection was probably cured before it resulted in scarring.

In general, women who have had pelvic inflammatory disease are at high risk for ectopic pregnancy, especially if the disease was brought on by gonorrhea. The gonorrheal bacteria eat into the Fallopian tubes, damaging the linings and often causing the fimbriated ends to stick together in ways that make the tubes completely useless as conveyors of a fertilized egg. After an STD, the chance of an ectopic pregnancy increases.

Ms. C. did not have an STD, however, and her present pain might be from her monthly ovulation. Other sources of abdominal pain are adhesions or endometriosis, which could cause damage and are more serious considerations than ovulation aches. Or, she might be so concerned about the possibility of an ectopic pregnancy that she is feeling psychosomatic pain. It is difficult to diagnose her pain from her letter. An X ray of her tubes might put her mind to rest. This X ray would expose her only to a tiny amount of radiation, and it would be scheduled right after her period, when it is certain that she is not pregnant. The dye injected prior to X ray might free the tube from a small adhesion, cleanse it, and make it a less likely environment for an ectopic pregnancy.

If an X ray indicates minimal damage in the tubes, Ms. C. might attempt to become pregnant, but she should be aware that there might be an ectopic complication. She and her doctor should try to identify an ectopic pregnancy as soon as possible in order to save her tube through microsurgery. In all likelihood, however, since Ms. C. was rapidly treated for her IUD infection, she will probably be able to conceive a healthy baby that grows to term inside her womb.

Can an Abdominal Pregnancy Be Carried to Term?

Is it true that a woman can carry to term in her abdomen? A few of us had a discussion about it over lunch the other day and we're divided. Half of us can't believe that a baby can grow outside the womb.

—T.G., Kearny, New Jersey

Abdominal pregnancy, a rare condition, occurs when the placenta implants itself outside the uterus, usually on the bowel or behind the womb. The placenta will get its blood supply from the surrounding tissue and it will produce the progesterone needed to maintain the pregnancy. The fetus grows because it is self-sustaining inside the embryonic sac, which will expand just as if it were in the uterus.

Even the abdomens of men might be suitable for abdominal pregnancies. Under experimental conditions, pregnancies have been carried to term by male animals (see chapter 10). The problem facing a man who might bear an abdominal pregnancy, however, is the same one that confronts a woman.

The risk is that the fetal membrane (the water bag) might break and cause a woman to have internal bleeding that could lead to shock and subsequent death. If the bag ruptures before term, she might die. Assuming that the expectant mother survives the gestation, the baby might be delivered by cesarean section, but the placenta from an abdominal pregnancy would have grown into the abdominal tissue from which it would not be able to detach itself like a normal afterbirth. Removing the placenta is very tricky. Surgery is needed, internal bleeding could result, and a woman might never recover. Fortunately, as mentioned before, abdominal pregnancies are extremely rare.

ABORTION—WHEN A WOMAN ELECTS TO END HER PREGNANCY

Of the three ways that pregnancy might not be carried to term, abortion is by far the most controversial. Miscarriages and ectopic pregnancies usually disrupt pregnancies that women would like to see continued, but abortion is a voluntary interruption of pregnancy—or VIP, as it is called. It is fraught with religious, political, and emotional questions which warrant thoughtful discussion too extensive to be dealt with here. Within the frame of this book—a health guide—abortion is viewed as a medical technique that is neither condemned nor condoned. On these pages, abortion is, like every other topic in *Listen to Your Body*, a health concern.

Before the Supreme Court made abortion a constitutional right in 1973, the effects of pregnancy interruption by illegal abortion created a very difficult area of medicine.Women, either by themselves or with aid, would inject fluids into their uteri, insert nonsterile implements into their vaginas, and end up with uterine infections and uncontrollable bleeding, on their backs in hospital beds. Sometimes a woman would have to face a hysterectomy, and many doctors remember cases in which women died from septic shock or internal hemorrhage. If a woman requires an abortion today, she can travel to an established hospital or medical center where abortion is performed under safe, sterile conditions. An illegal means of abortion remains a dangerous alternative.

For the good health of a woman, an abortion should be performed as early as possible. The best time for VIP is before the twelfth week of pregnancy, because later on an abortion procedure becomes more costly, more difficult, and more highly emotional. When a woman waits beyond the twelfth week of pregnancy, she faces the possibility of seriously damaging her cervix. A late abortion could also lead to future problems with miscarriage, incompetent cervix, and premature birth. It is important that pregnancy interruption be attempted early, and, indeed, statistics show that more than 90 percent of all abortions are performed in the first trimester.

About 1.2 million abortions are performed each year in the United States. That number represents a slight increase after years of decline, but according to the Centers for Disease Control's latest (1996) figures, this is still a 15 percent drop from former abortion numbers. The rate of abortions per 1,000 women aged fifteen to forty-four continues to be 20, the lowest rate since 1975. Teens, who used to be one third of the total, are now only one fifth. Among the reasons for the decline in abortions might be a decrease in the number of unintended pregnancies and the frequent use of condoms by young women. Also, there have been shifting attitudes toward abortion and, in some areas, limited access. Many women choose to have abortions because their pregnancies are accidental—either they are using contraception during sexual intercourse and have become pregnant inadvertently, or they are using contraceptives improperly or are having unprotected intercourse, believing that they cannot become pregnant.

Since the legalization of abortion, researchers using modern technology have refined and improved abortion methods. Today, women face septic abortions and fatal complications with far less frequency. Still, abortion is not simple. There continue to be medical risks and emotional difficulties any time a woman involves herself in the procedure.

All girls and boys, women and men, should be taught to protect themselves with contraceptives before intercourse. An abortion should not be thought of as a contraceptive. *Contra-* is a prefix that means "against." A contraceptive is something opposed to conception, used *before* conception. Abortion is a medical procedure that should be used in emergency cases when a woman's health is at stake, when there is an abnormality during pregnancy and fetal damage, when a woman can offer a less-than-secure home for the child, or when conception occurs due to failure of a contraceptive or as a result of rape.

Most doctors hope for a drop in abortion figures, but this cannot be anticipated until more thorough teenage health education is instituted and sexually active people begin to take a greater command over their own bodies.

Teenagers and Abortion

One fifth of all abortions are sought by teenage girls, and most states now have laws that require them either to notify their parents or to have parental consent. From state to state, the laws for girls under eighteen vary. When they are counseled afterward, most young women admit that they never used any form of contraception. One problem is that some teenagers have sexual intercourse, do not become pregnant, and decide that they are infertile. They then continue to have sex to test their fertility. Sometimes a young woman hates school and, fantasizing a marriage with her boyfriend as an escape, allows herself to become pregnant. Of course, this wishful thinking is rarely fulfilled. I have seen teenage girls carry their babies to term and their boyfriends always seem to disappear by the time of childbirth.

Contraception should be shared by young women and their boyfriends (see chapter 12). Parents of teenagers, or teenagers who are reading this book, should know that it would benefit a young woman and her boyfriend to visit a doctor or a clinic together to discuss contraception. Medical and health professionals want to reduce the abortion rate among teenagers, and they will never be judgmental toward a young woman and a young man who are taking care to prevent pregnancy.

Often when teenage girls do become pregnant they are afraid to tell their parents. They are worried about recriminations and they try to hide their pregnancies. By the time the pregnancy cannot be denied, a teenager might be in the third, fourth, or fifth month, and then she wants an abortion. An abortion at this stage is much more difficult and potentially more harmful than an early abortion. If a teenager is pregnant, she should not wait. As soon as she misses her period, she should have a pregnancy test through a doctor, a clinic, or a women's health collective. Pregnancy interruption is less risky if it is performed early.

How Safe Is a Legal Abortion?

In the early 1970s, before the Supreme Court decree, it was estimated that approximately 50 to 150 deaths occurred for every 100,000 illegal abortions performed in the United States. Most often, death was caused by infection from the contaminated instruments used for the procedures. Today, with legal abortions in sterile facilities, the death rate has dropped to 0.7 deaths per 100,000 first-trimester abortions. The death rate increases, however, for abortions during the later trimesters. For abortions performed during the thirteenth to fifteenth weeks of pregnancy, the death rate is 7.5 per 100,000 cases. For pregnancy interruption at twenty-one weeks or more, there are 22.9 deaths per 100,000 abortions.

The fatal outcome of an infection-ridden septic abortion was much more frequent when an illegal abortion was the only alternative to childbirth from an unwanted pregnancy. A septic abortion can still occur with a legal abortion, but it is much less likely. (See below, "How to Avoid a Septic Abortion.") However, the further along in pregnancy an abortion is performed, the more chance that infection, internal bleeding, and death might ensue. Even in clean hospital surroundings with the latest equipment and the best doctors, internal bleeding might begin with a late abortion. *The safest legal abortion is one that is performed as soon as pregnancy is verified, which should be within a week or two of a missed period.* But every woman should know that no matter when she has an abortion, she risks some chance of:

Uterine perforation. During an abortion, when a doctor inserts instruments into the uterus, he might, if he is inexperienced, rupture the womb and cause internal bleeding. A woman whose uterus has been perforated must be admitted to the hospital immediately for a laparoscopy, which is one way a doctor can evaluate the extent of the damage. The abortion must be completed at this time. If uterine laceration is extensive, an exploratory laparotomy must be conducted to suture the perforation. Sometimes, if the perforation is very wide and has torn uterine vessels, a hysterectomy must be performed to stop the internal bleeding and save the woman's life.

Laceration and tearing of the cervix during cervical dilation might lead to an incompetent cervix and miscarriage during future pregnancies. The chance of cervical damage is lessened, however, if an abortion is performed during the first few weeks of pregnancy when minimal or no dilation is needed.

Endometritis, infection in the uterus, appears in approximately 5 to 7 percent of the women who have had abortions. The pain, bleeding, and fever of endometritis can only be cured with the appropriate amount and type of antibiotic.

Syncope (sweating, a drop in blood pressure, and fainting) might be brought on by the stimulation of vaginal nerves during an abortion. A woman might need to be observed in the hospital or at a clinic until she stabilizes and her symptoms disappear.

Internal bleeding, as previously mentioned, becomes a much greater risk when an abortion is done after the first trimester, but that risk diminishes when a skilled physician at a reputable hospital or clinic conducts the procedure. Bleeding complications are quite serious, because if they're not controlled, they might lead to shock and, possibly, the end of a woman's life.

How to Avoid a Septic Abortion

A septic abortion is an infection in the uterus and pelvic organs after an abortion. Usually, nonsterile, germ-ridden implements used for a procedure introduce the infection.

Before 1973, when abortions were illegal, septic abortions were much more common, and even today, if a legal abortion is not performed in a first-rate facility, a septic abortion might still occur. Bacteria might enter the uterine environment from tubes, catheters, and needles that have not been properly sterilized. Once in the uterus, the infection-causing germs can climb into the Fallopian tubes and render a woman infertile.

After an abortion, if a woman develops a low-grade temperature combined with pain or discomfort and, occasionally, bleeding, she should see her doctor immediately. She might need rapid treatment with antibiotics to cure the infection. Sometimes a woman is admitted to the hospital and placed on high doses of antibiotics to stop the infection from spreading any farther—and to save her life. A septic abortion, if not treated, can be fatal. A woman must be very aware of her body after pregnancy interruption to make sure that a septic abortion does not start and spread.

Even if an abortion is performed under perfect conditions, if a woman does not follow her doctor's advice afterward, a septic abortion might take hold. A woman must try to keep her organs free from germs. A man's penis can push bacteria into the uterus, so a woman should not have intercourse for at least three or four weeks, or until all bleeding has stopped and her doctor has given her the okay to have sex. Also, during this celibate period, baths should be avoided and tampons should not be used. Nothing should be inserted into the vagina until the healing process is over, and any fever or pain in the aftermath of abortion must be evaluated by a doctor.

Today's Options: Medical or Surgical Abortion

A medical abortion uses drugs to stop the development of a pregnancy and expel it. A woman can terminate an unwanted pregnancy from the moment she learns she is pregnant up to seven weeks from her last menstrual period.

A surgical abortion is an extraction of a conception that can be performed from early to late pregnancy. Surgical abortion (see pages 347 to 351) remains the most available, most used method, while the two most effective medical abortions continue to generate controversy:

- *Mifepristone (RU486)/misoprostol prostaglandin.* The RU486 pill has been FDA-approved as safe and effective (92 percent) but it has not found a manufacturer in the United States. A 600-mg dose of mifepristone, followed two days later by a vaginal insert of the prostaglandin misoprostol, will result in a bleeding out of the conceptus.
- *Methotrexate/misoprostol prostaglandin.* On the market for treating other conditions, these drugs are available for medical abortions and might be up to 96 percent effective. A woman receives an injected dose of methotrexate according to her height and weight, and five to seven days later she uses vaginal inserts of misoprostol to help expel the pregnancy.

Emergency contraception, or the morning-after pill, is not a medical abortion but has been linked to it (see pages 354 to 355).

QUESTIONS ABOUT ABORTION

Even though abortions are regularly performed in this country, the controversial nature of the procedure overshadows information about the actual medical steps that are taken to make pregnancy interruption possible. Answers to questions in the following letters might help to clear up confusions over the way abortion is performed and the effects it has on a woman's body.

What Is the Best Surgical Abortion Method?

I am a counselor at a family planning clinic, but I am not a doctor. I keep up with the latest medical journals but sometimes I feel like I'm reading conflicting information. I want to provide my patients with good advice about the safest and best abortion methods for them, but I'm not always sure what to suggest.
—N.D., Fresno, California

The safest abortion is the earliest possible abortion. While a medical abortion (see above) exists, a surgical abortion remains the most available option. Up to six or seven weeks from a woman's last menstrual period, a pregnancy may be surgically interrupted in an outpatient clinic or in a doctor's office without the need for general anesthesia or cervical dilation, the opening of the cervix with anatomically designed dilators of increasing size. The office procedures performed during early pregnancy carry far less risk than the hospital methods used to interrupt later pregnancies.

Ms. D.'s question about the safest and best abortion methods cannot be simply answered. A doctor's choice of abortion technique depends on how far into the pregnancy a woman is when she seeks its interruption. My previous book, *It's Your Body: A Woman's Guide to Gynecology,*[1] contains detailed descriptions of the latest abortion methods, which, in response to Ms. D.'s question, are summarized here in the order of their preferred use from early to late pregnancy:

Up to six or seven weeks: Menstrual extraction (miniabortion) or manual vacuum aspiration (MVA) are used up to six or seven weeks after a woman's last menstrual flow. A California psychiatrist coined the term "menstrual extraction" as a way of easing the fact that an abortion was being performed. In association with other physicians and women's groups, he developed a catheter that could be inserted into a woman's uterus to extract its contents. The procedure continues to be used as a safe form of pregnancy interruption, although many medical institutions prefer to call it a *miniabortion* rather than a *menstrual extraction.*

During a *miniabortion* a woman is on the examining table with her feet resting in the stirrups. A doctor performs a pelvic examination and determines the size and position of her uterus. He cleanses her vagina and usually administers a tranquilizer or painkiller about half an hour before he inserts a small tube into her womb. At the end of thirty minutes, he injects Novocain around the cervical area and places forceps into the numbed cervix to steady the uterus. Then the Karman catheter is inserted into the uterus and suction is placed on the tube. The vacuum process loosens the uterine lining. When the catheter is turned in a circular motion, the contents of the uterus are aspirated. The cervix will not have to be dilated and the uterus will remain in perfect shape for childbearing. A woman usually experiences minimal pain during a miniabortion, and she might be crampy, faint, or dizzy for thirty to sixty minutes afterward, but once she feels strong enough to go home, she should be fine.

A *manual vacuum aspiration (MVA)* is an old-fashioned method that has come into vogue again. It can be utilized as early as eight days after ovulation, when the gestational sac is smaller than a pencil's eraser. MVA is quieter and gentler than the suction method, but so newly reborn that less than 10 percent of the 1.2 million yearly U.S. abortions are performed this way. MVA employs ultrasound and takes only five to fifteen minutes. A woman's cervix is dilated (widened), the vacuum tube is inserted into her uterus, and the doctor manually tugs on an attached 60-cc syringe. The force of the suction is enough to dislodge a fetus of up to ten weeks' gestation.

Seven to twelve weeks: The *suction method* is preferred when gestation has advanced from seven to twelve weeks. Since local, or sometimes general, anesthesia is used during the suction procedure, the abortion must be conducted in a hospital or an outpatient facility.

Anesthesia might cause an allergic reaction, or there might be complications if too much or too little is given. If a woman is in a hospital or at an outpatient clinic with a trained staff, an emergency team can bring her back to good health if she falls ill from anesthesia.

Before the suction begins, a woman's cervix is opened with dilators, smooth metal rods that come in increasing sizes. Starting with a small size, a dilator is inserted into the cervix. Then, larger and larger dilators are introduced until the cervix has stretched wide enough to accommodate a suction catheter of a diameter corresponding in millimeters to the number of gestation weeks; in other words, an 8-millimeter catheter would be used for an eight-week pregnancy. After the catheter is placed within the uterus, the contents of the womb are aspirated into a suction machine that works like a vacuum cleaner. The suction technique is the preferred, gentle method of withdrawing uterine tissue. The alternate procedure, which involves mechanical scraping, might result in excessive removal of a woman's uterine lining and the formation of adhesions in her womb.

NOTE: Due to the potential damage that mechanical cervical dilations might do to a woman's cervix and uterus, a number of teaching hospitals and university medical centers are using a new cervical dilation technique: *cervical priming with a prostaglandin suppository before suction abortion.* A prostaglandin suppository is placed in the vagina one to four hours before the abortion. Prostaglandins enter a woman's system and cause a mild uterine cramping that slowly softens and opens the cervix. Using this method, a doctor can avoid forceful dilation and possible injury of the cervix. Since the prostaglandins cause uterine contractions, the pregnancy interruption becomes more like a miscarriage followed by suction completion. There is less bleeding and less chance of infection. A woman who needs a suction abortion might call the major teaching hospitals or university medical centers in her area to find out whether cervical priming with prostaglandins is available to her.

Twelve to sixteen weeks: A few major hospitals allow a *dilation and evacuation (D & E)* to be performed between the twelfth and sixteenth weeks of pregnancy as calculated from a woman's last menstrual period. This is the "gray zone," when the fetus is too large for suction removal but not developed enough to respond to intraamniotic injection, a method used from about the sixteenth to the twentieth week of pregnancy.

At this D & E stage, the cervix must be widely dilated in order to remove the uterine contents. The expansion of the cervix might be hastened by priming the cervical area with vaginal prostaglandin suppositories or *laminaria digitala* (dried seaweed stem), which is inserted the night before pregnancy interruption is scheduled. The laminaria thickens cervical fluid, which expands and dilates the cervix. It is removed immediately before the abortion, which is performed with the aide of a vacuum aspirator and tissue forceps.

A D & E is much more dangerous than a miniabortion or the suction method because there is a greater chance that the cervix and uterus will be lacerated during the process and that there will be rupture and bleeding. *After the twelfth week, a pregnancy interruption moves into the sphere of mid-trimester abortion, which is always more complicated and less safe than a first trimester abortion.* A woman should seek an abortion as early as possible. As her pregnancy advances, the risks to her well-being multiply.

From the twelfth to the sixteenth week the fetus might be too small to respond to an intraamniotic injection designed to bring on labor, and at this time a prostaglandin suppository might be the most desired method of pregnancy interruption. Vaginal suppositories of prostaglandin E2 melt in the vagina. The prostaglandin content is absorbed into the body, where it results in uterine cramping. Every two or four hours, as the uterus continues contracting, the suppositories are replaced. Within twelve to fourteen hours the uterus expands, the cervix opens, and the uterine product expels itself. This is a safe procedure, although a suction curettage might be used as a follow-up to remove any remaining placental parts.

Sixteen to twenty weeks: A few years ago, when a woman sought pregnancy interruption between the sixteenth and twentieth weeks of gestation, she would receive an *intraamniotic injection of saline.* The hypertonic saline would be shot into the amniotic sac, the fluid environment surrounding the fetus. As the concentrated saline penetrated the uterine cavity, it caused the uterus to expand and contract as it would during labor. After a day to a day and a half of these contractions, the fetus would abort.

The laborlike process could be speeded up, it was found, with an *intraamniotic injection of prostaglandins* instead of saline. The prostaglandins bring on immediate uterine contraction, followed by expulsion, and they decrease the possibility of infection, bleeding, and the rare ruptured uterus. For these reasons, prostaglandins have replaced saline in most institutions.

Twenty to twenty-four weeks: With prostaglandins alone, all works well before the twentieth week, but at the twentieth week the intraamniotic injection shifts to a combination of prostaglandins and urea or prostaglandins and saline, which are considered safe and fast-acting. If prostaglandins alone are injected from the twentieth week on, the aborted fetus might not die before expulsion. Urea and saline in conjunction with prostaglandins will cause a definite demise of the fetus.

The procedure that a woman undergoes often depends upon her doctor and his affiliated hospital. Institutions may pick and choose the procedures they permit. And even deadline dates for allowable abortions can vary. The twenty-fourth week of pregnancy is the cutoff point for a legal abortion, but some hospitals might set twenty weeks as their limit, while others decree a twelve-week maximum. Planned Parenthood might be able to locate a hospital or clinic that will conduct an abortion up to twenty-four weeks, but a woman should not wait to make her appointment. The institution might be booked, and the longer she remains pregnant, the more difficult she will find her abortion.

My Blood Is Rh-Negative; Does That Mean That an Abortion Will Be Dangerous?

I became pregnant with an IUD and I am going to have an abortion. I have Rh-negative blood and I've heard that this might cause a problem. Will I need a transfusion or something equally horrible?

—T.E., Dallas, Texas

About 15 percent of white women and 5 percent of black women have Rh-negative blood, which means that they don't have the Rhesus antibody, so named because it was discovered during a study on Rhesus monkeys. The term does not signify any connection between monkeys and humans, except a similarity in physiological functions.

There is usually no problem if a woman with Rh-negative blood has an abortion early in pregnancy, while her doctor can perform a menstrual extraction or miniabortion. At that point, blood antibodies have not formed in the embryo. However, if the fetus has Rh-positive blood, a pregnancy interruption after the sixth or seventh week might cause some of the positive blood from the fetus to enter the mother's bloodstream. Nature will protect the mother by causing her to develop an immune reaction against the Rh-positive blood. But then, if she conceives an Rh-positive fetus again, her own bloodstream might reject and kill the baby.

The good news is that fetal rejection can be avoided if an Rh-negative woman receives an injection of *Rhogam,* an anti-Rh-positive vaccine, within seventy-two hours of her abortion. Then, if any Rh-positive blood enters her system, the Rhogam will form antibodies and a fetus will be fine in future pregnancy.

Could My Past Abortions Have Harmed My Body? Can I Have a Healthy Child?

I'm thirty-one years old and I've had three abortions. The first one was when I was eighteen. I got pregnant because I wasn't using any form of birth control. The last two times I was in my twenties and on both occasions I was wearing a diaphragm. I don't know what went wrong. I thought I put it in correctly. Anyway, now I'm married. My husband and I have been having intercourse without contraception for two years and I'm still not pregnant. I can't believe all those times I got pregnant without trying and now I'm trying and nothing happens. Do you think all those abortions harmed my body? Will I ever get another chance to have a healthy child?

—K.M., Larchmont, New York

The fact that this woman has not become pregnant for the past two years might mean that her uterus and/or her tubes were damaged as a result of her abortions. Perhaps too much uterine tissue was scraped away during one of the procedures. If that happened, adhesions could grow on the uterine walls and prevent the development of placental tissue in which a fertilized egg might nest. If an egg cannot implant itself in a uterine lining, a pregnancy cannot develop. It is also possible that after one of her abortions an infection entered her tubes and caused scar tissue that thwarts conception.

Ms. M. needs a hysterosalpingogram, an X ray of her uterus and tubes, to see if there are adhesions in her womb or blockages in her tubes. Adhesions would require her to have a D & C. Damaged tubes can be repaired by microsurgical techniques, as described earlier in this chapter. Ms. M. might also consider in vitro fertilization (IVF), as explained in chapter 10, to help her conceive.

Repeated abortions are potentially harmful to a woman's cervix, too. The more times a doctor forcefully opens a woman's cervix to perform an abortion, the more chances she has of having her cervix torn or rendered incompetent, unable to close properly. An incompetent cervix, as explained in the miscarriage section of this chapter, cannot stand the pressure of a growing fetus. Slowly, the cervix opens and allows the pregnancy to escape prematurely. A woman miscarries.

More than one abortion is physically destructive to a woman, and unfortunately, Ms. M. might have serious reproductive difficulties. After a woman has undergone one pregnancy interruption she should be extremely protective of herself because the infertility problems and emotional suffering brought on by multiple abortions are more than any healthy woman should endure.

Is the Abortion Pill the Same As the "Morning-After" Pill?

When I was in college we all knew about taking birth control pills after sex so we wouldn't get pregnant. Now with all the publicity about an abortion pill I'm wondering: Were we giving ourselves abortions with what we called the "morning-after" pill? Are these two pills the same?

—Y.J., Columbus, Ohio

In a word, no. Emergency contraception (EC), historically known as the "morning-after" pill, has been available through the use of regular birth control pills, taken as soon as possible within seventy-two hours of unprotected intercourse. Different brands of pills work at different dose levels, so usually two or four pills are taken, and then twelve hours later are taken again. Progestin-only minipills have also been used. These cause less nausea than the combination birth control pills, but you must take about twenty pills at once for effectiveness. In 1998, the FDA approved the *Preven Emergency Contraceptive Kit,* four pills available by prescription, the first designated EC.

Unlike abortion medications, emergency contraceptives cannot be used if a woman is already pregnant. EC prevents a pregnancy by inhibiting ovulation, blocking fertilization, and/or stopping a fertilized egg from implanting itself in a woman's uterus. Gynetics Inc., the makers of Preven, state that when Preven is used according to directions, only 2 out of 100 (without contraception, 8 out of 100) women might become pregnant after a single act of intercourse.

On the other hand, the insertion of a Copper-T intrauterine device (IUD), is a 99 percent effective EC. The IUD disrupts fertilization and prevents an embryo from implanting itself in a woman's uterus, but it is painful to insert at mid-cycle and is not recommended for women who have multiple sex partners or are rape victims—situations creating a higher than average risk of contracting a sexually transmitted disease.

If a woman does not have a doctor she can turn to for EC, she can call the EC hotline, 1-888-NOT-2-LATE, or visit the web site: www.opr.princeton.edu/ec, for information and referrals to doctors who can write prescriptions for EC.

What Happens When Abortion Is Denied?

A close friend of mine became pregnant when she was eighteen. My girlfriend's boyfriend refused to marry her and for religious reasons her family prevented her from having an abortion. She became an unwed mother. After a day of labor she finally had the baby by cesarean section. She eventually got married and we became neighbors. I love my friend but the daughter she had out of wedlock is a real troublemaker and I don't want my children around her. This girl is flunking out of school and she has been picked up by the police twice. Her life seems to have been doomed from the start. Is it possible that she knew she was unwanted before she was even born? Could this girl be as bad as she is because my friend was so unhappy during her pregnancy?
                                              —G.P., (name of town withheld)

According to some studies, when a woman is forced to carry a baby she does not want, her attitude during the pregnancy might affect the child's personality. In Czechoslovakia, a long-term investigation was undertaken in the early 1960s when a study group of 220 children born to women who were twice denied abortions for the same pregnancy was matched with a control group of 220 children born to mothers who wanted to be pregnant. The children were followed until they were sixteen to eighteen years old.

Throughout the years of the study, the children from unwanted pregnancies, although they were equal in intelligence to the control group, deteriorated in school performance. The study group had more behavior problems, were less sociable and more hyperactive than the controls. They required more educational and psychological therapy than the wanted children, and a significant number of them did not continue their schooling to the secondary level.

This study definitely suggests that a pregnant woman's lack of desire for motherhood can become a significant risk factor in the future life of a child. In fact, a woman's attitude during the pregnancy might even prevent a child from having a life.

In California, 8,000 women who received the same basic health care during their pregnancies were subjects in an attitude study. It was found that the death rate for fetuses of women who resented their pregnancies was 60 per 1,000, twice as high as the death rate for fetuses of women who favored their pregnancies. The negative women also had more accidents and infections during pregnancy and their babies had one and a half times more congenital abnormalities than the newborns of happy mothers.

The California study was conducted between 1959 and 1967, before the abortion laws were revised. Today a woman has a choice. If she feels she can cope with parenthood, she should never be forced into pregnancy interruption—but she can find a safe, legal abortion in an accredited hospital if she does not want to bear a child.

Abortion and Future Childbearing

Before I slept with my boyfriend in college I was a virgin. I was very scared but he used a condom and told me everything would be all right. It wasn't. I got pregnant and had to have an abortion, which made me very unhappy. When my husband and I decided to have a child last year, I went to my doctor and told him about the abortion because I was so afraid that I wouldn't be able to become pregnant again. I thought the abortion would have screwed up my insides and I guess I was guilty about it too. The doctor was very sympathetic and told me that my pregnancy had been an accident, that it wasn't my fault. He also said that my pregnancy proved that I was fertile and that all my organs were working well. I felt much better after our conversation and I conceived about a month later. Now I have a beautiful son and I'm thrilled with my life. I wish you would tell other women that an abortion isn't the end of the world. It's sad but it's not the end.

—E.L., Los Angeles, California

I appreciate this woman's letter. She apparently found a competent, caring doctor who understood her stress. If a woman has her pregnancy interrupted under safe, sterile conditions, the abortion should not harm her body at all. Indeed, women who have never been pregnant by the time they are thirty might have difficulty conceiving for the first time at this older age.

After she has had one abortion, a woman is usually in good physical condition, but she should not endanger her health with another unwanted pregnancy. Repeated abortions wear on the reproductive organs. Later on, sterility and miscarriage might be the unfortunate outcomes. However, a woman who has experienced a safe, legal abortion should feel heartened when she wants to become pregnant. She should know that if she conceived once, she probably will conceive again. Ms. L. is right. An abortion is not the end of the world; it's a reminder that fertility exists for life to begin.

12.

What Is the Best Contraceptive?

SHE OR HE? WHO IS RESPONSIBLE
FOR BIRTH CONTROL?

Before the birth control pill brought on the sexual revolution, men seemed to be more concerned than they are today about preventing conception and they appeared to be willing to assume a great deal of the responsibility during lovemaking. The condom was ever-present for birth control, and men joked about the circular impressions that contraceptives left on their wallets. Sexually active singles were always prepared, and even most husbands were ready to share the burden of contraception. It would be nice to suppose that this was so because men really cared about women, women's bodies, and whether women wanted to become pregnant, but when the truth is revealed, the opposite seems to have been the case, namely that men wanted to be in charge of contraception for their own reasons, not because they were sensitive to women.

It used to be that if a woman got pregnant a man considered himself "stuck." Either he would be forced into a "shotgun wedding" or he would be tracked down by the woman's family and saddled with child support. There was no legal abortion, and to end a pregnancy clandestinely meant to risk a woman's life. Illegal abortions were dangerous, sometimes fatal, always criminal affairs. A man who arranged an illegal abortion for his girlfriend not only played god with her survival but became an accomplice in a crime. When a man weighed the alternatives, taking part in contraception was definitely preferable to enforced marriage or police arrest. For years, men were worried and contraception-conscious.

Then the sixties arrived. The birth control pill and improved intrauterine devices made contraception invisible and much more a woman's domain. Both married and single men grew to assume that women would "take care of it." With the threat of pregnancy basically removed, sexual freedom flowered.

Sometimes a single woman who did not want to take the pill or wear an IUD felt embarrassed by her diaphragm. Sex was supposed to be spontaneous and since she would have to interrupt the act to insert her diaphragm, she just skipped the procedure. From the sixties on, most men never asked women if they were using contraception, since the unwritten rule became: "Birth control is the woman's responsibility." If a woman did not "take care of it" and she became pregnant, as many women did, it was also her responsibility to eliminate the unwanted conception.

Better education, more understanding between women and men, and advanced contraception methods were encouraged by everyone in the health field, but in spite of the effort to help people take charge of their bodies, there are today over a million abortions a year resulting from unwanted pregnancies. If, as a caring society, we aim to make modern contraception work, to *want* the children we conceive, we are far from our goal.

If a woman and a man are partners in sex, they should be partners in contraception. Although it has been well over a decade since birth control was, more than ever before, made into a woman's task, a man must now be ready to share the job. The rise in sexually transmitted diseases needs recognition and openness that should start with good communication about contraception.

The ideal contraceptive has still not been developed, and most effective methods of birth control continue to be the ones that are designed for women. Aside from vasectomy sterilization and the time-honored condom, male contraception remains in the research

phase. Although improved contraceptive techniques for women are
being studied, for the woman of today who wants easily controllable
fertility, the pill, the intrauterine device, and the diaphragm still
remain her top three choices in order of effectiveness. The potions,
pessaries, and magical rituals that used to be thrust upon women
have been abandoned, and thank God such things as an elephant-
dung-and-honey suppository are in the past. Our current contraceptives might someday seem just as antiquated, but most women find

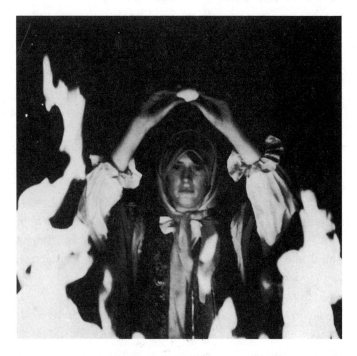

12-1 **Russian Contraceptive Ritual.** South Russian women on the Skalar Mountain range
practice a bizarre contraceptive ritual. A young girl, to avoid pregnancy, was admon-
ished to take a few drops of her menstrual blood and let it flow into a hole in the egg
from a young hen. She was then to bury the egg for nine days and nights. After this
period, she was to dig up the egg and count the number of worms inside. The number
of worms was supposed to represent the number of children she would bear if she so
desired. If she wished to have children, she was to throw the egg into the water. If not,
she hurled the egg into the fire, thus destroying her ability to bear children. *Reproduced
by permission. From the series Contraceptive Curiosities Art, Syntex Laboratories Inc., Palo
Alto, California.*

that at some time or another they must choose one from among those that exist. Ideally, a woman and a man should make the choice together, be partners in pregnancy prevention as well as in sexual intimacy.

I strongly encourage a man to accompany his wife or girlfriend when she goes to a gynecologist or a family planning clinic. In this way, a caring couple learns the basics of contraception and how to share in the decision about what contraceptive will be best suited to them. A couple who favor natural family planning or a contraceptive

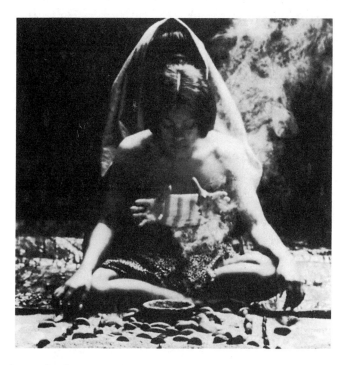

12-2 **Ancient Sterilization Ritual.** One tribe from British New Guinea believed the powers of inducing sterilization were held by women of their group. According to legend, these powers were passed from mother to daughter, from generation to generation. To induce sterility, the women of power would sit behind those desiring to be free of pregnancy and make passes over their abdomens while uttering incantations and at the same time burning roots and herbs, the smoke of which the women would inhale. *Reproduced by permission. From the series Contraceptive Curiosities Art, Syntex Laboratories Inc., Palo Alto, California.*

that is timed for effectiveness could greatly benefit from a joint consultation with the woman's doctor. I am convinced that contemporary men like to be included in this health issue.

It has been gratifying to speak to men's groups and to answer their questions about how different contraceptives might affect the women they love. Complicating relations is that the condom remains the best protection against the spread of the HIV/AIDS virus and other sexually transmitted diseases, but it is not the most effective contraceptive. A woman must be willing to educate a man with gentle affection, to teach him that he is not invading her privacy if he becomes involved in her choice of contraceptive. It is really *their* choice of contraceptive. More important than giving their bodies to each other, couples must be willing to share their hearts and minds.

THE BEST CONTRACEPTIVE IS THE ONE THAT FITS YOUR LIFESTYLE

A teenager is very different from a woman in her thirties. These two females will not regard sex in the same way, they will not be equally fertile, and they might hold divergent views about pregnancy interruption. Yet they both might want contraception.

The type of contraceptive any woman, from her teens to her early fifties, chooses should depend on her partner, her age, and her lifestyle. As a woman changes, so might her contraceptive.

Teenage Birth Control

As reported in chapter 11, one fifth of all abortions are performed on teenage girls. Researchers at Johns Hopkins University surveyed 1,200 teenagers in the 1980s and found that only 14 percent of them sought birth control information before they had intercourse for the first time. Barely twenty years later, at the end of the twentieth century, teenagers have grown more sexually enlightened. With the growth of the information age, households of working or single parents, and sex education that deals with preventing the spread of the deadly HIV/AIDS virus and other sexually transmitted diseases (STDs), today's teenagers are more sexually aware than any generation of young people before them. More than 50 percent of the females and 75 percent of the males ages fifteen to nineteen have experienced sexual intercourse. The average age for first-time sex is seventeen for girls and sixteen for boys. That said, sexually active teens are behaving more responsibly.

Declining numbers of teens are contracting STDs and becoming pregnant. The 1991 teen pregnancy high of 62.1 births per 1,000 teenage girls has dropped 12 percent to 54.7 births per 1,000. Surveys also show that about two thirds of teenagers use condoms, a jump three times higher than figures from the 1970s. Many teens are insisting on the use of condoms, the best protection against exposure to the HIV/AIDS virus during sexual intercourse, and even are abstaining until marriage. Still, a largely sexually active teenage population needs birth control more effective than, and in addition to, the condom. Since an adolescent boy is likely to have a more uncontrollable orgasm than a mature man, a condom might easily slip off his penis. I am also concerned about the girl who continues to test her fertility because she has unprotected sex once or twice and does not conceive.

Teenage girls who have regular sexual activity would be much better protected if they used the low-dose birth control pill. Recent research has indicated that currently available low-dose birth control pills do not cause cancer or any other harmful side effects because they contain less than 50 micrograms of estrogen.

A low-dose pill will provide a young woman with almost 100 percent protection against pregnancy—and peace of mind. A teenage girl who is involved in unprotected sexual intercourse should be nervous. The pill can alleviate her anxiety without causing negative repercussions within her body. Quite the contrary, the pill is often positive. It can decrease cramps, regulate her menstrual cycle, and make her breasts less cystic. (In some studies, smoking has been found to worsen the cardiovascular side effects of the pill, but no physical differences have been discovered among teenage smokers who take the pill. Still, smoking is terrible at any age and should be stopped.) When she becomes sexually active and starts taking the pill, a teenager must see her gynecologist twice a year for a complete physical examination, blood pressure check, and guidance.

I would not recommend an IUD for a teenager, especially for a girl who has more than one boyfriend, because she has greater occasion to pick up an STD, which, when an IUD is present, spreads more rapidly. Also, an IUD increases the chance of contracting pelvic inflammatory diseases that carry potential sterility, a traumatic condition for a woman who has never borne children.

A diaphragm is only recommended for a young woman who is extremely familiar with her body and is unafraid to explore herself internally. Most teenagers do not know their bodies well, nor are they usually disciplined enough to insert a diaphragm when passion is driving them to action. Thus, the low-dose birth control pill is probably the best contraceptive advice for a young couple. Norplant (six silicone rods, each about the size of a matchstick, implanted in the upper arm) releases synthetic progesterone and offers birth control for five years. (Depo-Provera injected every three months is also recommended for long-term contraception; see pages 419 to 420.) Norplant might cause progesterone overload for young teens, so I do not consider it until a girl reaches eighteen, when her periods are more regular.

The way to curb the continuing presence of teenage pregnancy is to teach young women and men how to care and share. A couple who want to experience sexual intimacy should make an appointment with a doctor or a clinic for contraception. A young woman who decides to become sexually involved must consider herself an adult with an adult responsibility to take care of her health. She should visit a doctor or a family planning clinic every six months for contraception consultation, and STD and cancer checks.

Women in Their Twenties

During her twenties a woman is still very fertile, but she might no longer like the pill as a continuing form of contraception. If she needs only occasional protection, she might want to use a diaphragm or a cervical cap, or she might rely on the effectiveness of an STD-protecting condom. However, if a woman must not become pregnant, the pill will offer her almost 100 percent effectiveness. In fact, there is no reason why she could not stay on the pill as long as she continues to have biannual medical checkups and remains healthy.

The switch from the pill to a barrier method works best when a woman is self-confident. A man interrupts sex to put on a condom, so a woman should not be shy about taking a minute to insert a diaphragm. If she chooses barrier contraception, a woman might involve her partner in her birth control process, whether or not he is her steady mate.

An IUD is usually not recommended for a young woman who has never borne a child, particularly if she has a very active sex life. The device is linked with infections, most especially among women who are exposed to many lovers. If a woman has only one sex partner or is married, the chance of infection is reduced and she might well be a candidate for an IUD. However, if she uses one she might listen to her body and not dismiss any abnormal pain or bleeding. These could be signs of an infection taking hold. She must immediately consult her doctor for an examination, diagnosis, and treatment.

If a woman who is wearing an IUD develops an infection, the contraceptive must be removed and she should be treated with antibiotics. Her reproductive system will then probably not be harmed on a long-term basis.

A woman who has given birth generally tolerates an IUD better than a woman who has not. An IUD is a recommended method of contraception for a woman who wants to space her childbearing.

Women in Their Thirties

Once a woman who smokes reaches thirty-five, she must give up either smoking or the pill, because if she does not her chances of having cardiovascular disease skyrocket. A healthy nonsmoker, however, could conceivably stay on the low-dose pill well into her forties. Low-dose pills, typically containing less than 35 (some as low as 20) micrograms of estrogen and 1 milligram of progestin, are now being used to help women through *perimenopause*, the years approaching menopause, when hormones are erratic. These pills also help women retain bone mass at a crucial time.

A woman in her thirties who has not had children might still be able to use an IUD if she is in tune with her body and alert to signs of infection. However, at this time of her life, a woman usually has a more defined sense of herself than she did in her twenties and she is less reticent about using more obvious forms of contraception. The diaphragm, cervical cap, or natural family planning, if her menstrual cycle is regular, might perfectly suit a woman in her thirties.

As she nears her forties, a married woman who has completed her family might find that her husband wants to have a vasectomy to lift their contraceptive worries. Male initiative in the area of contraception is growing. A woman might not want her husband to have a vasectomy, though. She might prefer to be sterilized herself. However, tubal ligation is not without side effects, and a woman should not elect this form of birth control until she knows all the pros and cons and is absolutely sure that she would never be interested in further childbearing.

Women Over Forty

A woman over forty is less fertile than she used to be, but she still needs contraception. If she is a healthy nonsmoker without diabetes, high blood pressure, or certain rare types of heart disease, she may take a very low dose type of pill or use an IUD or a diaphragm. Tubal sterilization might be suggested at this time, but a woman should know that this procedure changes the blood supply to her ovaries, which might throw off her hormonal balance. The surgery has also been known to increase the incidence of fibrocystic breast disease and premenstrual syndrome.

At this age a woman should be familiar with monitoring her body. Since her fertility is diminished, the rhythm method might be a form of contraception to be considered. If she chooses to use an IUD, any problem related to the device should be easy to recognize. The diaphragm, which allows her to control her contraception at will, might be even more preferable to the ever-present IUD.

The relationship a woman has with her partner is a big factor in her choice of contraceptive. A woman should tailor her birth control method to her living situation and her needs. She should use the form of contraception that gives secure protection when she's young and extremely fertile and vary her birth control as her age and lifestyle change. The diaphragm might be the best bet for the single, widowed, or divorced woman in her forties who has intermittent sexual contact. She should be prepared for contraception, but she does not need around-the-clock protection. A woman's personal intimacies, however, are her own to share with her partner and to regulate as they see fit.

All forms of birth control have pros and cons that are discussed in the following sections. A woman and a man should carefully analyze the available methods and, together, reach a decision about contraception. Loving and caring can greatly help to enhance an understanding of the contraceptives we have to live with until newer types are developed.

THE BIRTH CONTROL PILL

The idea behind the creation of the first birth control pill was that when a woman was pregnant she could not be impregnated again. The hormones estrogen and progesterone both increased during pregnancy, and researchers discovered a chain reaction. The high levels of estrogen and progesterone blocked the release of the brain hormones LH and FSH, and without these hormones an ovary was not stimulated to release a monthly egg. Without ovulation, there could be no pregnancy.

The original birth control pills were manufactured with the same amounts of estrogen and progesterone that were found in women during their pregnancies. These high amounts caused unhealthy side effects, among them high blood pressure, blood clots, and cancer, which resulted in death in some cases, and many women threw out their pills and looked for other kinds of contraception.

By the time the pill's drawbacks became apparent, women had begun to change their roles in society. This convenient form of contraception had liberated them. It is my belief that the original birth control pill was a great sociological asset even though it was not a medical success. Quite understandably, women felt betrayed by their doctors and all men involved in contraceptive studies.

The IUD seemed the logical alternative to the pill. Eventually, however, the scare stories of infections and infertility that came from IUD use lessened the popularity of the device and led to more studies on how to improve the birth control pill. The estrogen-free mini-pill was devised, but it had a pregnancy rate of 3 to 5 percent and frequently caused irregular spotting or steady bleeding, which is why its use continues to be limited. Many women did not like the mini-pill, and they welcomed the improved pill, which combines estrogen and progesterone in low doses.

The combined low-dose birth control pill inhibits pregnancy in two ways, first by preventing ovulation, and second by thickening cervical mucus so that it acts like a diaphragm. A woman who is a candidate for the birth control pill should be started on the kind with the lowest hormonal content. Generally speaking, no woman should be on a birth control pill that contains more than 50 micrograms of estrogen, and she should know that there are many different kinds of pills that do not all act identically. My previous book, *It's Your Body: A Woman's Guide to Gynecology*, contains a comprehensive breakdown of brand-name birth control pills and their hormonal ingredients. If a woman experiences adverse effects on one pill, she might switch to another. However, if a woman develops high blood pressure, diabetes, fibroid tumors, or other serious medical problems, she should be taken off the pill immediately. Furthermore, if a woman is a heavy smoker she should stop the pill when she is thirty, and definitely not be given a prescription for any type of birth control pill after she is thirty-five.

Should a Woman Still Be Afraid to Take the Pill?

Many women were justifiably frightened during the early seventies when the news broke about all the cardiovascular damage the pill might do to their bodies. For a while, it seemed that every day someone was discovering something scary about the pill. The stories of how the pill can afflict a woman have lingered from the past even though the pill itself has changed. Studies indicate that the modern, low-estrogen-containing pill is much safer than the old high-estrogen-containing pill. Still, every woman taking the pill should know its positive and negative effects:

Cancer and the Pill. The birth control pill does not cause cancer. Thousands of reports analyzing a possible link between the pill and ovarian, endometrial (uterine), and breast cancers show that today's low-dose pills are not the risky pills of yesterday. Some reports linked the original high-dose pills to cancer, but considering the millions of women who took these contraceptives, it's amazing how few people actually developed problems.

There were reports that the sequential birth control pill, which is now off the market, contributed to some cases of endometrial cancer. Women who were on the sequential pill took estrogen during the beginning of their cycles and/or progestin at the end. In a 1976 report, there were twenty-one cases of endometrial cancer found among all women in the United States under age forty who were taking oral contraceptives, and thirteen of these women were using the sequential pill. The other women were on pills with high estrogen contents that overstimulated their uterine linings. This was thus a very low incidence since at least 20 million women took the pill yearly. With the current low-dose birth control pill, the uterine lining has only a minimal buildup each month, so women have less menstrual bleeding and reduced risk of endometrial cancer. We now know that taking the pill at some point during the childbearing years can cut the risk of endometrial and ovarian cancers by almost half. For deadly ovarian cancer, that protection increases the longer a woman stays on the pill. Ten or more years might cut her risk by almost 80 percent.

As for a connection between the pill and breast cancer, the news is better than it used to be. After decades of investigations looking into whether the amount of estrogen in a birth control pill can stimulate breast cancer, the end result, basically, is that the pill does not raise the risk of breast cancer for older women; in fact, some researchers have found that the pill slightly decreases the risk after age 50, but there is some question about a link for younger women.

A 1995 study conducted by the National Cancer Institute (NCI) found that women under thirty-five had almost twice the breast cancer risk of women who had used the pill for less than six months or not at all, and women who started taking birth control pills before age eighteen, and used them for more than ten years, had three times the risk. In 1996, a study of 50,000 women found breast cancer diagnosed slightly more often in women who start on the pill as teenagers or in their early twenties. Experts say that the increase in breast cancer might be due to better screening, or the pill might have caused a breast cancer that might have appeared later in life to appear earlier, and since early-onset breast cancer is rare, the increased risk might mean only one more case per 100,000 women. On the "up" side, it is clear that the pill decreases the incidence of benign fibrocystic breast tumors, but the unclear "down" side is whether it increases your breast cancer risk if you start young and continue for more than ten years.

High Blood Pressure and the Pill. Women who have high blood pressure should never be on birth control pills, and women who take the pill should have their blood pressure checked by their doctors every six months. It has been found that sometimes women on the pill get high blood pressure. A large, respected study reports "reversible increased risk" of hypertensive disease among pill users, which means that if a woman's blood pressure increases when she is on the birth control pill her pressure will return to normal when she goes off the pill. She will be in perfect health once again. If a woman stays on the pill after she has been told that her blood pressure has risen, she is also risking kidney damage. Women who had high blood pressure while on the pill have often developed toxemia during subsequent pregnancies, which might indicate that these women have abnormal reactions to hormones in general.

Due to the risk of pill-induced hypertension, every woman on the pill should remind her doctor to check her blood pressure during each six-month visit. Sometimes a physician is so rushed, he forgets. Remember, persistent high blood pressure could lead to stroke.

Cysts, Fibroids, and the Pill. The incidence of benign growths in a woman's reproductive system is generally lower with the pill. While helping to prevent ovarian cancer, the pill also lowers the risk of developing benign ovarian cysts. Benign breast tumors and breast cysts are seen much less in pill takers, and fibroids, benign uterine growths, are less common.

Blood Clotting, Heart Attack, and the Pill. Blood clots remain an area of concern. Women on the pill have, on average, double the risk of developing deep-vein blood clots in their legs than women not on the pill. Those at greatest risk are pill takers who have predisposing conditions such as varicose veins, obesity, and a family history of blood clots. Still, relatively speaking, the risk is considered low. As one expert pointed out, the highest risks detected are only half of the thromboembolism (blood clot) risk that a pregnant woman faces. If a woman feels a leg pain or any strange sensation that could indicate a blood clot, she should stop the pill, take an aspirin to thin her blood, drink extra fluid, and visit her doctor immediately.

Heart attacks and strokes are not common among young and middle-aged women. The greatest risk of heart attack or stroke is among women already at risk, those who smoke or have high blood pressure. The pill appears safe for healthy women who are not in high-risk categories.

Part of choosing a contraceptive is learning the pros and cons of the method. A woman who is in good health and is screened by her doctor twice a year should remain fit on the pill. A woman must be aware, however, that along with the good feeling and effective pregnancy protection she receives from the pill, she might be one of the rare women who experience cardiovascular side effects. If a woman notices anything irregular in her circulation, even though she is enjoying the safety of the pill, she must still listen to her body and report any changes to her doctor.

Bladder Infection and the Pill. Generally, the pill does not cause bladder infections, but a woman who takes birth control pills might get yeast infections because the pill can give her a somewhat higher blood sugar level and can also alter her vaginal environment. During intercourse, it is possible for the yeast to be pushed into the bladder, where it might cause irritation. Some women on the pill complain about bladder pain, but when a culture is taken, there usually is no infection.

A bladder infection is more likely to occur when a woman is using a diaphragm. However, no matter what kind of contraception she chooses, a woman should urinate before and after intercourse to prevent any urinary problems.

Gallbladder Disease and the Pill. Studies have indicated that the birth control pill does have some effect on the gallbladder and the kidneys, particularly on the gallbladder. There has been some suggestion that the hormones in the pill might increase a woman's cholesterol level and lead to more gallstones. Women who are taking oral contraceptives also appear to run a higher-than-average risk of needing cholecystectomy—surgical removal of the gallbladder.

Benign Liver Tumors and the Pill. There have been reports that benign liver tumors have been noticed in women on the pill, but these findings, which were rare, were associated with pills containing high amounts of estrogen.

Amenorrhea and the Pill. Sometimes a woman develops amenorrhea, no menstrual period, when she takes the pill because the amount of progesterone in the pill she is using, in relation to the estrogen content, is too potent for her system. Her uterine lining is not thick and rich enough to create a menstrual flow because the progesterone has inhibited the buildup of her endometrium. She should stop the pill until her menstrual cycle returns. Then, if she wants to resume the pill, she should use another type.

Many studies have shown that the woman who misses her period while she is on the pill will regain her fertility when she goes off the pill. Sometimes a woman must be given either progesterone alone or a combination of estrogen and progesterone to stimulate her period again, but even if she must take supplementary hormones, amenorrhea is not a serious problem.

Many of the available low-estrogen-containing birth control pills can cause cessation of menstruation. If this happens, as already mentioned, a woman must stop the pill immediately. However, if she experiences even a minimal amount of spotting or bleeding every month, a woman can safely remain on the pill.

Acne and the Pill. If a woman has acne and she takes a birth control pill with a potent progesterone, she is likely to get a worse case of acne. A woman who has complexion problems might improve her skin if she takes a pill with a high estrogen/low progesterone combination. Estrogen has the power to clear up blemishes and make a woman's skin smooth. A pill with 50 micrograms of estrogen might regulate a woman's hormonal balance while it removes her acne.

QUESTIONS ABOUT THE PILL

I Don't Want to Go off the Pill

A year ago, when I was thirty-three, I had surgery for an ectopic pregnancy and my left tube was removed. I could have died because the pregnancy ruptured and I was bleeding internally. After the surgery, my doctor gave me birth control pills and I've never felt so wonderful. Even the people I work with say that I've changed, that I'm in a much better mood lately. My husband and I used to be afraid to make love because we were scared that I would become pregnant again. The pill has freed me. We have no more worries. I have read that when a woman reaches thirty-five she should stop taking oral contraceptives, but I don't want to go off the pill. Do I really have to stop?

—T.H., Oxford, North Carolina

This woman feels better on the pill because it eliminates all the fears she has about contraceptives failing. If she is in good physical health and does not smoke, according to studies, there is no reason why she cannot stay on the pill well into her forties. However, she might need a switch to a very low dose pill as her hormones change. She also needs a blood pressure check twice a year, because the chance of developing a cardiovascular abnormality, such as thrombophlebitis, increases somewhat after thirty-five.

If Ms. H. notices anything abnormal—if she skips periods or has a pain in her leg, arm, or any other place that should not be hurting—she must immediately stop the pill, take an aspirin to thin her blood, drink extra fluid, and visit her doctor. If she smokes, on her thirty-fifth birthday Ms. H. will have to give up either cigarettes or the pill, because a combination of the two could cause serious cardiovascular problems.

I'm Getting Married; Should I Go on the Pill?

I'm a thirty-two-year-old woman who is engaged to be married this year. I've used the diaphragm for four years, but I've never lived with a man before. I know my sex life will be more regular after I'm married and I'm wondering if I should go on the pill. Do you think it's a good idea for me to switch contraceptives?
—W.S., St. Paul, Minnesota

If this woman is healthy, there is certainly no reason why she should not go on the pill, at least at the start of her marriage. The pill will regulate her periods and free her from any pregnancy worries until she and her husband have established their new life together. After the wedding, she probably will have sexual intercourse more regularly than she used to during her single days, so for those first few years of marriage, the birth control pill would be perfect.

If Ms. S. decides she wants to become pregnant, she should stop the pill about three months before she tries to conceive, to clean out her system. Studies have shown that the pill has a positive effect on a woman's fertility, and after her three-month cleansing, Ms. S. might not have to wait long at all to bear a child.

I Got Pregnant on the Pill

I took a pill for a few months and then I got pregnant and had an abortion. I'm nineteen years old and I have a steady boyfriend. My doctor wants to put me back on the pill, but I'm worried that I might get pregnant again. What should I do?
—L.U., Newport, Rhode Island

It is not clear whether this young woman was taking the pill properly when she became pregnant. Generally, a woman should try to take a pill at about the same time every day in order to maintain a steady concentration of hormones in her bloodstream. If she misses the pill one day, she must immediately double up on the following day. If she forgets the pill for two days, she should take two more pills on the next day. If a woman overlooks more than three pills, she should stop, wait until her period arrives, and start a new pack of pills on the fifth day of her period.

The birth control pill is considered 99 percent effective, so pregnancy can in rare instances occur, but usually only when the pill has not been properly taken. If a woman becomes pregnant when she is on the pill, pregnancy interruption should be encouraged since medical experts do not know what effect the extra estrogen and progesterone will have on the conceptus.

This woman followed the advisable course of action by having her pregnancy interrupted. If she returns to the pill and takes it according to her doctor's instructions, it is highly unlikely that she will become pregnant again.

I Developed Breakthrough Bleeding on the Pill; What Should I Do?

I started taking the pill four months ago and now, for the second month in a row, I've had spotting before my period is due. Could this be a sign of cancer? Could the pill be giving me cancer? What should I do?

—P.D., Centereach, New York

Breakthrough bleeding while on the birth control pill can always happen, and is most commonly seen when a woman first begins to take oral contraceptives. *She does not have cancer.* An irritation in her vagina or cervix, or breakthrough bleeding from the uterus, might be the cause, and she should visit her doctor for an examination.

Often the low-dose pills used today are not strong enough to prevent breakthrough bleeding, which might occur any time during the cycle while a woman is on the pill. If a woman begins to stain, she should open another pack of pills and take two pills a day until the bleeding stops. Sometimes two pills are ineffective and three pills are needed. Two or three days later, if the bleeding stops, a woman may return to one pill a day. If spotting occurs during her next cycle, she should double up on the pills again. A woman's body should get used to the pills she is taking. If breakthrough bleeding continues to occur, her body is not adapting to her birth control and she might be wise to ask her doctor to prescribe a different pill for her.

Should I Take Vitamins with the Birth Control Pill?

I'm a very athletic twenty-five-year-old woman who has been on the pill for a few years. I'm wondering if my system needs extra vitamins since the pill, I know, changes my body. I've been running in races and training every day and I want to be in absolutely perfect physical condition. What vitamins would be good for me?
—K.H., Cambridge, Massachusetts

Some studies indicated that woman on birth control pills might benefit from extra vitamin B_6, which has usually been removed from refined foods. During pregnancy and while taking oral contraceptives, which create a pseudopregnant state, a woman might take 50 to 100 mg of vitamin B_6 daily.

To feel really good, in addition to taking B_6, Ms. H. might cut down on her salt intake, since the estrogen contained in the pill binds salt, which in turn binds water and causes swelling and edema. Ms. H. might also include zinc, which helps to strengthen the body and prevent infection, in her daily vitamin plan. A proper diet, vitamin B_6 and zinc supplements, and low sodium intake should keep Ms. H. in prime condition.

How Long Can a Woman Stay on the Pill?

My seventeen-year-old daughter is going steady with a boy in her class and, with my approval, she was placed on the pill. Lately I'm not sure this was a good idea. She's so young. If she starts the pill now, how long is it safe for her to stay on it? Will she really be all right if she takes the pill for years?
—K.B., Tucson, Arizona

As already mentioned, today's low-dose pill is considered one of the safest, most reliable methods of contraception for healthy teenagers. I am pleased that your daughter realizes that she needs protection now that she is going steady.

A young woman might begin her contraception with the pill, but as mentioned on pages 369 to 370, if she becomes a pill taker in her teens and continues for more than ten years, she might slightly increase her risk of developing breast cancer. Even before this finding was known, I was advising a break from the pill after about five years' use. Ms. B.'s daughter might also discover as she matures into her twenties that a different method of contraception is more appropriate. It is believed that a woman might stay on the pill during her twenties and thirties without difficulty, but if any abnormalities are found during a biannual checkup, her doctor might suggest a break from the pill.

THE INTRAUTERINE DEVICE

The intrauterine device (IUD) has between 97 and 99 percent effectiveness if it is fitted properly. However, less than 2 percent of the women in the United States use an IUD because they fear pelvic inflammatory disease (PID), which can infect their uterus and Fallopian tubes and result in infertility. Over 10,000 lawsuits faced the makers of the Dalkon Shield, which was taken off the market in the seventies due to its high risk of PID. Today two IUDs are available in the United States: the Copper Y-380A, which lasts for ten years; and the Progesterone-T, a progesterone-releasing IUD that must be replaced every year. These newer, safer, T-shaped IUDs are recommended for women who have given birth and are married or in a steady relationship with one partner.

A woman should visit a competent physician who probes her uterus and measures its depth before he fits her with an IUD. A device that is too big for a uterus might cause cramping, bleeding, expulsion, and other difficulties. An IUD that is too small or is wrongly placed within a woman will not be an effective contraceptive, and it might also cause pain and bleeding, and possibly be expelled.

An IUD should always be inserted during a woman's menstrual period, when her uterus is open. Usually on the second or third day, when a woman's flow begins to slow down and her cervix is still open, a skilled physician can most easily place the device in the right spot, which is as high as possible inside the uterine cavity. Remember, the fertilized egg travels down the Fallopian tube to the womb, entering the womb at the top, so if an IUD is placed too low, if it is too small, or if it has slipped, the conceptus might have room to implant itself at the top of the uterus.

It is theorized that the intrauterine device prevents pregnancy by separating the inner walls of a woman's uterus and making it impossible for a fertilized egg to implant itself in the uterine lining. The egg disintegrates instead. The presence of copper from the copper-type IUDs and progesterone from the Progesterone-T will change the uterine environment and make implantation more difficult. Another theory is that the IUD causes a woman's body to produce more prostaglandins. When prostaglandins increase, there is cramping in the tube and ovary, and an egg is squeezed out of the tube without ever having had a chance to be fertilized.

Studies have shown that pregnancies can sometimes occur when women are wearing IUDs. (See chapter 11, pages 318 to 320, for information about the possibility of miscarriage with an IUD and the question of abortion after a woman who is using an IUD becomes pregnant.) To gain the best birth control from an IUD, a woman must start by choosing a doctor who is experienced in inserting them.

Never permit a physician to insert an intrauterine device in the middle of your cycle unless your cervix has been primed with prostaglandin suppositories, as described below. Women have reported that they have been ill and vomiting for days after they had their IUDs inserted at times other than during menstruation. Any woman who goes through such an ordeal after an IUD insertion should have the device removed and replaced during her period. About half an hour before her visit to the doctor, she might take two aspirins or two Midol tablets to lower her prostaglandin level and to reduce cramping.

There are several studies aimed at finding easier ways of inserting IUDs on days when a woman does not have her period. Prostaglandin suppositories that soften and dilate the cervix can be inserted into a woman's vagina an hour or two before IUD placement. As the cervical area relaxes, positioning of the IUD becomes less painful. Unless a doctor uses prostaglandin suppositories or a similar technique to prime a woman's cervix, a woman should not permit him to place an IUD in her body when she is not menstruating.

Inserted at the right time by a knowledgeable physician, an IUD can be extremely effective in preventing pregnancy.

How Safe Is an IUD?

Even if an IUD is properly inserted, there might be potential problems. A woman must be sensitive to any signs of infection or abnormality in her abdomen, and as soon as she has the slightest inkling that something might be wrong she should visit her doctor. As long as she pays immediate attention to her symptoms, she can avert all crises and feel safe with her IUD. She should be on the lookout for:

Pelvic Inflammatory Disease (PID). At least since 1974, it has been recognized that an infection in a woman who uses an IUD can be very damaging. During that year it was reported that a number of women who were wearing Dalkon Shield IUDs—which were subsequently removed from the market—suffered severe infections and septic abortions. The connection between pelvic inflammatory disease (PID) and the intrauterine device was made.

Today, studies have indicated that the chance of an IUD user's developing PID—an infection in the uterus, Fallopian tubes, or ovaries—is not greater than in women using other forms of contraception. Researchers linked the PID complication to the tail of an IUD, which acted like a wick and provided a way for bacteria to enter a woman's body. (Most harm was found with PID-causing chlamydia bacteria in the uterus. Women who have pain with an IUD should be checked for chlamydia.) The tail of the Dalkon Shield was a braided string made up of multiple filaments that probably enhanced bacterial migration. The tail of today's IUDs is a single monofilament that won't absorb bodily fluid. However, the presence of bacteria is still a problem, and a woman who has an active sex life with different partners risks more exposure to bacteria than a woman who has only one partner.

Once germs are introduced into the womb, a woman must be alert. She must be treated with antibiotics at the earliest sign of trouble, because a pelvic infection can be insidious. An infection might come and go, and seemingly leave no ill effects, but then, when a woman tries to conceive, she cannot. Her infertility might result from the fact that her body, when it effectively fought off the infection, produced scar tissue in her tubes or on other sites of the disease.

Scar tissue in the Fallopian tube can prevent an ovulated egg from entering the tubal passage. Scar tissue can also prevent an egg that is in the tube and has been fertilized from completing its journey to the womb. When blocked, a fertilized egg might implant itself right where it is, and a tubal pregnancy will occur. If a fertilized egg successfully travels through a tube but then encounters scar tissue in the uterus, it might be unable to implant itself in the womb and a woman might miscarry.

A woman who is wearing an IUD must be particularly sensitive to any changes in her body. An infection might start slowly and be symptomless and silent like chlamydia, or show only a few signs. Abnormal bleeding or low-grade pain should send a woman to her doctor immediately. A woman who does not investigate her pain permits a pelvic infection to spread to the point where she might need hospital care. Some women wearing Dalkon Shields ended up with hysterectomies after their infections had overtaken their organs.

When a woman reports her bleeding and pain right away, her infection can be stamped out quickly with potent antibiotics, possibly penicillin in association with, for example, Cleocin, a medication that kills most of the dangerous bacteria that are impervious to penicillin. A mild, properly treated, quickly cured infection might not require the IUD to be taken out. A lingering inflammation tells a doctor that IUD removal is a must. A woman with a prolonged pelvic problem might need a hospital stay to receive sufficient intravenous antibiotic treatment. Sometimes triple therapy—a combination of three antibiotics—is the best way to conquer the disease. Women who have been treated with only one antibiotic have often remained infected until hysterectomies were needed to save their lives.

When the advice a doctor gives is hysterectomy after antibiotic treatment, a woman should still seek a second opinion. Whenever a hysterectomy becomes a possibility in a woman's life, she should talk to more than one physician. I can remember one woman who had a bad infection and received triple therapy, but in spite of it all her doctor said, "I want to do a hysterectomy." Against her doctor's advice, she signed herself out of the hospital and went for a second opinion that same day. The second doctor did not concur with the first. A year later I saw her holding an infant, her son. "If I had agreed to the hysterectomy the doctor urged me to have, I would never be looking at my little boy," she said. I watched her smile and I could not stop staring at her as she walked away with her baby. I was smiling too. She had listened to her body.

Ectopic Pregnancy. In the past, women using IUDs have faced a higher-than-average likelihood of conceiving ectopically. Actually, it was the high risk of infection with an IUD that caused the greater chance of ectopic pregnancy. With current IUDs, a woman's risk of infection is lower, and primarily linked to her exposure to sexually transmitted diseases (STDs). The rate of ectopic pregnancy, particularly for women using the Copper T-380A, is lower than the rate for women using no contraception.

If there is a sign of infection, before scar tissue forms, a doctor might diminish the possibility of ectopic pregnancy. As a partner in her own health care, a woman must move fast whenever she notices symptoms. Abdominal pain or vaginal bleeding might be portents of a pelvic infection or an ectopic pregnancy. An immediate visit to a doctor is in order.

A woman who has recovered from PID should have a hysterosalpingogram, an X ray of her uterus, to make sure that her tubes are open and healthy, in good shape to function for her future childbearing.

Uterine Perforation. In a case of uterine perforation, an IUD travels through the wall of a woman's womb, but considering that T-shaped IUDs of today do not have sharp edges, this should not be a major concern. Usually, when perforations have occurred, they have happened when IUDs were being inserted. Rarely has an already inserted IUD moved through the wall of a uterus without provocation.

If a skilled physician inserts an IUD during a woman's menstrual period, or after he has primed her cervix with prostaglandin suppositories, the chance of uterine perforation is practically nil. A doctor who is going to give a new mother an IUD should wait a few months after her childbirth before he inserts the device. This delay allows the uterus to heal. As the muscular wall of the womb strengthens, the chance of perforation diminishes.

If a woman or her doctor suspects that an IUD has perforated her uterus, the woman should be X-rayed. On X ray, if an IUD appears outside the uterus, abdominal surgery—a laparoscopy or a laparotomy—should be performed to remove the displaced IUD before intestinal harm occurs.

Bleeding and Cramping. Since an IUD is a foreign body that a uterus, by nature, will try to expel, menstrual bleeding and cramping often increase when women use IUDs. As long as infection can be ruled out as the cause of excessive bleeding and cramping, women can now be successfully treated with prostaglandin-blocking drugs such as Motrin and Anaprox. One to two tablets of prescription Motrin or Anaprox taken four times daily as soon as bleeding begins and throughout the menstrual flow should considerably reduce bleeding and cramping. The fact that antiprostaglandin medication affects IUD-instigated bleeding and cramping is terrific. A woman who is concerned about heavy bleeding and severe cramping might ask her doctor to prescribe either Motrin or Anaprox to relieve her condition.

QUESTIONS ABOUT IUDS

Should I Use an IUD or the Pill After the Birth of My Child?

I'm twenty-three years old and just gave birth to my first child, a daughter, three weeks ago. I had a natural delivery with no problems. I never used contraceptives because my husband and I wanted a family right away. Now I'm wondering what would be best for me. Should I use an IUD or the birth control pill?
—E.J., Ville Platte, Louisiana

Ms. J. might easily space her childbearing with an IUD. An IUD is best tolerated by women who have had children because their uteri seem to accept the device better after pregnancy.

I suggest that, first, Ms. J. give her womb a chance to return to its normal size and strength. She should wait a few months after her delivery and use foam or condoms during the interim. After Ms. J.'s uterus heals and her period resumes, she might have an IUD inserted on the second or third day of her menstrual flow. If she is breast-feeding and not menstruating, she is still a good candidate for an IUD because the chance of pregnancy during breast-feeding, although slim, does exist.

If a physician fits the device carefully, Ms. J. should have very little problem with an IUD, although she might have heavier periods.

If she does, as mentioned before, she should see her doctor immediately. The possibility of pelvic infection should occur to every woman who has pain while wearing an IUD.

My choice for Ms. J. is an IUD, but if she does not like this form of contraception, or if her monthly flow is extremely heavy, then, providing she is in good health, there is no reason why she cannot take the pill.

An IUD, My Last Resort

I was on the pill for six years, from when I was eighteen to twenty-four years old. My doctor thought it would be a good idea for me to give my body a "rest," so I went on contraceptive foam for a few months before I resumed the pill. I never got my period when I went back to the pill because I was pregnant with my first daughter. After I finished breast-feeding, I started the same pills I was taking before I got pregnant but eight months later, I was pregnant again. This time I had an abortion because my husband and I could not support another child either emotionally or financially. I tried a diaphragm but I spent more time picking it up off the bathroom floor than getting it inside me. My doctor put me on new birth control pills. He was trying to find the pill with the right strength for me when I became pregnant with my second daughter. My baby is now four months old. I've had an IUD for two months and I've been spotting at different times and sometimes bleeding quite heavily. Is this normal? Am I going to be able to use an IUD? This is my last resort. I don't want to have my tubes tied because I'd like a son someday, but I can't risk any more birth control methods that don't work.

—L.C., Charleston, South Carolina

This woman certainly has had her share of difficulties with contraception, but I believe that since she has given birth to two children an IUD should be able to work for her. For the first couple of months with an IUD, it is often normal for a woman to notice some spotting. Initially, a uterus will try to expel the contraceptive, and a woman might see staining and feel cramping. If a doctor has inserted an IUD during a woman's period, she should have fewer bleeding problems.

After a few months, a uterus usually adjusts to the presence of an IUD and intermittent bleeding and cramping stop. If Ms. C. finds that her bleeding problems intensify after a few months, or if she feels any pain or notices any discharge, she should report her symptoms to her doctor. If there are signs of infection, she needs immediate treatment; however, if she has been fitted with the proper size IUD and she has no sign of infection or abnormality, the doctor might elect to observe her for another cycle. If the mid-cycle bleeding recurs the following month, the doctor should try to curb the bleeding with progesterone tablets, such as Provera. She might take one 10-mg tablet twice a day for five to ten days.

I Bleed Very Heavily with an IUD; What Should I Do?

I've had an IUD for about four years. It has always increased my periods, but lately I seem to bleed heavier and heavier each month. Should I stop the IUD and use something else? What should I do?

—M.H., Higganum, Connecticut

Women who use intrauterine devices always have heavier periods than women who choose other forms of contraception. The IUD is a foreign body that the uterus will attempt to expel through contractions. The uterine contractions will create heavier periods.

Also, an IUD increases the secretions of prostaglandins, the hormonelike substances that bring on more cramping and bleeding. New studies have indicated that IUD users who take prostaglandin-blocking drugs such as Motrin or Anaprox will lessen their bleeding. A doctor who does not prescribe antiprostaglandins for a woman who is bleeding heavily is perhaps unaware of the benefits that these medications offer. A woman might suggest that the doctor prescribe one of these drugs for her. One or two 400-mg Motrin tablets taken four times a day for the duration of her bleeding should reduce her flow significantly. She might also benefit from vitamins C and K.

A woman who flows for more than five days might benefit from a progesterone medication like Provera, 10 mg twice a day for five to seven days starting on the fifth day of her period.

Ms. H. should be able to slow down her bleeding and feel better with her IUD when prostaglandin-blocking drugs, possibly in combination with progesterone, are used. If this regimen does not curb her heavy bleeding, the IUD should be removed.

I've Had an IUD for Nine Years; Is That Safe?

I had an IUD inserted after the birth of my second child and I've been wearing it for nine years. I've had no problems, but I wonder if it's healthy to have a foreign object inside me for so long. I don't want to do anything that is unsafe.
—F.B., New Hope, Pennsylvania

Because Ms. B. has had two children, her uterus has easily accommodated an IUD. If a woman has no difficulty with an IUD, if she watches for any signs of infection such as bleeding and pain, there is no reason why she cannot continue using this form of contraceptive. A woman who uses an IUD without problems can use it until menopause. Plastic devices that do not contain copper or progesterone need not be changed if they create no problems.

As mentioned before, a woman's uterus seems to adapt more readily to an IUD after pregnancy, and Ms. B., a mother of two, has—like many other women—demonstrated that an IUD can be used continuously for many years without harm. I do not foresee any IUD problems in her future; however, I recommend a yearly medical checkup with a Pap smear.

THE BARRIER METHODS OF CONTRACEPTION

Barrier methods of contraception block sperm that are trying to get into a woman's uterus and tubes. The diaphragm, the cervical cap, the sponge, and the condom set up actual physical blockades, while spermicides—contraceptive jellies, foams, creams, vaginal film, and suppositories—create chemical obstacles.

The Diaphragm

The increasingly popular diaphragm is one of the more effective barrier methods. Many women who are concerned about side effects from IUDs and birth control pills have turned to this soft rubber, dome-shaped device.

A woman puts a sperm-killing jelly into a diaphragm's dome and, with or without the aid of an introducer (a long-handled hook for inserting the diaphragm), she inserts the device into her vagina before intercourse. A spring-tension rim around the diaphragm holds the spermicide in place in front of the cervix, the mouth of the womb. Not an effective contraceptive by itself, the diaphragm must be used with a spermicidal jelly or a woman will have only slim protection.

The diaphragm, which rests between the rear wall of the vagina and the upper edge of the pubic bone, covers a woman's cervix. It comes in various sizes, and a woman must be anatomically fitted by her doctor. After a doctor positions a diaphragm for his patient, she, in association with him or his nurse, should be instructed on how to remove and reinsert the device. If a diaphragm feels uncomfortable during intercourse, or if it irritates a woman's partner, she might seek a new fitting from her doctor or visit a family planning clinic for a second opinion.

After a woman has had an abortion, given birth to a baby, or gained or lost weight, her diaphragm should be checked for fit. When the vaginal structure changes, a diaphragm can lose the snug muscular niche it once had to keep it in place, and it could become dislodged during intercourse.

Any alert woman who knows her body can easily use a diaphragm. Some women have short fingers or long nails and they occasionally have difficulties with insertion, but if their doctors take time to teach them about diaphragms, they usually can overcome any problems. A woman who has an anatomical abnormality such as a tilted uterus might not be able to wear a diaphragm well and her body might be better suited to another form of contraception. A woman who has no anatomy problems might find the diaphragm so perfect for her lifestyle that she has diaphragms to meet her needs wherever she might be—traveling, in the city, in the country, and so forth.

Basically, an aware woman with a knowledge of her body is a good candidate for the diaphragm. For the most part, sensible women who are not afraid to touch themselves have few problems with diaphragms. A teenager who falls into this category might also be able to use a diaphragm to its best advantage, but in general I do not recommend diaphragms for teenagers because many young women become pregnant with diaphragms; either they insert them incorrectly or they fail to place additional contraceptive jelly inside their vaginas before they repeat sexual intercourse.

When Is a Diaphragm Most Effective?

When a diaphragm adequately covers a woman's cervix and she can feel the good fit with her fingers and know that the device never moves during intercourse, contraception should be very effective. Of course, a woman can only count on a diaphragm to be reliable if she uses it according to instructions.

Before she inserts the diaphragm, a woman should squeeze about a teaspoonful of contraceptive jelly into the inner portion of the diaphragm. A thin layer of spermicide might also be spread around the diaphragm's edge. Then, with the device pressed between her fingers or hooked onto an introducer, a woman should insert the diaphragm into her vagina no more than two hours before (but as late as up until the moment of) intercourse. The diaphragm must always remain within a woman's vagina for at least six hours after intercourse, which is the life span of sperm in the vaginal environment.

If sexual intercourse is repeated more than two hours after a woman inserts her diaphragm, more contraceptive jelly should be placed inside her vagina with the aid of an applicator. The diaphragm stays in place during jelly augmentation.

If the diaphragm is inserted in the right way at the right time, and is left in long enough, contraceptive effectiveness might be as high as 97 to 98 percent. However, if a woman does not use the diaphragm exactly as her doctor tells her, the contraceptive might fail from 5 to 20 percent of the time.

QUESTIONS ABOUT THE DIAPHRAGM

My Diaphragm Is Like a Frisbee; How Can I Make Insertion Easier?

The illustrated instructions for inserting the diaphragm that you get with a tube of contraceptive jelly make the whole process look so simple. I've never had an easy time. Usually I get the jelly all over my fingers and the diaphragm slips out of my hand. Once I got the thing halfway in and the spring action make it pop out like a Frisbee in flight. Another time I was struggling to get it in and just as I was almost finished I coughed and the diaphragm shot out of my vagina and stuck on the bathroom wall. I got so disgusted that I didn't use the thing for a long time. Isn't there any way that inserting a diaphragm can be made easier for women?
—G.A., Boulder, Colorado

This woman's experiences with the diaphragm could be script for a comic movie made by the enemies of diaphragms. Insertion certainly need not be quite as bad as she portrays it.

First, before a woman attempts to insert a diaphragm she should wash her hands to prevent contamination. Second, she should completely dry her hands to strengthen her grip on the diaphragm. Some of the devices have soft springs or so-called flat springs that make the diaphragms easier to bend and insert into the vagina. Ms. A. might request that her doctor prescribe one of these types of diaphragms to make her contraception less frustrating. Also, a diaphragm introducer—a long-handled hook that eliminates the need for a woman to insert the contraceptive with her fingers— might help.

By relaxing her vagina or shifting into a new position, a woman can usually insert a diaphragm without enduring disasters like the ones Ms. A. experienced.

Can I Use a Diaphragm During Menstruation?

I'd like to use my diaphragm to have sex during my menstrual period, but some of my friends have told me that the blood will back up and give me endometriosis. Is that true?
—M.W., Santa Fe, Tennessee

A diaphragm can be used at any time. Naturally, during menstruation a woman is not fertile and she does not need contraception. However, if a woman does use a diaphragm during her period to make intercourse less messy, the blood will stay in the upper portion of her vagina. Her flow will not back up and lead to endometriosis. If a woman is flowing heavily, the blood will run over the edge of her diaphragm.

A woman might want to douche away the excess blood in her vagina after she inserts a diaphragm in order to make her period totally unnoticeable. After intercourse, when she removes her diaphragm, a woman should expect to see it filled with blood. The diaphragm should be carefully washed, first with cold water and soap and then with a long warm-water rinse. The diaphragm, if it is not perfectly cleansed, might stain after it is used to block a woman's menstrual flow.

Why Does Spermicide Taste So Terrible?

Why can't science invent a contraceptive jelly that is pleasant for both partners? The spermicide I use with my diaphragm turns off my husband so much that he does not want to have oral sex. One day, out of frustration, I went to the drugstore and bought a bunch of different contraceptive jellies just to taste them and see if one was better than another. The flavors varied, but they all tasted terrible. I want effective contraception. I buy my jelly for its sperm-killing ability, but I would like to have it just a little more palatable. Why don't they make a spermicide that is easier on the taste buds?
—V.N., Venice, California

This woman's letter is a good one. Science has finally begun to realize that oral sex is not a sin, and new, flavorless contraceptive jellies are being marketed. A woman might ask her pharmacist to point out these flavorless jellies or she might do what Ms. N. did and comparison-shop.

Sometimes creams and jellies are manufactured in fruit flavors such as strawberry and raspberry, but you might not find them in your local drugstore. These specially flavored jellies are often sold through mail-order houses, and I don't know the extent of their effectiveness.

Of course, during oral sex no one should be consuming chemicals, and sometimes a couple who uses a diaphragm for contraception should wait until after foreplay before inserting the diaphragm. In such a situation, a woman should not rush to the bathroom for her contraceptive but should insert the diaphragm in bed. Her husband might even insert it for her.

The Cervical Cap

Like a diaphragm, a cervical cap used with a spermicide establishes a physical barrier that prevents sperm from entering a woman's womb. However, the device, usually made of soft rubber, sometimes of hard plastic, is smaller in diameter than a diaphragm, and it is deeper. In shape, the cervical cap has been likened to a thimble.

The cervical cap slips directly onto a woman's cervix, which extends into her vagina. The inner lips on the rim of the cap form an airtight suction seal that stops the cap from moving around. Then, uterine contractions keep the suction grip constant.

Cervical caps have been worn by European women for more than a century, and it used to be that women would keep the caps in place for months. However, today's rubber caps can develop an unpleasant odor if they remain in vaginas for more than forty-eight hours. Doctors advise that the cap be removed at least every forty-eight hours, washed, and reinserted as needed.

Before a cap is put back into position, it is suggested that it be one-third filled with contraceptive jelly. When placed over the cervix, the cap retains the jelly with no leakage. The jelly does not

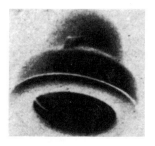

12-3 **The Cervical Cap.** The cervical cap, a classic contraceptive, has been recently rediscovered. Like the diaphragm, the cervical cap establishes a physical barrier that prevents the sperm from entering the uterus. Unlike the diaphragm, which is held in the vagina by spring tension, the cervical cap stays in place through suction. The photo shows the British Prentif Cavity-Rim Cervical Cap. There are several other types of cervical caps, but the Prentif is, at present, the most popular.

drip out and interfere with oral sex the way it might with a diaphragm. Also, no additional jelly need be applied. Intercourse can
occur any time within the forty-eight hours without extra concern
about conception. After a final intercourse, however, the cervical cap
must remain in place for at least six hours, until any sperm remaining in the vagina would have died.

How Available and Effective Is the Cervical Cap?

The cervical cap has gained much attention because many women
do not like the diaphragm, with its requirement of extra jelly for
repeated acts of intercourse, and they are concerned about side
effects from the IUD or the pill. These women want a safe form of
contraception that will be more effective than the condom or spermicide. The cap offers 82 to 94 percent protection, and there are few
anatomical difficulties in fitting the device. Even a woman who has
a tilted uterus can wear a cervical cap.

Although it is known that women can have cervical irritation and
erosion while on the birth control pill, that the tail of an IUD might
cause irritation, and that a diaphragm sometimes causes vaginal erosion and bleeding, the cervical cap has not been shown to create any
cervical irritation or abnormality. Studies in Iowa, New York, New
Hampshire, and Boston have not produced any complaints from
women about cervical inflammation.

In my own studies, I have fitted more than a thousand women
with cervical caps and have not found cervical inflammation to be a
problem. Sometimes women have had slight bleeding after intercourse, but on examination no harm was ever done to their cervixes.
The bleeding might just have been due to stimulation of the uterus
during intercourse. There does not seem to be a physical problem
with the cervical cap. In fact, women who use diaphragms often
complain about recurring urinary cystitis that happens because the
diaphragm rests against the urethra. The cervical cap will not cause
this problem, either. Cervical caps are available in various sizes, and
a woman must be fitted by a doctor.

The Female Condom

Made by the Female Health Company, the Reality female condom, which offers 79 to 95 percent protection against pregnancy, is a lubricated polyurethane sheath about six and a half inches long. It looks like a long, floppy tube with flexible rings at each end. One end is closed, and the other open. The closed end is inserted high *inside* the vagina and the ring at the open end remains *outside* the vagina.

The promise that the nonprescription female condom held when it was introduced in 1993 has not been fulfilled. It is unpopular because women report an undesirable squeaking sound during intercourse; it is also not widely available. Still, it is an option. The female condom can be inserted from eight hours before up to immediately before intercourse. Each condom has a one-time use and must be removed before a woman stands after sex. The male condom, described on pages 398 to 399, is still the more effective barrier for preventing pregnancy and the spread of HIV/AIDS and other STDs.

The Return of the Contraceptive Sponge

The Today contraceptive sponge, a well-liked over-the-counter birth control device sold from 1983 to 1995, was removed from the market due to manufacturing problems. In March 1999, a New Jersey company, Allendale Pharmaceuticals Inc., announced that it had purchased all rights to the Today sponge and would return it to the market.

Millions of women used the soft, cushiony circle of polyurethane foam treated with a high concentration of spermicide with nonoxynol-9. Sperm meet the physical blockage of the sponge itself and the chemical blockade set up by the spermicide. In the past, the "down" side of the sponge was its variable—76 to 92 percent—rate of contraceptive protection. It offers twenty-four-hour birth control, however, after which a woman easily removes it by pulling the loop that crosses its diameter and hangs down. Then it is discarded.

QUESTIONS ABOUT THE CERVICAL CAP

Could I Use My Diaphragm as a Cervical Cap?

I have wanted a cervical cap ever since I read about it in a magazine article, but no doctor in my area has one. Suppose I asked for the smallest-size diaphragm? Would the tiniest diaphragm work like a cervical cap?

—F.H., Soldier, Iowa

A cervical cap fits over the cervix and is held on by suction, a vacuum, rather than by spring tension, which keeps a diaphragm in position. Sometimes a woman has a uterine abnormality like a tilted uterus and she is fitted with a small-size diaphragm. In such a case it has sometimes been found that uterine suction builds up and secures the diaphragm, but when contraception is most needed, during intercourse and orgasm, the diaphragm often does not hold.

So, although a small-size diaphragm can be fitted like a cervical cap, it might not work like a cap during sexual activity.

My Dripping Diaphragm Is Making Me Crazy; Will a Cervical Cap Be Better?

My fiance and I are madly in love. We're planning to be married in a few months, but we are so hot for each other right now that we have sex all the time. I'm using a diaphragm, which has always worked well for me, but I have to inject so much jelly that I'm running around with this glob dripping out of me constantly. It's making me crazy. Is there any way I could use a cervical cap and avoid this mess?

—W.D., Chicago, Illinois

Contraceptive jelly need be placed inside a cervical cap only once before the cap is inserted for forty-eight hours. If a cervical cap fits well, there is no reason to inject additional jelly before the cap is removed; in fact, some women's health groups feel that the cap and jelly can remain within a woman even longer than forty-eight hours.

Ms. D. might try the cervical cap if she can find a doctor who is fitting women with this contraceptive. (As mentioned before, a local chapter of NOW or Planned Parenthood might help her locate such a physician.) The cap will certainly be less messy than her diaphragm, and her active lovemaking will have no unpleasant aftermath.

My Cervical Cap Slipped Out During Sex; Do I Need a Different Contraceptive?

> *I've been using a cervical cap for the past year and I've been very happy with it. Lately I've been a little worried though, because the cap slipped out twice during sex. Do you think I need a different contraceptive?*
>
> —Y.P., West Haven, Connecticut

Every woman has different uterine contractions and suction capabilities that keep the cervical cap on her cervix. Every man makes love to a woman differently. The penis thrust of some men might not affect a cap's placement, while other men might dislodge the device if the uterine suction is not especially strong.

If a woman has a new partner, she should check her cervical cap after lovemaking to make sure that the device is still in place. In Ms. P.'s case, the cervical cap came off. Perhaps her cervix has changed size and she needs to be fitted for a new cap, or perhaps she did not place it properly. If her doctor tells her that she is already wearing the appropriate size and she is placing it correctly, she might have to inquire about other forms of contraception. The suction from her uterus might have diminished and she might no longer be a candidate for a cervical cap.

One Condom, Two Kinds of Protection

Condoms are sheaths for the penis. Most are made of thin latex rubber, although some are made from the intestinal tissue of sheep. Centuries ago, the condom was originally used for protection against venereal disease; then it gained notoriety as a contraceptive device. Today, while it still traps sperm and prevents pregnancy, the condom has had a comeback as a protector against sexually transmitted diseases. There are currently about thirty STDs, with the fatal HIV/AIDS virus the most serious, and condoms keep them at bay.

Of all the types of condoms available, *I feel that the one that offers the greatest protection against pregnancy and exposure to STDs is one made of thin latex, lubricated with sperm-killer nonoxynol-9.* Whether contoured, ribbed, nubbed, or colored, with a plain or a reservoir tip, the uniformly manufactured latex condoms block the smallest microbes, while the natural condoms made from sheep's intestinal tissue might have porous, weak spots. As for nonoxynol-9, this spermicide increases the antipregnancy factor of a condom and also kills the bacteria that cause gonorrhea, syphilis, and chlamydia. Condoms that are lubricated with gels or silicone-based products do not destroy living organisms.

NOTE: A couple should never try to give more lubricating power to a condom with oils or oil-based products. In less than a minute a lubricant with oil, such as baby oil, mineral oil, petroleum jelly (like Vaseline), cold cream, and hand or body lotions, can make a condom leak. The safe lubricants are water-based: K-Y Lubricating Jelly, Today Personal Lubricant, Corn Huskers Lotion, and any spermicidal cream or jelly made for use with a diaphragm or cervical cap.

A condom has 84 to 98 percent effectiveness as a contraceptive, but even so, I recommend that women who are having sexual relations with men who use condoms continue to use other forms of birth control, perhaps the pill, a diaphragm, cervical cap, vaginal film, or spermicidal jellies, creams, or foams. Even if the condom is a couple's chosen contraceptive, and they would use a condom whether or not it offered protection against STDs, I still recommend backup birth control to increase the rate of protection. Sometimes a condom can be a problem because it falls off a man's penis during the thrusting action of intercourse.

During sexual activity, after a man has an erection, he holds the tip of the condom, unrolls the sheath to the base of his penis, and holds it there when he ejaculates. This way sperm are contained in the condom and are not released into his partner's body; also, there is no exchange of bodily fluids, with their risk of containing STDs.

After intercourse, before a man loses his erection, he should disengage from his partner, immediately remove the condom, and wash his genitals in case there is semen around the area. If a man permits his penis to become limp before he withdraws from a woman, there is a good chance that the condom might slip off. This allows sperm to escape and forfeits any protection against exposure to STDs. The condom is preventive medicine for those women and men who have more than one sexual partner.

Vaginal Contraceptive Film

Vaginal Contraceptive Film (VCF) is a small, thin, translucent square sold in packets of twelve as small as matchbooks. It is an ideal contraceptive to use in combination with a condom. VCF contains nonoxynol-9 spermicide, which offers 70 to 97 percent pregnancy protection. One square wafer of film offers two hours of birth control, but a new square must be used for every intercourse. At least five, but preferably fifteen, minutes before sexual intercourse, a woman folds the wafer over the tip of her middle finger and places it high inside her vagina, near her cervix. There it dissolves into a gel that coats the vaginal canal and chemically kills any sperm. If intercourse occurs more than two hours after inserting a square, another one must be used. After intercourse, the film washes away with natural body fluids. No douching is needed, but if a woman desires douching, she must wait at least six hours after intercourse to make sure all the sperm have died off.

Spermicides

Spermicides come in five different varieties: jellies, creams, injectable foams, foaming tablets, and suppositories. They usually contain one or the other of two sperm-killing chemicals—nonoxynol-9 or octoxynol—which stay close to a woman's cervix when combined with an inert substance. Both nonoxynol-9 and octoxynol are considered safe by the FDA. Spermicides, however, are problematic because their effectiveness varies from study to study, and most of the time their failure rates are high.

In a survey of U.S. women, about 15 percent of women using spermicides became pregnant during a one-year period, compared to 2 percent of pill users, 4 percent of women with IUDs, and 10 percent of women whose partners were wearing condoms. The unwanted pregnancies occurring with spermicides might be due to the fact that many women became confused about how to use the different products or sometimes do not regularly employ them.

It is usually advised that creams and jellies be used along with the physical barrier methods—diaphragms, cervical caps, or condoms. Foams and suppositories are often not thought of in connection with other barriers, but these spermicides will also increase in effectiveness if paired with diaphragms, cervical caps, or condoms. All spermicidal products effectively incapacitate sperm for one hour after they have been inserted into the vagina, but the timing of insertion is sometimes tricky.

Creams, jellies, and injectable foams from pressurized containers are effective as soon as they are introduced into a woman's vagina. Foaming tablets and suppositories need at least fifteen minutes to dissolve or they will be totally useless sperm-killing agents. All five kinds of spermicides should be inserted not more than twenty minutes before intercourse. After a woman has inserted a spermicide, she should remain in a reclining position. If she stands, the jelly or foam might drip from her vagina.

As mentioned before, spermicides are effective for up to one hour after they have been inserted, and each time intercourse is repeated additional spermicide must be applied. A woman should avoid douching for at least six to eight hours after her last intercourse because live sperm, which cannot survive in the vagina longer than that, will have died by then.

If spermicides are properly and consistently used, their effectiveness might increase to as much as 95 percent, but there have been reports that more and more women who are seeking abortions at clinics have become pregnant with spermicides. Women who use spermicides for contraception must be highly disciplined individuals with cooperative, understanding partners.

My Foaming Tablets Burned My Boyfriend

The other night I inserted a foaming tablet and right after intercourse, my boyfriend withdrew, said he was hurting, and dashed to the bathroom to wash his penis. The foam had burned him and he asked me never to use it again. Could I have seriously harmed his genitals with my contraceptive? I wasn't burning at all.
                                        —R.E., Detroit, Michigan

Foaming tablets are inserted at least fifteen minutes prior to intercourse to give them time to melt and effervesce within a woman's vagina. The foaming action is heat-producing, and couples, both women and men together, have been known to complain of burning sensations.

Since Ms. E.'s boyfriend is particularly sensitive to her contraceptive, she might try a suppository like Semicid, which does not effervesce. A spermicidal cream or jelly used in conjunction with a diaphragm or a condom might be even easier on the organs, while providing more effective contraception. The irritation Ms. E.'s

boyfriend experienced was only momentary. She can feel assured
that he will not have any lingering pain.

Spermicide Warning

The Boston Collaborative Drug Surveillance Program conducted
an eighteen-month study of babies born to 4,772 women in Seattle,
Washington. There were 763 women who had used spermicides at
or near the time of conception. The babies born to these women had
twice as many (2.2 percent) unusual, severe birth defects as the newborns of women who had relied on other forms of contraception. In
a control group of babies born to almost 4,000 women, only 1 percent had birth defects.

The study also revealed that the chance of late miscarriage for
women who used spermicides was almost twice what it was for
nonusers. Sperm that are not killed by spermicides might be damaged by the contraceptives before they proceed to fertilize the eggs.
When conception occurs with an imperfect sperm, there is a strong
possibility that an abnormal embryo will be created and, following
nature's way, the embryo will spontaneously abort.

A woman who becomes pregnant while using a spermicide alone,
or a spermicide with a diaphragm or a cervical cap, must realize that
she might face a higher incidence of either miscarriage or the birth
of a malformed child. These findings are very new and somewhat
scary. If a woman does not want to be pregnant under these conditions, she might be advised to consider a pregnancy interruption.
Certainly, if she wanted to continue the pregnancy, she should seek
genetic counseling about the potential problem of birth defects.

NATURAL FAMILY PLANNING

Perhaps because the adverse side effects of chemical and mechanical
birth control methods have been so well publicized, natural family
planning is gaining favor among women. A woman who chooses

natural family planning as her method of contraception should have a real understanding of her menstrual cycle. A cooperative partner helps, too.

Natural family planning relies on a woman's judgment of the fertile and infertile days of her cycle. She can calculate these days by using any of three methods:

1. *The Ovulation Method.* A woman gauges her ovulation by using her fingers to feel the position of her cervix and the changes in her cervical mucus, as described in the mucus checks in chapter 3 (see pages 61 to 63). Intercourse might take place until the day that a woman notices her cervical wetness increase. Then she and her partner must abstain until the evening of the fourth day after her secretion has peaked. Usually, abstinence lasts from a week to ten days during the middle of the month.

The Drs. Billings, an Australian husband-and-wife team, formulated the five-stage Billings method of monitoring cervical mucus, which might be explained to a woman who inquires about the technique at her local Planned Parenthood clinic. Also, the book *The Billings Method* should be available at local bookstores.

Sometimes an ovulation predictor kit, when used for two or three cycles, can help in gauging "safe" days.

2. *The Temperature Method.* The "I've Had Every Test Imaginable . . ." section of chapter 8 (see pages 213 to 218) explains how a woman might determine her ovulation by taking basal body temperature readings and charting them over four to six months. A special ovulation thermometer makes it easy to register the slight dip in temperature that occurs at the time of ovulation. A woman's temperature will rise a day or two after ovulation and remain high until immediately prior to menstruation, when it drops. A woman's "safe" days will occur from three days after her temperature rises until seven days after menstruation begins. Please note, however, that *the temperature method is not an aid in calculating "safe" days* before *ovulation.*

3. *The Symptothermal Method.* Women who use this method combine the ovulation method and the temperature method with the calendar rhythm method that women have used for generations. In the calendar rhythm method, which is no longer considered effective by itself, a woman judges her first "unsafe" days before ovulation by subtracting twenty-one days from the shortest cycle, in the previous six months. Using the symptothermal method, a woman figures out her first fertile "unsafe" day with the calendar method but double-checks her calculation by monitoring her cervical mucus. If mucus appears earlier than her estimated "unsafe" date, she must abstain at the sign of the mucus.

At the same time that a woman is assessing her "unsafe" time before ovulation, she is taking her temperature to determine the beginning of her safe days after ovulation, when abstinence may be lifted. As mentioned before, a woman's "safe" days will be from three days after her temperature rises until her period begins. This is an infertile interval in her cycle.

A California study that compared the ovulation method with the symptothermal method found that, for reasons not yet determined, pregnancy rates were significantly higher for those couples using the ovulation method.

QUESTIONS ABOUT NATURAL FAMILY PLANNING

Is Research Being Done on Natural Family Planning?

I cannot take the pill and I have had numerous side effects from other forms of contraception. My husband and I have been unsuccessful in preventing pregnancy and I am having my second child in two years. Financially, we cannot keep up this pace. I am determined to make natural family planning work, but I wondered why it's so difficult for me to get information about the latest findings. I'd like to stay informed because the minute an easy, natural method of contra-

*ception is discovered, I want to be the first to use it. Is research being
done on natural family planning?*

—N.C., Jamestown, New York

Natural family planning has been promoted and taught through
church groups throughout the country. Ms. C. might learn about the
latest methods by contacting a parish priest or minister in her area
or by contacting the Billings Ovulation Method Association, 316
North 7th Street, St. Cloud, MN 56303, toll-free phone: 888-637-
6371. The Billings Association, also called BOMA-USA, will direct
a woman to a local method teacher. A helpful source affiliated with
BOMA-USA is: Natural Family Planning Center of Washington
DC Inc., 8514 Bradmoor Drive, Bethesda, MD 20817-3810,
phone: 301-897-9323. If Ms. C. has irregular periods, natural family
planning might be difficult, but if she is regular this might be a good
contraceptive choice.

Does the Rhythm Method Result in Babies with Birth Defects?

*I have heard what I hope is an old wives' tale. I heard that
if a woman becomes pregnant while she is practicing the rhythm
method she stands an above-average chance of bearing an
abnormal baby. Could this be true?*

—I.B., Russellville, Arkansas

An Australian researcher pointed out that in western Australia
there were 1.137 cases of Down's syndrome for every 1,000 live
births from 1966 to 1975. However, among Catholic women the
rate was 1.935, which was more than twice the .842 rate for women
of other religions. The higher incidence of Down's syndrome among
Catholics, it was theorized, might be due to the rhythm method of
contraception, which requires self-control and abstinence. In fact,
researchers in Great Britain have suggested that there is a link
between infrequent intercourse and an increased incidence of Down's
syndrome.

Couples using the rhythm method do not have intercourse in the middle of the month, during a woman's ovulation. If an egg is available for fertilization at an odd time of the month, it might be abnormal. Also, a woman who conceives when she is trying to avoid pregnancy might be an older woman whose chance of carrying a Down's syndrome child is normally higher. It might be, too, that women who use the rhythm method do not believe in pregnancy interruption and so their Down's syndrome babies are born, whereas women using other birth control methods might choose to terminate unwanted pregnancies, especially if they know they are carrying a Down's syndrome child.

STERILIZATION

While natural family planning, birth control with no medical intervention, is enjoying new popularity, on the other end of the contraceptive spectrum is the popularity of surgical sterilization. Sterilization through vasectomy or tubal ligation is the most common method of contraception among all U.S. couples. Yearly, about 500,000 vasectomies are performed on men and 640,000 tubal ligations on women. Vasectomy, with a 1 percent failure rate, is by far the more effective birth control. The 1997 CREST study of over 10,000 women found an 18.5 percent rate for tubal ligation over ten years' time. Still, women's sterilization numbers jumped from 9 percent in 1973 to 18 percent in 1990, while male sterilization stayed at 11 percent. Among U.S. women using contraception, more than 50 percent of those over age forty choose sterilization.

Tubal Ligation—Sterilization for Women

Often women who have one or two children early in life think that their desire for childbearing has been fulfilled and they choose tubal ligation over other forms of contraception. Only later, when they are older, and possibly remarried, or after they have suffered the loss of a child, do woman realize that they might have acted in haste. Then they want their sterilizations reversed. In chapter 8, the sections "Can My Tubal Sterilization Be Reversed?" (page 245) and "The Ends of My Tubes Were Crushed" (page 247) contain information about how complex these reversals are. The microsurgery involved is lengthy, expensive, difficult, and offers women at most a 70 to 80 percent chance of fertility.

Before a woman agrees to a permanent sterilization, she should attempt other forms of contraception, at least give available types of contraceptives a try before she decides against them. If she has used different contraceptives already and she is in her late thirties or early forties, and she is a woman who can say without a doubt that she does not want future childbearing, only then should she consider tubal ligation. And still, before she permits herself to be scheduled for surgery she should be counseled and evaluated by her doctor. Too many women rush into tubal sterilization.

A law in many states requires a woman to sign a complex consent form at least thirty days prior to tubal sterilization. A woman is informed that the chances for reversing a tubal sterilization are very slim. She must know that she is probably choosing a one-way street. Then, in front of the doctor, a nurse, and a witness, she signs the form and has thirty days to reflect on her decision.

Often a woman feels less inclined to submit to surgery after she has had thirty days to think about it. Almost 50 percent of the patients in my practice who sign up for tubal sterilization cancel. If future pregnancy would endanger a woman's health, or if a woman has a sufficiently large family and she finds other forms of contraception unsuitable, sterilization might be in order. Otherwise, I would encourage a woman to examine her options. The thirty-day consent form, although annoying to some people, is probably a good idea.

What Is the Best Form of Tubal Sterilization?

"Tubal sterilization" is a phrase used synonymously with "tubal ligation." In the past, women were sterilized by only one method—

ligation, in which a thread is tied around the tube. To ligate technically means to bind. When a woman says that she has had a tubal
ligation today, she has probably had her tubes rendered nonfunctional, but she might not have had them tied at all. Today there are a
variety of techniques for tubal sterilization that involve more than a
suture. Still, in a throwback to the original method, the surgery is
often called a tubal ligation. If a woman's doctor indicates that she
needs a tubal ligation, he most likely means a sterilization.

A healthy woman who has never had surgery might find that
sterilization by laparoscopy is the best method of tubal ligation for
her. During this procedure, a doctor will make a small incision
inside her navel through which he will pass a laparoscope, a medical
periscope designed to afford him a view of a woman's internal
organs. (A doctor should make an "invisible" scar by placing his incision deep inside a woman's navel. A woman might discuss the incision procedure with her doctor before she undergoes surgery. She
should ask him where he intends to place the surgical cut. There is
no reason why a physician cannot make an incision in such a fashion
that it will hardly be visible. Later on, when she is wearing a bikini, a
woman need not display a visible scar that shows she has been
"fixed.") Then, after inserting the laparoscope, a doctor will guide
abdominal forceps through the instrument and, by manipulating the
forceps, he will pick up a portion of the Fallopian tube and use one
of two methods to make the tube nonfunctional. He will either *cauterize* (burn) the tube with special instruments or he will close the
tubal passage with a *Falope ring,* or a *Hulka clip,* or a new *Filshie clip.*
A Falope ring or a Hulka clip is much easier to reverse than a cauterization since, generally, less tissue has been damaged.

Cauterization can be risky. Sometimes doctors burn too large a
portion of a tube and reduce the blood supply to the ovaries.
Cauterization is advised only if surgeons use modern instruments
that burn just enough of the tube to adequately complete sterilization. If the latest electrocautery is not used, a physician could burn
the bowel or other internal areas and a woman might suffer severe
complications. If her doctor suggests sterilization through cauteriza-

tion, a woman should try to find out whether he has had extensive experience performing it before she submits to surgery. She might inquire about his ability by questioning his nurse, his patients in the community, and a few members of the hospital staff. She must have faith in his ability and she might, if she thinks she might ever want the surgery reversed, encourage him to burn only a small portion of the tube in an area approximately two inches from her uterus. Minimal altering of the Fallopian tube makes the possibility of reversal more hopeful.

Tubal ligation by laparoscopy is one of the more popular and safer methods of sterilization if performed by a skillful physician. A woman has only a short hospital stay, and the incision and her scar are small. However, if a woman is overweight, or if she has undergone previous surgery that might have left adhesions that might make laparoscopy dangerous, she is better suited to tubal sterilization by laparotomy or mini-laparotomy. These two abdominal operations differ in complexity. The mini-laparotomy is much simpler and faster than the laparotomy. Both surgeries expose the abdominal cavity and require incisions in or about the pubic hairline, but with a mini-laparotomy the cut is only one inch in length, one third the size needed for a laparotomy.

In a laparotomy, a woman is given general anesthesia and a doctor uses special instruments to enter her abdomen and locate her Fallopian tube. Then, following what is called the modified Pomeroy technique, he lifts a portion of the Fallopian tube and sutures the tube shut at two different points approximately one and one half inches apart. He then cuts and removes the portion of the tube between the two sutures. During a mini-laparotomy, a doctor identifies and exposes the Fallopian tube with instruments designed to be used during surgery with a tiny incision. When the tubes are identified and brought into the surgical field, a similar modified Pomeroy technique is carried out.

A postpartum tubal ligation is a tubal sterilization undertaken in association with a cesarean section or immediately after a vaginal delivery. During a cesarean section, when the uterus, tubes, and ovaries are already exposed, a tubal sterilization is a simple procedure that takes less than five minutes. The modified Pomeroy technique is generally the procedure of choice. For a woman who delivers a strong, healthy baby by cesarean section and is definitely sure that she does not want any more children, a tubal ligation at the time of her surgery would certainly be appropriate.

A woman who delivers prematurely by cesarean section might have a child who cannot survive in the world. Sometimes a newborn appears to be hearty but her or his internal organs are not fully developed. Such a woman should postpone her sterilization if her baby is premature. It is terribly tragic to see a woman who lost her premature son or daughter want another pregnancy and be unable to have her sterilization reversed.

Laparoscopy, laparotomy and mini-laparotomy, and postpartum tubal ligation in association with a cesarean section are the most widely used and probably the safest forms of tubal ligation and permanent contraception. Tubal sterilization can also be performed via the vaginal route, when a surgeon exposes the Fallopian tubes to an incision inside the vagina. (Since tubal sterilization through the vagina is rarely performed, however, even a woman who undergoes tubal sterilization a day after a vaginal delivery will usually have the operation performed abdominally.) The tubes are then cut using the modified Pomeroy technique or by placement of the Falope ring or the Filshie or Hulka clip. Since the doctor is entering the less-sterile vaginal area, the risk of infection is much higher with this operation. Overall, the vaginal approach to sterilization has declined in popularity and is performed with considerably less frequency. However, a revolutionary new reversible technique currently under investigation—tubal occlusion—which will be described on pages 415 to 416, is performed during a vaginal procedure. Women and doctors are still learning ways to make tubal sterilization work.

QUESTIONS ABOUT TUBAL STERILIZATION

I Haven't Been the Same Since My Tubal Ligation

During my cesarean section for my third child I had my tubes tied. That was almost three years ago. Every month since then, when my period is due, I have an excruciating pain on my right side in the area of my tube. I never had menstrual problems before and I wonder if the tubal ligation has something to do with my pain. If the pain never goes away, will I have to have a hysterectomy?
—N.C., Marshfield, Missouri

I had a tubal ligation six months after my second child was born and ever since then I have been in unbelievable pain and discomfort during my periods. My doctor just says, "Some women must suffer." He assures me that my pain has nothing to do with the surgery, but I never had menstrual cramps or pain before. I want someone to tell me the truth. Does a tubal ligation give you cramps and pain afterward?
—E.P., Troy, Michigan

I'm a healthy thirty-two-year-old woman. After my second child, my husband and I decided that I would have my tubes tied. The operation was fairly simple, although it took me much longer to recover than I thought it would. Since the surgery, which was about eight months ago, my periods have been very light and two weeks before I'm due to menstruate I become very depressed and lethargic. I don't want to get out of bed. I used to be nicknamed "the sunshine kid." but now my children are starting to call me "the Grinch." I don't feel like myself at all. In fact, I haven't been the same since my tubal ligation. Could something have gone wrong?
—J.H., Brooklyn, New York

Up to 15 percent of the women who undergo tubal ligations report complications during the first month after the operation.

Certainly, many women feel terrific after tubal sterilization because they are no longer worried about pregnancy and they are able to enjoy sex with more freedom, but what about that 15 percent? Since millions of women choose to be sterilized, this percentage represents a significant number of women.

Researchers who continue to study the aftereffects of tubal sterilization have named the postoperative condition post-tubal-ligation syndrome (PTLS). Women who experience this syndrome after surgery might have pelvic pain, irregular menstrual bleeding, severe premenstrual syndrome (PMS), and galactorrhea (a milky discharge from the nipples). Sometimes women are so incapacitated by the pain of PTLS that they undergo further surgery. Women have had D & Cs, additional laparoscopies, removal of their ovaries, and even hysterectomies to rid themselves of this syndrome. Tubal ligation should not be considered minor, inconsequential surgery. Tubal sterilization can bring on the pain and misery of post-tubal-ligation syndrome.

Most likely, PTLS is caused by hormonal imbalance. If a physician cauterizes, removes, or damages too large a portion of the Fallopian tubes and their blood vessels, he will reduce blood flow, the ovaries might shrink, and women might bleed less during menstruation. A hormonal imbalance might result in abnormal ovulations with irregular menstrual bleeding. When ovulation is off, there can be decreased progesterone production, which brings on premenstrual syndrome with its excessive mood swings and depressions. The PTLS hormonal imbalance can also result in ovarian pelvic pain, which can become so unbearable that patients agree to unnecessary surgery.

A woman must realize, *before* she submits to tubal sterilization, that this is not problem-free surgery. Even if many doctors are not aware of or dismiss the fact that pelvic pain and depression symptoms have been linked to tubal ligation, women should know that there is a direct relationship between the surgery and the symptoms. As mentioned before, sometimes when the pain becomes excruciating, women undergo D & Cs or further surgery. Ms. H., the author of the third letter, seems to be suffering from the depression of pre-menstrual syndrome. She might refer to chapter 4, "Premenstrual Syndrome—the Monthly Malady," for ways to alleviate her "dragged out" feeling. She might also take extra vitamin B_6, which seems to promote neural transmissions and regulate monthly periods.

Considering the recognized postoperative complications of tubal sterilization, I must emphasize all the more that women who elect this surgery should not rush into it. They should try to wait until they are in their late thirties or early forties before they make sterilization their method of contraception. Even if a patient has the procedure done later in life, she can still be a victim of post-tubal-ligation syndrome. However, if the sterilization has been properly performed with minimal tubal damage, her symptoms should be less severe. If symptoms occur, they should be recognized as PTLS and treated conservatively rather than radically.

Should I Be Sterilized or Stay on the Pill?

I'm twenty-eight years old and I have been taking the birth control pill since I was nineteen. I stopped the pill to have a baby three years ago, but otherwise I have been taking it almost nonstop for nine years. I think it's time for me to quit and I told my doctor that I want my tubes tied. I do not want more children. My mother is very upset about this and she is causing me to have second thoughts about the operation. What do you think? Should I be sterilized or stay on the pill?

—V.R., Toledo, Ohio

This woman does not say whether she is married or single. If she is divorced, she might remarry and change her mind about children. At twenty-eight she is still, in my opinion, too young to be sterilized, since her life might go through changes she cannot predict right now. If she wants to go off the pill because she is worried about side effects, then I refer her to the birth control pill section of this chapter. Recent studies have indicated that a healthy woman, a nonsmoker, who has no history of diabetes or high blood pressure, can safely remain on the pill for years.

Since Ms. R. has borne a child, she might also be a good candidate for an IUD because her uterus might tolerate the device better than the uterus of a woman who has never given birth. An IUD might be her alternative to the pill. An IUD is linked to problems of infection, but if Ms. R. is aware of her body, she might be able to use an intrauterine device without problems. If she at least tries another form of contraception before she decides on tubal sterilization, Ms. R. will regain a few years for reflection.

I do not believe Ms. R. should be sterilized right now because, as mentioned in the previous section, the operation is not without complications. Why make thing worse?

What Is the Best Type of Tubal Sterilization for Joggers?

I'm an active forty-year-old woman who is the mother of four children. I definitely don't want any more children and I'm thinking about having my tubes tied. Could you tell me if there is a type of tubal sterilization that is best for joggers? I run about five miles a day and I've been wondering if there is a way to tie my tubes that's better for my organs when they bounce during running.
                                   —M.F., Cazadero, California

Women, and also men, who are serious joggers probably do not even need sterilization, because extensive jogging lowers fertility. In women, jogging inhibits the brain hormones that stimulate ovulation, so female joggers often have very light or absent periods. In men, jogging lowers sperm counts.

However, since Ms. F.'s jogging schedule might vary from day to day, she might want tubal sterilization anyway. If there is no dissuading her from the surgery, I believe that a laparoscopic sterilization performed by a skilled surgeon who uses either a Falope ring or a Filshie or Hulka clip, or minimal cauterization on her tube, would probably be the safest and easiest procedure. Ms. F. is a healthy woman and sterilization by laparoscopy should cause few problems for her.

Vasectomy—Sterilization for Men

Vasectomy is fast. It takes fifteen minutes in a doctor's office and requires only local anesthesia. A doctor makes a small incision in a man's scrotum and finds the vasa deferentia, the tubes that carry the sperm from the testes to the penis. Then the physician cuts, ties, cauterizes, or clips the tubes to prevent the release of sperm. This is

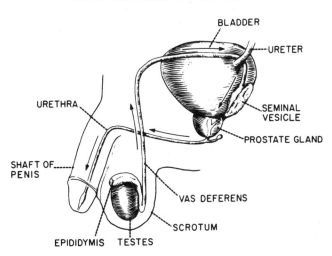

MALE REPRODUCTIVE SYSTEM

12-4 **The Male Reproductive System.** The sperm are produced in the testes and stored in the sperm collection system (the epididymis). After maturation, the sperm move up and into the vas deferens. They then travel past the bladder and the urethra. As the sperm reach the junction of the vas deferens and the seminal vesicle, they mix with seminal fluid, which now makes the so-far infertile sperm fertile. The sperm continue their course in the vas deferens and pass through the prostate gland. The vas deferens meets the urethra, the tube that transports urine from the bladder, in the prostate gland. During ejaculation, the sperm will be propelled through the urethra. When a vasectomy (male sterilization) is performed, a portion of the vas deferens is tied and cut. The vasectomy incision is made at the top of the scrotum, approximately at the point where the line indicating the vas deferens is located in the illustration.

not a castration operation because a man's hormonal and bodily functions will not be altered. A man will still ejaculate semen, but his semen will not contain sperm.

Generally, there is no infection or undue pain attached to a vasectomy. A man can usually return to work in a day or two without feeling any discomfort. The only problem with vasectomy is that there is a chance that the sperm ducts will spontaneously reunite if the sterilization has not included removal of portions of the tubes. When tubes are tied and cut the failure rate tends to be higher than when the tube is cut and a segment is removed. A man who is considering a vasectomy should ask his doctor about the particular method that the physician intends to use, and question what chance there is that the procedure might reverse itself. The experience and skill of a physician are essential to success because there have been cases in which doctors have made the wrong cuts. Such mistakes are easily detected by sperm counts.

In fact, even after a proper vasectomy a man might have a sperm count for a while because some sperm might have been alive in his reproductive tract before surgery. A man and his partner should use birth control until the man has had at least two negative sperm counts. Then, vasectomy is almost 100 percent protection against pregnancy. Women report that their men have become more sexually desirous after vasectomies. Perhaps the surgery leads to a surge in testosterone, or perhaps men are more relaxed in bed because they are controlling contraception; whatever the reason, men seem to feel more sexually positive after vasectomy. Of course, a number of men do worry about their masculine self-images and might experience the opposite effect, but they are in the minority.

Men who want their vasectomies reversed do not have the odds in their favor. In chapter 8, the section "Can I Have My Vasectomy Reversed?" (see pages 250 to 251) contains a discussion of the reversal procedure. The reverse sterilization is best performed by a specialist experienced in the delicate microsurgical technique required. Reports on reversal to fertility range in success, from 16 to

85 percent, but less than 50 percent of wives achieve healthy pregnancy. If he chooses to leave his vasectomy intact, a man can become a father through the ICSI method (see page 273).

Does Vasectomy Cause Heart Attack?

My husband got a vasectomy five years ago. A few weeks after his operation he started getting pains in his legs. He thought he needed more exercise until a checkup a few years ago revealed that he had atherosclerosis. His arteries are blocked from the abdomen down. The doctors say that there is no connection between his vasectomy and the condition, but we think there is. He is trying to build himself up through vitamins and swimming. We know the bleak prognosis for vasectomy reversal and I don't think we will attempt further surgery. However, we just want to know if there is some connection here.

—D.F., Cannon Falls, Minnesota

Ms. F. has touched on a controversy. The notion that vasectomy might cause heart attack comes primarily from the studies of Dr. Nancy Alexander, a physiologist at the Oregon Regional Primate Research Center in Beaverton, and Dr. Thomas Clarkson, a veterinary pathologist at Bowman Gray School of Medicine in Winston-Salem, North Carolina. Drs. Alexander and Clarkson fed ten monkeys a high-cholesterol diet for six months. Then they gave vasectomies to five of the monkeys while continuing to feed a high-fat diet to all ten animals. At the end of ten more months, the monkeys were killed and their organs were closely examined. All the animals showed fatty lesions, but the five vasectomized primates were more extensively damaged.

After further analysis the doctors discovered that the five sterilized monkeys had more sperm antibodies. It is known that when a vasectomy is conducted, sperm are still in a man's reproductive tract. These sperm are treated like foreign bodies, which are then attacked by antibodies. Since sperm cells are fat cells, the sperm antibodies are like fat antibodies. Drs. Alexander and Clarkson therefore set forth their belief that the sperm antibodies affected the arteries in ways that resulted in atherosclerosis, which can lead to heart attack.

In a follow-up study, Drs. Alexander and Clarkson compared the arteries of ten monkeys that had been given vasectomies nine to fourteen years earlier with those of eight monkeys that had not been sterilized. Even though both groups had been fed low-fat diets, the vasectomized animals had a greater amount of fatty deposits. The Alexander/Clarkson data, however, has created more questions than answers. A controversy now exists.

A study in *Lancet*, a British medical journal, found that the incidence of heart attack in almost 5,000 vasectomized men was no higher than it was for 24,000 men who were not sterilized. Several other recently conducted investigations on vasectomized men have also failed to show an increased incidence of heart attack as a result of vasectomy. One research team at Mt. Sinai School of Medicine in New York has investigated the relationship of vasectomy to heart attack by replicating the Alexander/Clarkson experiments. Ten monkeys were fed a "normal American diet" with a 35 percent fat content. After six months, five of the animals were given vasectomies. Following the surgery, all ten primates remained on the diet. After ten months, the animals were sacrificed and their organs were examined using the same method that Drs. Alexander and Clarkson did in their original study. Although the five vasectomized monkeys had more sperm antibodies, they did not have more extensive atherosclerosis than the control group. Fatty deposits were high in all the monkeys. The increased sperm antibodies in the sterilized group did not seem to have had any effect on the extent of the atherosclerosis. The results of this monkey study showed that vasectomy does not promote atherosclerosis and supported the findings of researchers who have conducted human studies. Recently, a large study found no association between vasectomy, cardiovascular disease, and other health effects. What remains inconclusive is whether there is any link between vasectomy and prostate cancer. Although several large studies found no connections, two reported a slight increase in risk. Most experts feel that a connection is unlikely. In regard to Ms. F.'s husband, if he is on a low-fat diet, following his present fitness regimen, with his current awareness, he is doing the best that one person can to stay healthy.

WIDENING THE RANGE OF CONTRACEPTIVE CHOICES

The number of birth control methods available in the United States expanded significantly during the 1990s with the FDA's approval of Depo-Provera, emergency contraception, and Norplant. Injectable Depo-Provera and the morning-after pill for emergency contraception were well-known but, until the nineties, unapproved. Now they are accepted choices. Here is how the latest contraceptives work.

Depo-Provera

Depo-Provera is an injectable synthetic progesterone called progestin depot medroxyprodesterone acetate (DMPA). A long-acting progesterone (because it is suspended in tiny crystals in a solution), Depo-Provera gives three months of contraceptive protection. The influx of progesterone, the pregnancy hormone, sends the brain a false message that pregnancy exists. The brain hormones respond by inhibiting ovulation and therefore stopping menstruation. A woman's ovaries relax. On occasion there might be breakthrough bleeding before the next three-month injection, so some doctors, to avoid a patient's staining, administer Depo-Provera every six to eight weeks.

Actually, a heavy woman produces a high amount of estrogen from her fatty tissue that might stimulate the buildup of her uterine lining. She might experience more breakthrough bleeding than the thin woman, who has less estrogen and less chance of increased endometrial tissue. The heavy woman might need an injection every six to eight weeks, while the thin woman might respond well to three-month doses.

Depo-Provera was available in ninety countries before it was approved in the United States in 1992. Debate over its cancer-causing potential was at the heart of the delay. Today, it has been found that Depo-Provera does not increase a woman's risk of developing PID, benign fibrocystic breast disease, and ovarian cysts.

On the "down" side, however, Depo-Provera might slightly increase the risk of breast cancer for women who begin taking the contraceptive when they are under age thirty-five. Other side effects that might be experienced by some women include weight gain, depression and mood changes, breakthrough bleeding, and abnormal bone loss in women over age thirty-five who have taken the drug for more than five years. Depo-Provera is not the contraceptive of choice for every woman, but if a woman is taking injectable Depo-Provera under the supervision of a doctor, her health should not be threatened. Here is a three-month contraception option requiring only one dose.

Emergency Contraception—the Morning-After Pill

For years, women and their doctors have been aware of emergency contraception (EC), better known as the morning-after pill, which is really two large doses of regular birth control pills taken within seventy-two hours of unprotected intercourse. Depending on the brand, two or four pills are taken, and then twelve hours later are taken again. In 1997 the FDA sanctioned six brands of birth control pills for morning-after use. Then, in 1998, the agency approved the four-pill Preven Emergency Contraceptive Kit, available by prescription and the first pills solely designated for EC. This is a historic approval.

As with traditional EC, Preven works by inhibiting ovulation, blocking fertilization, and/or stopping a fertilized egg from implanting itself in a woman's uterus. Preven pills have the same hormonal contents (ethinyl estradiol and levonorgestrel) of oral contraceptives already on the market. They are 75 percent effective in preventing pregnancy (only 2 out of 100 women become pregnant as opposed to 8 out of 100 with no EC). In fact, before a woman takes Preven pills she must take a pregnancy test to make sure she has not conceived. The pills are effective after sexual intercourse, providing no pregnancy is confirmed. If taken after conception, the pills will not work. Women who suffer from liver disease, blood clots, cardiovascular disease, or other circulatory problems should not take the pills because serious side effects such as blood clot, stroke, or heart attack might occur. For a day or two after taking Preven, a woman might experience nausea and vomiting, but these side effects disappear. More information about Preven is available on the web at www.PREVEN.com or toll-free at 1-888-PREVEN2.

If a woman does not have a doctor she can turn to for EC, she can call the EC hotline (1-888-NOT-2-LATE) or visit the web site (www.opr.princeton.edu/ec) for information and referrals to doctors who can write prescriptions for EC.

Norplant

FDA-approved in December 1990, Norplant has a failure rate of less than 1 percent and is one of the most effective contraceptives ever put on the market. Norplant is comprised of six silicone rods, each about the size of a matchstick. In a fifteen-minute procedure using a local anesthetic, the doctor makes an incision one-tenth of an inch long on the inside of a woman's upper arm. He implants the six soft rods in a fanlike design under the skin. The rods release the synthetic progesterone hormone progestin, which provides birth control for five years.

Norplant has come under fire from women who reported that they suffered pain and scarring when the rods were removed. This has led to a drop in Norplant's popularity, but studies show that this problem is virtually nonexistent when specially trained doctors and nurse practitioners perform the removal.

Norplant is effective birth control with side effects similar to Depo-Provera's. Norplant's most common side effects are a change in the length and intensity of menstrual flow and breakthrough bleeding during the first year. Other less frequent side effects include weight gain, headaches, mood changes, and depression. Researchers are still investigating Norplant's relationship to reproductive cancers, but it is expected that Norplant will lower rates of PID, benign fibrocystic breast disease, and ovarian cysts.

Women who are interested can locate trained doctors by contacting Norplant's maker, Wyeth-Ayerst, toll free at 1-800-934-5556, or by calling their local chapter of Planned Parenthood.

INTO THE FUTURE

The Chinese Birth Control Pill for Men

Contraception for woman is aimed at controlling the release of one egg a month. In men, contraception means controlling the release of millions of sperm, produced daily.

In the United States, scientists have experimented with injections of antibodies to the brain hormones LH and FSH, which are responsible for the production of both testosterone, the male hormone, and sperm. Administered to rats, such vaccines have lowered sperm counts to zero, but they have also eliminated the secondary sex characteristics. Male rats have shrunk and lost their hair, their aggressive instincts, and their potency.

Researchers have also attempted to use danazol, the synthetic male hormone used as treatment for endometriosis in women, in combination with testosterone for contraception in men. Sperm counts have dropped; however, the combination of these two drugs is very expensive and has never gained popularity. Studies with the danazol compound have been stopped. Other research continues, but a big problem with sterilizing a man is that it is difficult to lower sperm production without seriously tampering with the secretion of testosterone and altering masculine traits.

The solution might come from China, where *gossypol,* an extract from the seeds of the cotton plant, has been rendering Chinese peasants infertile for years. U.S. scientists have recently discovered that gossypol inhibits an enzyme that is essential to the function of sperm. Gossypol supposedly decreases sperm maturation. If this maturation is slowed, the sperm will not grow to become fertile. Thus, gossypol attacks sperm but does not affect the male hormone. Virility remains while fertility drops. The Chinese claim a 99.8 percent rate of effectiveness with gossypol.

Unfortunately, the men in China's Hebeth Province who were taking the gossypol, while they were infertile, were also suffering from heart irregularities. Cardiac arrests and deaths occurred. Gossypol is a fatty substance, a lipid that can accumulate in the tissue for a long time and thus possibly build up and cause problems. The Chinese feel that the substance, still, is safe. It has not been found to be cancer-causing. Tests for acceptability have shown that in high doses the gossypol can cause cardiac irregularity and, sometimes, death, while low doses might lead to loss of appetite, anemia, reduction in growth rate, vomiting, and diarrhea.

The world production of cotton seed equals approximately 78,000 tons of gossypol a year, which means that mass production certainly could be cheap and enough gossypol could be produced to create birth control for all the men on the planet. Perhaps the future of male contraception, however, will come from the male contraceptive pill being tested in Scotland, China, South Africa, and Nigeria by Organon Pharmaceuticals. This pill has no circulatory side effects as it introduces hormones into the bloodstream that stop the production of sperm. It is predicted to be available in 2005.

The Contraceptive Ring

Studies are under way for the contraceptive vaginal ring, which releases the same hormones contained in birth control pills, estrogen and synthetic progesterone, progestin. Developed by Organon Pharmaceuticals, the contraceptive ring remains in a woman's vagina for three weeks out of the month and offers pregnancy protection similar to that of the pill. Women who have participated in a study report that the ring is easy to insert, comfortable, and not at all noticeable during sexual intercourse.

The contraceptive ring is said to have fewer side effects than the pill, but it might bring on more pronounced ovulation pain, as well as occasional vaginal discharge and irritation. Women over thirty-five who smoke and cannot take the pill might be candidates for the contraceptive ring.

THE IDEAL CONTRACEPTIVE

There is a continued search for safer and more effective methods of contraception, but the ideal contraceptive still does not exist. Steroid implants, vaginal rings, antipregnancy vaccines, techniques to destroy the corpus luteum after ovulation, and prostaglandins for menstrual induction have been and still are under investigation. Future research is focusing on inhibiting sperm or egg maturation with as few side effects as possible.

Scientists at the University of Maryland School of Medicine are analyzing a natural protein produced by the body that curbs the development of the oocyte, the female egg cell. This "oocyte maturation inhibitor" (OMI) does not damage egg cells but permanently arrests their growth. Women ovulate, but the released egg is immature and unable to be fertilized. However, with ovulation actually taking place, neither the menstrual cycle nor the hormonal balance is affected, as they have been with the birth control pill. OMI might also work to inhibit sperm growth without affecting a man's hormonal balance.

It is impossible to predict how people will prevent pregnancy in years to come. The creation of an OMI-type contraceptive appears very likely, but it might be some time before such a product is on the market. Today a woman and her partner must, with all their awareness, choose from the available contraceptives the one that fits their lives. There is no reason for a woman to conceive an unwanted pregnancy unless her contraceptive fails her, and the responsibility for contraception should not be hers alone.

Effective birth control needs a combined effort from a woman and her man. In this age when sexual relations involve a condom for prevention of sexually transmitted diseases, choice of birth control is more easily and openly discussed between partners. For pregnancy prevention and STD protection, trust and support are needed more than ever before.

13.

Menopause—How to Demystify This Natural Process

JUST ANOTHER PHASE

After passing through adolescence, most adults can look back on difficult but memorable times. We might view menopause as being, like adolescence, just another phase, another life passage with highs and lows but without the confusion. As adults with awareness, women and men need not be as baffled by the changes of menopause as they once were by the early signs of their sexuality. Today, there is increased medical knowledge about the natural process of menopause, which is why we know, for instance, that menopause is not a passage for women only. Men are not spared the physical and emotional changes of a menopause, which for them is often called the midlife crisis. In fact, considering that menopause is inevitable, both sexes might decide to enjoy themselves, to think positively about this phase, which has been historically and mistakenly regarded as "terrible."

DEFINING MENOPAUSE

Menopause, which comes from the Greek *mens,* meaning "monthly," and *pausa,* meaning "stop," is the time when a woman's monthly menstrual period comes to a halt. When we speak about menopause, we are talking about the changes that occur in a woman after she stops menstruating.

Menopause can last anywhere from one year to several years, varying from one woman to another. It is the time when a woman might experience well-known change-of-life symptoms such as hot flashes, hot flushes, dry skin, backaches, and other problems associated with declining estrogen levels. Some women, particularly women who have no obvious symptoms of menopause, might never know when menopause begins and ends because they are able to pass through this phase with little or only minimal discomfort.

The time prior to the complete cessation of menstruation, when a woman is noticing a change in her menstrual pattern due to the natural decline in her female hormones, is called *perimenopause*. This is a time when a woman might see irregular or so-called dysfunctional uterine bleeding. During the perimenopause, a woman might also experience mild menopausal symptoms—hot flashes, hot flushes, depression, aches, and pains. The perimenopause can last anywhere from a few months to several years, although some women never experience this phase at all—one day they just stop menstruating and enter menopause.

The *postmenopause* begins after menopause and lasts the rest of a woman's life. This is the time when all the physical and emotional change-of-life symptoms have completely disappeared and a woman feels that her body is maintaining a steady, even balance.

Many women today are pleased when menopause arrives because they are no longer burdened with pregnancy worries and they are free from the hassle of monthly menstruation. Men in their corresponding "menopauses" have reached maturity, acquired knowledge, and, one hopes, "found themselves."

Since both sexes undergo changes in midlife, a comparison of the events that men and women might experience seems appropriate. Although a man's change-of-life is not quite as apparent as the change-of-life in a woman, when cessation of menstruation is a clear sign, we must realize that everyone shares an evolution into maturity.

The male hormone testosterone peaks in a man during his early twenties. Then, testosterone slowly decreases until a man reaches the age of forty, when the hormone rapidly begins to drop. Some men might feel the effects of the diminishing testosterone while they are in their thirties, while others experience nothing until their forties. Eventually, a man might feel that he is becoming weaker, more tired, less virile. He might become afraid of growing old. Men usually are much more worried about aging than women. In fact, often men can fearfully describe the approach of their fortieth birthdays as the coming of "the Big Four-Oh." Unsure of what will happen to him, a man views that fortieth birthday with trepidation. And his nervousness might be justified, because if he is not willing to take care of himself he might develop the so-called middle-aged spread and even lose interest in sex. With all his fretting, however, a man never has to rise above all the change-of-life "scare" stories that haunt women.

Myths about female menopause abound. Negative descriptions of "the change" are passed down through generations, and it's about time we begin to demystify these tales. Proper nutrition, exercise, and a healthy, positive mental attitude can help women overcome change-of-life difficulties and, indeed, eliminate them. The real facts about the menopausal phase of life should actually create a peaceful state of mind. Women do not have to steel themselves for menopause. They can relax into it.

The word *climacteric* has been used to describe all the physical, emotional, and psychological changes that a woman was expected to experience during menopause, but this term is extremely negative. *Climacteric* implies that a woman, before menopause, has reached the culmination of her potential and thereafter can expect to drop to a terrible low. After a climax in her life, a woman is expected to settle into some over-the-hill phase! This is not true, and the word *climacteric* should no longer be used. One should speak optimistically about reaching menopause, or maturity, without surrounding those words with negative jargon.

Menopause is, if it is not surgically induced, a gradual process that, like adolescence, takes some time, possibly from one to ten years. In the past, women would often experience menopause in their late forties, but more and more women today are not noticing signs of menopause until they are in their early fifties or older. Improved nutrition, exercise, and healthier mental outlooks are keeping women in better condition. A woman today can expect to menstruate longer than the women in previous generations of her family used to.

By the time menopause arrives, as mentioned earlier, many women feel that the life change is liberating—no more birth control. And women who are busy, who have positive attitudes, many interests, or engrossing jobs, and who are physically and sexually active, have no or only minimal discomfort. They are able to move through menopause without physical or emotional difficulties. Remember, contrary to most myths, many menopausal women feel pleased and relieved. They need no longer worry about menstrual problems and birth control. They know menopause is not an illness, misfortune, or disability. Menopause is just another phase of life that should be enjoyed as much as any other phase.

WHEN MENOPAUSE IS UNNATURAL

There are two occasions when the change-of-life is induced and definitely not natural: surgical menopause and traumatic menopause.

Surgical Menopause. Surgical menopause can be a horrifying event in a woman's life if she is unprepared because her doctor never informed her about what would happen when she underwent an operation that involved surgical "castration." A hysterectomy (removal of the uterus) in which both ovaries are also removed is just such an operation. Female ovaries and male testicles are both gonads, sexual glands responsible for vitality, potency, and the essence of feminine and masculine traits. If the gonads are removed during castration, strength, energy, and the typically masculine or feminine physique will diminish and potency will disappear. A man will develop feminine characteristics and a woman will lose the fullness of her breasts and hips—and she might even begin to grow a beard.

Men are extremely aware of and worried about their testicles. They protect their genitals and safeguard their masculinity because they fear castration. They know what eunuchs look like. However, when it comes to castration of women through oophorectomy, removal of the ovaries, very few women and practically no men understand the serious consequences.

After a woman has had her ovaries removed in combination with a hysterectomy,[1] she will instantly enter menopause. She will never again experience her menstruation. And if she is not given hormone replacement immediately, her symptoms might be much more intensified than those associated with natural menopause because the process is sudden and the effects are speeded up.

Once the ovaries, which produce female hormones and eggs, are surgically excised, female hormone production stops. A woman whose ovaries normally would have functioned into her mid-fifties will, if she has had an oophorectomy before then, find herself without natural female hormone production. She might have felt fine previously, but now she might find herself overcome with hot flushes, backache, and depression. Often women who are put into surgical menopause will gain weight because they are distraught, do not feel well, and have difficulty being disciplined about diet. Fatigue and loss of energy are also intensified after surgical menopause. Plus, a woman's metabolism changes, and normal calorie intake suddenly adds weight. Increased body weight might then lead to high blood pressure and even heart disease if care is not taken. Due to all the grave potential problems associated with surgical menopause, a woman should make every effort to keep her reproductive system intact. A premenopausal woman should explore every possible alternative before having her ovaries removed.

When the possibility of hysterectomy is presented to a premenopausal woman, she should always seek a second or even a third opinion, and she should always try, if possible, to hold on to her organs.

Traumatic Menopause. A crisis, severe stress, or the sudden loss of a loved one can send a woman into such a shock situation that her brain hormones, FSH and LH, stop functioning and give up directing the ovaries through a normal menstrual cycle. When this happens, a woman's ovaries will abruptly atrophy and no longer produce the female hormones estrogen and progesterone. Women in their thirties and forties, when thrown into such extremely stressful states, will, as the hormone production ceases, stop menstruating and often develop increased anxiety accompanied by such physical changes as sagging skin, aches, constipation, headaches, occasionally even hot flushes and other problems associated with menopause.

Knowing that traumatic menopause might occur, a woman who has been hurled one of life's horrible surprises might try to fortify herself with B-vitamin supplementation. The B vitamins, acting like coenzymes, help convey nerve transmissions that might aid in triggering the resumption of the menstrual cycle. An increase in vitamin B-complex containing vitamin B_6, in an amount of at least 100 to 500 mg daily, might help reverse traumatic menopause, especially if a woman is fit and follows a healthy diet. By realizing that cessation of menstruation could be induced by stress, a woman discovers a truth that will enable her to halt and even reverse the process. With proper nutrition, rest, and reduction of stress through exercise and meditation—possibly yoga—a woman might be able to resume her menstruation and end traumatic menopause.

WHAT HAPPENS DURING NATURAL MENOPAUSE?

Although improved nutrition and healthier lifestyles have somewhat lengthened menstruation in women, heredity still is a significant influence. A woman often begins menstruating at the same age that her mother did, and notices menopause at the same time that her mother became aware of the change.

In the natural course of life, the ovaries reach the end of their life spans and begin to decrease their levels of estrogen production in a woman's middle age. It is as if nature let the ovaries know that a woman's body is no longer strong enough to cope with the strain of childbearing. Menopause, actually, is preserving a woman's longevity by guaranteeing her a natural contraception. Anyway, as estrogen diminishes, the interaction that this female hormone usually has with the brain hormones FSH and LH changes. The brain hormones, which aid the timing of menstruation, flow differently during menopause and a woman might no longer experience her usual cycle. Her menstrual flow might thicken and the length of time between periods might become erratic. In some women, periods just become shorter and shorter until they disappear altogether. Menstrual patterns during menopause might be different altogether. Menstrual patterns during menopause might be different for different women, but every middle-aged woman thinks about menopause when she has skipped periods, irregular periods, prolonged bleeding, or continuing abnormalities in her menstrual cycle. Any of these menstrual changes represent the first sign of menopause.

However, women in their forties should be cautioned to refrain from concluding immediately that they have menopause if their cycles change. A woman of any age might experience menstrual irregularity when she is under stress, when she exercises, or when she gains or loses weight. Sometimes unusual menstrual patterns are signals of declining fertility but not necessarily the throes of menopause. A woman should examine other possibilities before she considers herself menopausal. If she still has good skin tone and does not have abnormal hot flushes, backaches, or increased arthritis, she is most likely far away from menopause. Her menstrual abnormality could be due to, among other things, a changing lifestyle or stress.

While periods are irregular and hormones are readjusting, some menopausal women might experience various emotional and physical symptoms. Some might have hot flashes[2] or hot flushes[3] along with an anxiety or depression reminiscent of premenstrual syndrome. It is estimated that approximately 75 percent of all women going through menopause experience some form of discomfort. Some of this discomfort is caused by the fluctuations of the brain hormones FSH and LH. These brain hormones probably have a direct effect on the involuntary muscles that have the power to constrict or expand the vessels controlling the blood flow throughout the body. The heart and the intestines might also be affected by these brain hormones.

As it decreases after menopause, estrogen, which generally controls the secretions of the FSH and LH (see chapter 3), can no longer regulate the production of these brain hormones. The brain, not understanding the biological goings-on, will increase the release of FSH and LH in order to spur the ovaries to produce estrogen. In a menstruating woman, the ovarian production of estrogen will block the brain hormone, but after menopause, the ovaries will not manufacture enough estrogen to block the FSH/LH. When there is no estrogen to curtail them, FSH and LH surge to higher and higher levels in extra attempts to increase the estrogen. It is these high levels of brain hormones that will trigger the hot flashes and hot flushes.

Woman on estrogen or hormone replacement therapy (ERT/HRT) can find relief from hot flashes and hot flushes because the estrogen will block the release of the brain hormones FSH and LH, which will then return to normal levels. (The safety of ERT/HRT is discussed later on in this chapter.) However, there are other ways to curb the surge of the brain hormones. A regular physical exercise routine such as swimming, bicycling, or jogging might, if it is performed with some exertion, decrease FSH/LH levels and subsequently reduce or eliminate menopausal symptoms. Furthermore, good nutrition might lead to conversion of the body's fatty tissue into estrogen and influence the adrenals to release estrogen. The female hormone might, in turn, curb the FSH/LH rush. A diet high in nature's phytoestrogens (*phyto* meaning "plant"), rich in soy, carrots, peas, beans, cruciferous vegetables, whole grains, berries, and flaxseed, has been reported to relieve hot flashes and help to improve cholesterol counts and increase bone density.

Generally, hot flushes might continue for years after menstruation stops, although the severity of the symptoms will vary from one woman to another. Subsequently, the FSH and LH might decline, but by then a woman's body will probably have adjusted to the presence of higher levels of these brain hormones.

Another effect of the cessation of menstruation is that the uterus and ovaries will shrink. The decline of estrogen will result in some sagging of the skin and some dryness in the vagina. More seriously, diminished estrogen can lead to a calcium depletion from the bones that could result in joint pain, back pain, and eventually *osteoporosis*, a weakness of the bones, particularly in the spine and the legs. Osteoporosis might bring on the collapse of the vertebrae and a compression of the spinal column, which puts pressure on the spinal nerves and causes increased backache and also causes a woman to appear to shrink in size. (Osteoporosis is discussed in more detail later on in this chapter.)

While a woman is going through menopause, she should use contraception. A period can sometimes occur almost a year after a woman has considered her menstruation over. In fact, some doctors ask their patients to use birth control for a year after they have what they think are the last periods of their lives to prevent conceiving a change-of-life baby.

It is important to emphasize that not every woman experiences every symptom of menopause, and in fact, some 25 percent of the women who go through menopause do not even know they're having a change-of-life. They're barely uncomfortable. Other women, through no fault of their own, must live with physical and psychological ups and downs that make them feel like they're strangers in their own skins. Sometimes, they might be. Adolescence sometimes makes teenagers crazy but they get over it, and women too will overcome menopausal unpleasantness. The symptoms of menopause are only temporary. They end after a time, and a woman who stays interested in life and activity will also travel through this life passage and begin her postmenopausal life with spirit.

Menopause in the Overweight Woman

Women of above average weight will usually experience less severe menopausal symptoms because the fatty tissue in their bodies will enhance production of estrogen, the female hormone. It's almost as if nature, in order to make menopause easier, changed the source of estrogen production from the ovary in a fertile woman to the body tissue and body fat in the menopausal woman. In this way, a woman still will have estrogen production to make her body function properly, but she will not run the risk of pregnancy.

In the overweight woman, estrogen is produced from the body's fatty tissue by conversion of a biologically inactive male hormone called androstenedione, which is available in higher concentration in obese or aging women. Androstenedione is known as an estrogen precursor because it is a hormone from which estrogen might be derived. In the menopausal woman, this androstenedione is converted, in body fat, into endogenous estrogen, which is estrogen produced by the ovaries. Another estrogen precursor, estrone, which is in cholesterol, activates the conversion of androstenedione, a derivative of cholesterol, into estrogen. In other words, cholesterol, which is in high concentration in fatty tissue, provides a great store of estrone, which, in turn, affects the androstenedione. The result is a constant supply of estrogen that lessens menopausal symptoms in the overweight woman. Estrogen from the ovaries might have stopped, but the overweight woman is producing so much of the hormone in other parts of her body that she is counterbalancing her loss. The change-of-life should be smoother for her than for a thin woman who is below the normal weight for her height.

Women should not rush to gain weight to avoid the symptoms of menopause, however, because the overweight woman runs a higher than average risk of developing both breast cancer and endometrial cancer. The estrogen converted from fatty tissue gives a permanent and continuous stimulation to the endometrium, the uterine lining. The lining can thicken into a condition called *hyperplasia*, which might precede cancer. The converted estrogen is also stimulating breast tissue continually. During a normal menstrual phase in a pre-menopausal woman's life, progesterone curbs this overstimulation, breaks down the uterine lining, and brings about menstruation, a natural cleansing of the uterus. Progesterone also gives the breasts a rest from continuous estrogen stimulation. However, during menopause, progesterone is no longer available to keep the hormonal balance.

Too much body fat is just as problematic as too little. Every woman should understand that to avoid unpleasant side effects during menopause, and to keep mind and body at their best, an average body weight, one that she knows is ideal, should be maintained.

Menopause in the Fit Woman and in the Thin Woman

Problems might arise for fit and thin women, depending on the fat-to-muscle ratio of their bodies. A moderate complement of body fat enables a woman to produce just enough estrogen to curb serious menopausal problems. A lack of body fat can inhibit estrogen conversion and stimulate symptoms.

A woman who is suffering severe menopausal symptoms, which can include hot flashes, vaginal dryness, urinary frequency, thinning skin and bones, and mood swings, can initially strive for hormonal balance and relief from debilitating conditions through natural means. A disciplined exercise regimen, which can include a combination of activities such as swimming, weight-training, bicycling, running, and workouts on cardiovascular exercise equipment for an hour a day, three times a week, can help with hormonal adjustment. Exercise can help the body create a hormonal balance that alters estrogenic activity.

The next variable is diet. Certain plant foods contain phytoestrogens, chemicals in plants that are similar in molecular structure to a woman's own estrogen. These phytoestrogens might be helpful in diminishing menopausal symptoms because they trick the body into recognizing them as human estrogens, and the body responds accordingly. Soy (tofu, soy milk, soybeans, tempeh) is high in phytoestrogens, but they also appear in a variety of fruits, vegetables, and whole grains. One daily four-to-twelve-ounce serving of a soy food seems to be enough to generate health benefits. Soy supplements, which might include calcium and vitamin D to battle bone-thinning osteoporosis, are available in health food stores, but I recommend eating whole foods, with their full complement of phytochemicals, as much as possible.

If a woman does not experience natural relief, some type of hormone replacement therapy might be an option (see pages 445 to 450 for the pros and cons of HRT). A number of estrogens and progesterones exist, and a woman who chooses HRT often finds herself mixing and matching different types to find the ones that make her feel best. Since taking estrogen alone increases a woman's chance of developing endometrial (uterine) cancer, only women who have had hysterectomies are advised to use estrogen replacement therapy (ERT), either through the pill or a skin patch. Other women who are interested in exploring HRT can elect *cyclical therapy*: daily estrogen through pill or patch, accompanied by a separate progesterone pill for a set number of days per month; or *continuous therapy*: estrogen and a low-dose progesterone combined in one or two daily pills or in the CombiPatch for the skin.

WHAT IS OSTEOPOROSIS?

If a woman has osteoporosis, her bones physically change. Estrogen stimulates a constant supply of calcium to the bones, and when the estrogen level drops after menopause a woman's bones might thin down and become fragile. The bones remain normal in chemical composition but they diminish in density. A progressive loss of bone mass can continue until the skeleton is no longer strong enough to support itself. When that happens, bones might begin to collapse and spontaneously fracture. A woman might appear to shrink.

About 25 percent of all postmenopausal women are affected by this disorder. Postmenopausal osteoporosis, in fact, accounts for most of the cases of osteoporosis that exist among both women and men. A reduction in testosterone after forty might encourage bone weakening and osteoporosis in a man, but his condition will not be as severe as a woman's can be. Ultimately, a man might lose about 20 percent of his bone mass, but a woman can lose one third. If her osteoporosis results from surgical menopause, a woman might suffer a more severe condition than if she had had a natural menopause. During natural menopause, bone mass loss is slow, but after surgical menopause everything happens quickly and in the extreme. Osteoporosis might also be much more severe among women who already have calcium deficiencies, who lead sedentary lives with no exercise, or who smoke.

Osteoporosis usually begins with low backache or increased incidence of fractures of the lower forearm, upper thigh, or vertebrae. Bones break more easily because, as mentioned before, calcium depletion has weakened them. A slight fall, one a woman might not have previously considered dangerous, might cause her limbs to fracture. Even if she is not troubled by breaking bones, a woman might experience increasing backache when she bends. She might also become an arthritis sufferer.

At first, osteoporosis is silent, thinning the bones before back pains and fractures surface. For every woman in menopause, I recommend a bone density test. One of the best is the dual energy X-ray absorptiometry (DEXA), a double beam of low-level X rays that picture bone density at two sites, such as wrist and hip. With certain machines, images can also be made of the hand and foot to determine the need for calcium.

Can Osteoporosis Be Prevented and Treated?

One of the best ways to prevent severe osteoporosis is to avoid hysterectomy with removal of the ovaries, which brings on surgical menopause.

During natural menopause, a woman might prevent a severe case of osteoporosis if she maintains a balance of calcium and phosphorus in her body. Certain foods such as cottage cheese, spinach, lobster, milk, and spaghetti contain varying quantities of these two minerals. In addition, approximately 1,500 mg of calcium carbonate should be taken daily in combination with magnesium, 750 mg; vitamin D, at least 400 units; and zinc, 30 mg. Fluoride tablets help strengthen teeth and bones, and vitamin E—800 to 1,000 units daily—might also improve the bones, although there has not been any documented evidence to prove that vitamin E works to combat osteoporosis. (If a woman chooses to take vitamin E, she should also add extra vitamin C to her regime since the body's supply of vitamin C is somewhat depleted by vitamin E.) Since most refined foods have been robbed of vitamin B, a vitamin B-complex containing vitamin B_6 would complete this supplementary regimen.

A woman might fight osteoporosis with a diet including the calcium-rich foods mentioned earlier; dairy products, sardines with skin, dark green leafy vegetables such as kale and collard greens, and bone-building soy foods (tofu, miso, tempeh, soy milk, and soybeans). Weight-training and resistance exercises are top bone builders, but any four-hour workout over the course of a week strengthens a woman's skeleton.

If a bone density test shows that natural measures have no effect on a woman's osteoporosis, she might choose ERT (if she has had a hysterectomy), HRT, or a therapy that minimizes the possible increased risk of breast cancer found with current ERT/HRT: a low dose (0.03 mg) of estrogen alone or in combination with progesterone; calcium carbonate, 1,500 mg; magnesium, 750 mg; and vitamin D, 400 IU. An exciting, targeted estrogen called raloxifene, brand name Evista (see pages 450 to 451), increases bone density and lowers the risk of breast cancer by 76 percent, but should only be used postmenopausally since it intensifies hot flashes. A nonhormonal drug, alendronate sodium, brand name Fosamax, cuts the risk of fractures in half, builds bone, and has no cancerous side effects (see page 451). Fosamax can be used by women whether they are on ERT/HRT or not.

QUESTIONS ABOUT MENOPAUSE

I have received a great number of letters from women who have asked questions about menopause. Their queries show that fears, confusions, and myths about the change-of-life are very deep-seated. I hope the answers to the following letters will help women of all ages to understand this time of life more clearly.

Does It Really Have to Be That Bad?

I am a thirteen-year-old girl who just read that when women reach menopause, they grow facial hair, gain weight, their voices deepen, their breasts dry up, and their genitals shrink. The book I am reading says that women were originally intended to live less than forty years, so that when modern medicine increased life span, they began to outlive their usefulness as women. The only answer is estrogen. I was naturally horrified to think that this is what awaits me. My mother and grandmother tell me it's not true, but they are not doctors, so maybe they don't know. I hope that you will answer this letter and put my fears to rest.

—S.P., Nashville, Tennessee

Menopause is a natural maturing process, a change in bodily function that until recently has been greatly misunderstood. The problems that might come from menopause must be demystified because there is no reason a thirteen-year-old like Ms. P. should think she has something so terrible ahead of her.

It is true that estrogen decreases during menopause. The male hormone testosterone, which every woman produces in her adrenal glands and ovaries, also drops, but at a slower rate. As a result of the reemphasis of the hormones, some women might notice that they are hairier than they used to be, but hirsutism and a deepening voice are not high on the list of menopausal symptoms. More women are concerned with hot flashes, night sweats, sleep deprivation, and vaginal dryness. Today's researchers have labored to find ways to treat these symptoms, and by the time Ms. P. reaches midlife the conditions of menopause might have been entirely eradicated.

At the beginning of the twenty-first century, women are more aware of natural ways of calming menopausal symptoms through vitamin supplementation, diet, and exercise (see page 439). Along with natural methods, ERT and HRT have good track records for relief, but estrogen taken alone increases the risk of endometrial (uterine) cancer, and whether taken alone or in combination with other hormones, estrogen slightly increases the risk of breast cancer. Researchers are busy creating selective estrogen receptor modulators (SERMS) such as raloxifene (Evista), which will offer the benefits of estrogen without the worries (see pages 450 to 451). A recent study shows that raloxifene actually reduces the risk of breast cancer by 76 percent. With all this, menopause is becoming a new and different passage in a woman's life. Most important by far is that Ms. P. stays fit and maintains a diet high in fresh fruits, vegetables, and whole grains. Feeling fit and eating healthfully are two powerful ways to minimize the effects of menopause.

How Early Does Menopause Start?

A year ago I started having muscle and joint pain in my limbs, lower back, shoulders, and neck. I am thirty-seven years old and up until this started, I considered myself healthy. I went to a family doctor who put me on Valium, which didn't help. Then I visited an orthopedist who fitted me with a cervical collar, took X rays, gave me Librium, and suggested a neurologist. Instead, I went to my gynecologist and asked him if I could be going through menopause. He laughed and said I was "far too young." I left and went to the neurologist, who admitted me to the hospital, did a G.I. series, diagnosed a pinched nerve, and put me on Valium again. Then I went to a chiropractor for the pinched nerve. None of these doctors know what is really wrong with me. But I do. I really think I might be going through menopause even though I still have periods. What else could be happening to me?

—N.N., Louisville, Kentucky

It is highly unlikely that a woman of thirty-seven would go into the change-of-life. Since heredity does have some influence on the process, if Ms. N.'s mother or other females in her family began menopause at young ages, there might be some possibility of an early start. However, as mentioned before, improved nutrition, advanced health care, and greater understanding of their bodies have caused women to enter menopause at older ages than in previous generations. If Ms. N. expects that she will go into menopause early because her mother did, the emotional stress alone could block her brain hormones so that her ovaries begin to produce less estrogen. Then she might find herself with some of the problems of menopause.

Ms. N. does not say whether her periods are irregular. If her menstrual pattern has changed at all, with the backache and, possibly, other symptoms, she might be suffering traumatic menopause, a stress-induced condition. She has been through a lot with all her doctor visits, and she might be able to reduce her stress with vitamin supplements. She might be helped by vitamin E, 800 to 1,000 units a day; vitamin D, 400 units a day; calcium, 100 to 500 mg a day; and possibly zinc, 50 mg a day, and vitamin C, 1,000 mg a day.

By taking extra vitamins and enrolling in exercise or relaxation programs such as stretching or yoga classes, she might change the way her body feels. I do not believe that a woman would generally have menopause at age thirty-seven, although it becomes a rare possibility when heredity is a factor. I think Ms. N., if she tries to combat her symptoms, might be able to reverse her situation.

How Long Does Menopause Last?

I am seventy years old and I have had hot flashes ever since I started menopause at age fifty. My doctor prescribed Premarin pills, but I stopped them because years ago I started to bleed and the flashes weren't affected. What can I do? How long does menopause last anyway?

—L.W., Columbus, Ohio

The symptoms of menopause vary from woman to woman, and they can last from one year to, as in this woman's case, twenty years. Some women, particularly those who are very busy with work and families, seem to sail through the change. A woman who is in her sixties or seventies today is biologically much younger than she would have been in the past. Ms. W. should try to counter her problem, because she certainly does not want her activities curtailed by hot flashes.

Vitamin supplementation, as described in the answer to the preceding letter, is the natural way to start attacking the symptoms. First, I would try this natural approach with a diet and exercise program as described on page 439. If that doesn't work, I would suggest low doses of hormones. Sometimes progesterone, such as Provera, one or two 10-mg tablets daily for a week to ten days, might help to alleviate symptoms. Progesterone does not cause uterine cancer, but instead shrinks the uterine lining. Then, there are cases in which women have benefited from a minimal amount of the male hormone testosterone, which keeps a positive bone balance by building calcium in the bones. The male hormone also strengthens a woman's body by increasing her metabolic rate. The natural approach, and then, possibly, hormones, might change Ms. W.'s twenty-year condition.

Sexual Desire and Menopause

I'm fifty-two and going through the change. Sometimes it seems as if my organs are turning around and my whole body is just worn out. I've been married almost thirty years and I love my husband very much, but I'm just not interested in sex much

*anymore. If we have intercourse once a month, that's fine with me.
I used to be more sexually active. Will I ever be that way again?*
—A.G., East Meadow, New York

Most women find somewhat of a decline in sexual responsiveness due to menopause, but their desires are usually not as diminished as Ms. G.'s. Since estrogen declines, vaginal tissue does not become as moist as it used to during sexual stimulation. A woman, therefore, might find that she occasionally takes longer than usual to achieve orgasm, but the difference is only between seconds and minutes. If a woman becomes exceptionally dry in her vagina, intercourse might not be pleasurable for her or her partner and she might try an over-the-counter lubricant such as Replens, Astroglide, or K-Y Jelly. Inserted vaginally, these lubricants last from forty-eight to seventy-two hours.

The Kegel exercise—squeezing together or tightening the vaginal muscles—should be a daily routine for menopausal women. Performed at least twenty times a day, this isometric exercise will strengthen a woman's vagina and tighten its grip on the penis.

Ms. G. might also consider a prescription vaginal estrogen cream such as Estrace or Premarin. A small amount of estrogen cream, inserted vaginally every day for three weeks, and then used continually two or three times a week, increases blood flow to the vagina, strengthens the vaginal walls, improves the pH balance, and relieves the pain of intercourse. Also available is a prescription doughnut-shaped device, Estring, which can be inserted vaginally for ninety days of continuous estrogen release. The level of estrogen is so low that experts do not believe it increases a woman's chance of developing endometrial or breast cancers.

If these measures do not affect Ms. G.'s diminished libido, then testosterone might help. Research shows that adding a little testosterone to estrogen can improve sex drive. Estratest tablets are a combination of esterified estrogens and methyltestosterone, and can be prescribed by a doctor as part of a woman's hormone replacement therapy. Unless a woman has had a hysterectomy, progesterone can be recommended to prevent increased risk of endometrial cancer. Testosterone's side effects might include acne and liver disease, so a woman should consult her physician about whether this hormone, in tablets or cream, is right for her.

What Vitamins Can I Take After Surgical Menopause?

A year ago I had a complete hysterectomy due to endometriosis. I am thirty-four years old and I've only been married five years. I am very worried about this change that is being forced upon me and I would like to know if there is anything I can do about it. Are there any vitamins I can take to help me with the symptoms of surgical menopause?

—C.B., Palm Springs, California

The vitamin regime explained in the "How Early Does Menopause Start?" section of this chapter (see page 441) is designed to boost the body's mineral level and to diminish the onset of osteoporosis, hot flashes, and anxiety. Ms. B. might follow this regimen, and she might also avoid coffee, tea, chocolate, and caffeine-containing soft drinks, since caffeine has been found to deplete calcium in the bones. And once a calcium loss sets in, so might osteoporosis.

However, Ms. B. might do all this and still experience severe symptoms from surgical menopause. It has recently been learned that 0.3 mg, a low dose, of estrogen (available in Estratab), along with calcium (such as in Tums tablets) and vitamin D supplements, offers the bone-building benefits of estrogen and lessens unpleasant side effects such as headaches, nausea, and breast tenderness.

Is Hormone Replacement Therapy Safe?

I am a fifty-five-year-old woman who has been in good health until recently, when I started going through the change. My menstruation has been irregular for the last year and I have not seen my period in six months. I'm beginning to feel hot flushes and sometimes I wake up in a sweat in the middle of the night. Emotionally, I'm like a walking disaster. I'm becoming depressed more and more frequently, and I'm very hard on my husband. He tries to be understanding, but how can he understand me when sometimes I don't even understand myself? I asked my doctor what I could do to find relief and he wanted to put me on hormones. I've heard so many bad things about hormones that I don't want to take them. However, my symptoms are getting worse and when I called the doctor the other day he said he would not see me unless I agreed to take hormones. Do I really have to take them?

—M.J., Boynton Beach, Florida

No woman should be forced into any type of treatment. If Ms. J. wants to agree to hormone replacement, the choice is hers. Her hesitation is understandable, however, because there has been much publicity about the association between ERT/HRT and cancer.

When estrogen replacement therapy was first popularized, women often were given synthetic estrogens indiscriminately. Women who were taking estrogen felt wonderful; they had good skin tones, moist vaginas, and no hot flashes or hot flushes. They would occasionally have menstrual-type spotting or bleeding during the ERT, but there *appeared* to be very few problems associated with the hormone treatment. Doctors began to prescribe hormones such as Premarin in high doses as soon as women complained of fatigue or other menstrual difficulties. *There is no doubt that too many hormones were prescribed in doses that were too high for too long.* At a time when almost every woman with menopause was given ERT, reports began to emerge that some women who were on very high amounts of estrogen for years without pause developed endometrial cancer (cancer of the uterine lining).

Eventually progestin, synthetic progesterone, was prescribed with estrogen to form hormone replacement therapy (HRT). Progesterone stimulated a sloughing off of the endometrial tissue (the uterine lining) built up by estrogen and prevented endometrial cancer from developing. Women experienced periodic vaginal bleeding similar to menstruation. A woman who has had a hysterectomy can remain on ERT-estrogen alone in a pill or a patch—since she has no uterus at risk.

Traditional HRT is cyclic. A doctor prescribes an estrogen replacement medication in pill or patch to be taken from the first of each month to the twenty-fifth. A pill form of progesterone is taken from the sixteenth to the twenty-fifth of each month. Then, from the twenty-sixth to the end of the month, no medication is taken, and a woman might bleed and release uterine tissue. Newer HRT is offered as continuous therapy, estrogen plus low-dose progesterone taken in one or two pills every day. A woman on continuous therapy does not bleed, but she might have a higher risk of endometrial cancer.

There are different types of estrogens and progesterones available for hormone replacement today. In patches worn on the skin, natural estradiol is available in the Alora, Esclim, and Vivelle patches, and new patches seem to appear on the market every day. In pills, Premarin is estrogen derived from the urine of pregnant mares; Estrace is a natural estradiol; Estratab comes from modified soy estrogens; Cenestin is a tablet of conjugated estrogens derived from plants. Provera is a synthetic progesterone synthesized from plants, while Prometrium is a natural micronized progesterone from a natural plant compound. Does a woman find relief from hot flashes but experience headache, nausea, dizziness, and bloatedness on a certain type of estrogen or a certain estrogen/progesterone combination? Women coping with menopause do not want to feel worse than they do, and often it takes a few months of working with their doctors and adjusting hormone levels before the right combination is found.

Once on ERT/HRT a woman can gain health benefits—and health concerns. As for benefits, estrogen brings relief from the symptoms of menopause such as hot flashes, mood swings, night sweats, vaginal dryness, thinning skin and hair; the hormone reduces bone loss and the risk of osteoporosis; favorably affects cholesterol, and might improve memory and mental functioning.

Health concerns include the issue of whether or not HRT protects against heart disease; an increased risk of endometrial cancer, which can be offset when progesterone is included in HRT; and an increased risk of breast cancer.

It is no longer certain that HRT protects against heart disease. In early 2000, in the Hormone Replacement Therapy trial of the Women's Health Initiative (a huge federal study of approximately 25,000 healthy, postmenopausal women), a surprising event occured. The women in the study were assigned to take either HRT or placebo medication, and those on the hormone replacement had slightly more heart attacks, strokes, and blood clots in their legs and lungs than those on placebos. The number of women who experienced these symptoms was small, less than 1 percent, but this was enough for the study's investigators to feel they had to inform the women and the public during the course of the study. Other studies have reported that the estrogen in HRT helps to protect against heart attacks, so this finding was surprising. The issue of estrogen's relationship to heart disease is a health concern to be weighed by any woman considering HRT. Whether a woman chooses hormone replacement is a matter of balance for her to decide. She will alleviate menopausal syptoms, but she must consider her health history.

Research studying breast cancer as a health concern has shown, until recently, that women on HRT for five years or less have a risk of developing beast cancer 1.8 times greater than women who never used HRT, and women on HRT for over five years have 2.65 times the risk. It was always thought that estrogen was the hormone having the greatest effect on breast cancer development, but now it appears the progesterone may have an effect as well. A study of over 46,000 women, conducted by the National Cancer Institute, has shown that women who take combination estrogen/progestin HRT increase their risk of developing breast cancer by 8 percent per year if they continue hormone use for four or more years. Women who take estrogen alone have an increased risk of only 1 percent annually.

However, in a study of over 37,000 women, researchers discovered that the breast cancers developed by women on HRT were less common, less risky types such as medullary, papillary, tubular, and mucinous tumors, which offer good prognoses. Estrogen might also stimulate existing fibroids and endometriosis; increase a woman's risk of developing gallstones and blood clots; and lead to weight gain.

Weighing the pros and cons is an individual balancing act for every woman. I feel that when ERT/HRT becomes necessary, a woman should be placed on the lowest dose of hormones that will control her symptoms. The natural approach to symptom relief, using diet, exercise, and vitamin supplementation, should always be tried first.

What Is the Best HRT?

I started menopause about five years ago when I was forty-five, and my doctor put me on hormones. He gave me .625-milligram tablets of estrogen, Premarin, along with progesterone. He told me to take this estrogen tablet alone for twenty-one days each month and then to combine it with the progesterone, Provera, a 10-milligram tablet, which he asked me to take for the last ten days of the cycle along with the Premarin. Then he said I should stop all the pills for one week before I return to my routine again. I did exactly what he said and I have felt terrific. In the week off I bleed. I have been on this regimen a long time. I understand there are now pills that don't cause a period. Should I switch?

                                              —A.D., Toms River, New Jersey

Ms. D.'s cyclical HRT, an estrogen/progesterone combination, mimics the hormonal fluctuation of a normal menstrual cycle and increases a woman's sense of well-being. When progesterone is given in the form of Provera, it will normally lead to a monthly bleeding when it is stopped. At the end of the twenty-one-day cycle of estrogen followed by estrogen/progesterone, a woman should expect to menstruate. This bleeding is actually beneficial because the uterine lining is being shed. If progesterone had not been given, the estrogen alone could thicken the uterine lining and this overstimulation of the uterine lining could possibly lead to endometrial cancer. Thus, Ms. D.'s periodic vaginal bleeding is healthy.

There is continuous HRT available today using estrogen plus low-dose progesterone daily in one or two pills or in a CombiPatch. A woman is said to receive some protection against endometrial cancer without the annoyance of monthly bleeding, although the amount of protection compared to that of cyclic HRT is not known since continuous HRT is relatively new.

The hormone replacement a woman chooses depends on her individual health profile and how she responds to different types of hormones. Ms. D. seems to have done well on her present regimen but I do not believe that a woman has to take hormones all the time. Ms. D. might stop HRT for a while, eat a well-balanced diet, exercise regularly, take vitamin supplements, and see how she feels. If she wants to return to HRT, she might try low-dose estrogen (0.3 mg) combined with 100 mg of natural progesterone, or 2.5 to 5 mg of Provera daily, supplemented with calcium, magnesium, vitamin D, and zinc (see page 442).

ABOUT "TARGETED ESTROGENS" AND MENOPAUSE

The terms "targeted estrogens" or "designer estrogens" or SERMS (for Selective Estrogen Receptor Modulators) all stand for man-made estrogens, tailored to do good without doing harm. The first approved targeted estrogen was tamoxifen, which blocks estrogen receptors in the breasts and lowers the risk of developing estrogen-dependent tumors.

In 1997, the FDA approved *raloxifene*, brand name Evista, for the prevention of osteoporosis. Raloxifene works by binding to estrogen receptors in bone. Its benefits also include a lowering of total and LDL (bad) cholesterol—and, amazingly, raloxifene has been shown to lower the risk of breast cancer by 76 percent (more research is under way to find out whether this effect is long-lasting). Yet while raloxifene is without estrogen's increased risk of developing breast cancer, it does not have many of estrogen's benefits. Raloxifene does not raise HDL (good) cholesterol, relieve hot flashes, help prevent memory loss, protect skin tone, or prevent vaginal dryness. Also, raloxifene cannot be used by women who have a history of phlebitis—in rare cases, it might lead to a potentially fatal blood clot. Yet for women who are not suffering hot flashes, and who want bone-building benefits without an increased risk of breast cancer, raloxifene is an option. It is a customized hormone, paving the way for more targeted options to come.

NOTE: Bone-thinning osteoporosis can also be battled with *alendronate sodium*, brand name Fosamax. This nonhormonal drug reduces the activity of the cells that cause bone loss and offers a bone-building effect comparable to HRT. Just how long the power of Fosamax lasts is under study. After menopause, no matter what option a woman chooses, she should be alert to her need for extra calcium, magnesium, vitamin D, and zinc (see page 442), and resistance exercise for her upper and lower body.

How Long Can I Stay on Hormones After a Hysterectomy?

I had a complete hysterectomy when I was thirty-six and I was put on Premarin. Now I'm fifty-four, so I've been taking Premarin for eighteen years. My skin looks good and I have no problems, but I'm worried about being on hormones for all these years. Once I tried to quit but my husband said my disposition was awful, so I went back on the pills. Will these hormones be harmful to me? How long can a woman safely stay on hormones after a hysterectomy?
—C.W., Anoka, Minnesota

This woman was subjected to surgical menopause after a hysterectomy with removal of both ovaries. By taking Premarin after her surgery she prevented her body from enduring abrupt change and she stopped osteoporosis from weakening her bones. She does not seem to have had any problems with the Premarin. Generally, the main worry with Premarin is endometrial cancer, but since Ms. W. does not have a uterus, she need not concern herself with uterine cancer.

However, since Ms. W. now is fifty-four she might not need hormone replacement anymore. She should try to stop the Premarin, use vitamin supplementation, eat well-balanced meals, and see if she can do without the hormones. Some women will experience no menopausal symptoms when they stop estrogen after the age of fifty, while others will feel hot flashes and hot flushes. Women who continue to suffer might need to resume ERT, but they can probably curb their symptoms by taking lower doses of the estrogen.

If Ms. W. does not think she can handle menopausal symptoms without estrogen, she might, for a short time, return to Premarin but in a lower dose than she had previously been taking. She may also try Cenestin, a natural plant-derived estrogen in patches worn on the skin. Hormones can be used for a few months and then stopped for a few months. They do not have to be taken all the time. A woman should judge how she feels when she is on and off hormones. Remember, though, studies show a slight increase in breast cancer with hormone replacement, and this remains a concern. When estrogen is taken for up to five years, a woman's risk increases 1.8 times more than if she never used hormones. After five years, she has 2.65 times the risk. The fact that the diagnosed breast cancers are more treatable is not necessarily comforting. On the other hand, the positive cardiovascular effects of hormones should be weighed.

In general, after hysterectomies women can safely stay on ERT, with estrogen given in the lowest possible dose, until they are fifty, the time when estrogen production would begin to decline naturally. After age fifty, a woman who has had a hysterectomy might follow the advice given to Ms. W.

Is Hair Loss a Part of Menopause?

I had a tubal ligation this year at age forty-two. Up until I was forty I took birth control pills. I stopped the pills, had my tubes tied, and now I'm starting to lose my hair. My doctor says he might have to put me on hormones. I don't understand. Is my hair loss due to my surgery or could I possibly be starting menopause?

—L.S., Blair, Nebraska

After years on the pill, it might take Ms. S.'s own hormones some time to return to normal. Her hair loss might be from her readjusting hormones, but it might also be due to her tubal ligation. When the tubes are tied, blood supply to the ovaries often decreases and causes some women to have menopausal symptoms earlier than they normally would.

Women with menopausal symptoms often do lose their hair. When a woman notices her hair falling out, she should tell her doctor, who should, before he does anything else, check her thyroid. A sluggish thyroid gland, which can be corrected with thyroid medication, might be the cause of the problem. Also, supplementary B vitamins, head massages, and exercise might improve the condition.

If a woman cannot stop her hair loss with natural measures, and if thyroid medication does not help, she might need a low dose of estrogen to aid in hormone adjustment. Even after childbirth, when hormonal levels are shifting, some women have tendencies to lose their hair. Women will not become bald, however. Hair might thin, but it will not disappear.

Menopause vs. Premenstrual Syndrome (PMS)

I am a forty-two-year-old woman who had tubal sterilization four years ago. My menstruation has become increasingly irregular in the last year and I haven't had a period in three months. I gained at least fifteen pounds in the last year and my stomach is bloated. I feel like all the blood is pushing my stomach out. I'm beginning to be depressed and I have hot, sweaty nights. What is happening to me? Could I be going through menopause?

—F.P., New Orleans, Louisiana

This woman is most likely *not* in menopause. Her menstrual irregularity could be the result of her weight gain, or it might be related to her tubal sterilization. Many women who experience menstrual irregularity, depression, and weight gain in the forties immediately assume that because they feel different they are in menopause. Usually these women are not premenopausal (or perimenopausal), but they are suffering varying degrees of premenstrual syndrome.

Women in their forties who have gained weight or who have had tubal ligations often experience the symptoms of premenstrual syndrome, because both weight gain and sterilization cause hormonal imbalances leading to PMS. It's important that women realize the difference between premenstrual syndrome and menopause, because the two conditions require opposing treatments.

Ms. P., who is probably experiencing premenstrual syndrome, might cut down her salt intake and take extra vitamin B-complex with B_6, or be prescribed progesterone medication, if needed (see chapter 4 for more details). When it comes to hormonal therapy, there is a marked difference in the way premenstrual syndrome and menopause are treated. When a woman is suffering from PMS, her estrogen becomes too potent in relation to her progesterone, and her hormonal treatment, if needed, should be progesterone. On the other hand, a woman with menopausal symptoms so severe that hormone treatment is indicated might need estrogen to curb her symptoms. Thus, if a wrong diagnosis is rendered and the wrong medication is given, a woman's condition might worsen rather than improve.

Therefore, a woman in her forties should consider the possibility of premenstrual syndrome before she concludes that she is entering menopause when she notices menstrual irregularity. When a woman in her forties has gained weight or has undergone tubal sterilization, she is more likely a candidate for PMS than for menopause.

My Doctor Cares and It Makes a Difference

I am in the change-of-life. My doctor is very understanding and when I first noticed menopause, he explained what was happening

in a way that I could understand. He encouraged my husband to
accompany me on office visits and he told my husband just what I
was going through. His patience has made this whole transition so
much easier for me. He has recommended HRT to me, but he never
pushes me to stay on medication. There is a wonderful communi-
cation between my doctor, my husband, and myself. Having my
husband in on the change is such a blessing. I hope other women
find understanding doctors who will include their husbands in
their changes.

—G.G., Banning, California

It is important that everyone in the family understand what a woman is going through when she enters menopause. A husband and wife might even try to diet, exercise, and take vitamins together during her change. Making it through menopause can be a mutual effort. It is encouraging to learn that doctors are bringing husbands into the change and are educating both partners together.

Every woman reacts differently to menopause, and every woman should be aware of her symptoms and know the latest ways to alleviate her problems. I encourage women to try natural methods of symptom relief through diet, exercise, and vitamin supplementation before turning to hormone replacement. If symptoms are severe, or if a woman's health history indicates a high risk of osteoporosis or heart disease, she might need ERT/HRT. She should be aware that there are several types of estrogen and progesterone to choose from, and she might require different combinations and dosages before she finds the right pairing for her. She should take her time. If her main concern is preventing osteoporosis, options such as raloxifene/Evista and alendronate sodium/Fosamax should also be on her list to consider.

The entire process of menopause must be viewed as a natural course of events, a maturing made easy when a woman's family, friends, and most of all, her doctor are communicative and compassionate.

14.

Vaginitis and Sexually Transmitted Diseases (Including HIV/AIDS)

Vaginitis is a catchall name for a variety of vaginal infections that are, at times, sexually transmitted. When a woman has a vaginal irritation with itching, burning, or odor, she might fear a sexually transmitted disease (STD), when, indeed, she might only be suffering from a more bothersome but less physically harmful vaginitis. In contrast, a woman who thinks that an STD could not happen to her might, with similar symptoms, be an unknowing carrier.

The confusion over whether a vaginal infection is an STD is created by the fact that the symptoms can be very vague. Then, there are the causes to consider. Vaginitis does not have to be related to sex; it can be triggered by a number of conditions, including emotional stress. On the other hand, a sexually transmitted disease—which in the past was always known as a venereal disease (VD)—is very rarely spread by anything other than sexual intercourse.

Symptoms and causes of vaginitis and sexually transmitted diseases might at first appear to be identical, but there are distinct differences, and treatments are far from matching. The only way we can achieve a complete cure of vaginitis and bring an end to the spread of STDs is through in-depth education, knowledge, and understanding of these diseases.

WHEN TO WORRY ABOUT
VAGINAL DISCHARGE

Most vaginal discharges are normal, physiologically necessary, and always changing due to hormonal fluctuations during the monthly menstrual cycle.

Right after menstruation, a woman will have little excess moistness in her vagina. A woman will be dry in comparison to other times during the cycle. However, as the middle of the menstrual month and ovulation approach, the female hormone estrogen increases and promotes vaginal secretion. A woman will be wetter, and sometimes she can have a discharge that is so abundant she must wear tampons or pads. Women who have high estrogen levels experience excessive secretions, but they usually know themselves so well that they do not worry when they notice heavy discharges once a month. Women who are in tune with their bodies correctly interpret their secretions as healthy signs, but other women, not understanding how their bodies function, become extremely concerned about vaginal secretions. The added wetness, which every woman experiences to some degree each month, is nature's way of enhancing the vaginal environment for the movement of sperm toward conception.

After ovulation, the progesterone hormone increases and inhibits the amount of vaginal secretion. A woman will feel less of a discharge and because her vagina is somewhat drier, she might have less natural lubrication during sexual intercourse. Every woman should make an effort to recognize her own vaginal changes in order to know when a discharge should be considered normal or strange.

Women who use IUDs usually have slight watery discharges in addition to the vaginal secretions that vary according to their menstrual cycles. An IUD irritates the uterus and leads to this increased secretion. A woman should not worry about the altered secretion unless the discharge becomes abnormal. Then, she might ask her doctor to treat the discharge or to remove the IUD, if the device is the cause of her problem.

Women who use diaphragms can sometimes have vaginal irritations and discharges if the contraceptive remains in the vagina for a particularly long time. A vaginal problem due to a diaphragm might be either cystitis or vaginitis. (There have even been a few cases of toxic shock syndrome in association with diaphragm use; see chapter 6.) Suspecting one of these conditions, a woman should have her doctor check whether the diaphragm is sized correctly. When cystitis or vaginitis persist with the use of a diaphragm, the size of the contraceptive must be changed, or if switching to a new-size diaphragm makes no improvements in the vagina, another form of contraception must be found.

A change in vaginal odor often causes a woman to think that she has caught vaginitis or a sexually transmitted disease when, in fact, this different smell could be the result of natural body odors from her present diet. Has she recently eaten spicy, garlic-seasoned foods? Exotic foods? Her whole aroma might change. The pores of the skin and all orifices emit odors from the foods we choose to consume. Urine will smell differently due to shifts in a woman's diet, and her vaginal secretions will respond in kind to what is put into her body.

Thus, any different smell or secretion should not immediately make a woman push the panic button. She should try to evaluate the causes of these conditions by educating herself to her normal vaginal secretions. When she notices changes in discharge or odor, she should consider the causes mentioned above before she becomes concerned about a sexually transmitted disease. She might also pay attention to her age, because as a woman grows older vaginal changes and menstrual irregularity are setting the stage for menopause.

If she cannot pinpoint any reasons for her vaginal changes, a woman should consider the possibility that she might have vaginitis or a sexually transmitted disease, and then she should contact her doctor for further tests.

WHAT IS VAGINITIS?

Vaginitis occurs when parasitic microorganisms such as fungi, protozoa, or bacteria invade the vaginal environment and irritate or inflame the sensitive walls of the vagina. As vaginitis takes hold, a woman will notice an excessive vaginal discharge which can cause pain and itching. The three most common types of vaginitis are: moniliasis, caused by the fungus *Monilia albicans,* also called *Candida albicans;* trichomoniasis, caused by the protozoan *Trichomonas vaginalis;* and bacterial vaginosis (BV), formerly called *Hemophilus vaginalis* (vaginitis), or *Gardnerella vaginalis* (vaginitis). These three kinds of vaginitis are easy to recognize and a woman should try to understand the characteristics of these infections in order to give herself some insurance against improper treatment.

Monilia or Candida Albicans, *the Most Common Complaint*

There are several fungi residing in the vagina, but only the *Candida albicans,* which is more commonly referred to as Monilia, has the potential for causing problems. In healthy individuals this organism is ordinarily found in the mouth and in the gastrointestinal and genital tracts. *Candida albicans* can be isolated from the vagina in approximately 25 percent of all women who have no symptoms of vaginal infection. It is only when the vaginal milieu is changed that the fungi begin to multiply and cause severe symptoms of infection.

The vagina houses a delicately balanced store of microorganisms, bacteria, and yeast. The *Candida albicans* is a gram-positive yeastlike fungus. The most common bacteria in the vagina is the Döderlein's bacillus and it is the stability of this bacillus that prevents the proliferation of the fungal yeast. The Döderlein's bacillus's main function is to keep the vaginal environment acidic, with a pH balance between 4.5 and 5.0. When acidity is maintained at this level, the spread of yeast is restrained. However, if the acid level in the vagina drops, the fungus begins to multiply and cause symptoms such as discharge, irritation, itching, or odor.

To prevent the spread of *Candida albicans,* a woman should make a mental note of the ways in which the vaginal acidic balance can be upset and cause problems:

- Antibiotics can change a woman's body chemistry and kill the Döderlein's bacilli. As the bacilli die off, the pH increases and the *Candida albicans* breed.
- A weight gain or an increase in the level of a woman's blood sugar can also affect her vaginal environment. Women who are prediabetic or diabetic have a high rate of vaginal infection due to their increased levels of blood sugar.
- The birth control pill, which creates a sort of pseudo-pregnancy state, might unbalance the vaginal milieu.
- Pregnancy, with its hormonal changes, makes a woman prey to the abnormal growth of *Candida albicans.*
- Stress might cause hormonal shifts that disrupt the vaginal situation.
- Women who are on hormone replacement therapy during menopause might find that their vaginas are more conducive sites for the breeding of Monilia.
- The constant wearing of airtight panty hose or tight pants might also promote the breeding of yeast.
- It must not be forgotten that Monilia/*Candida albicans* can also be sexually transmitted.

A fungal yeast infection, once it develops, has different symptoms and treatments than protozoan or bacterial infections.

*Symptoms of Monilia/*Candida Albicans. A woman can detect a Monilia infection by holding a mirror to her vaginal area and examining the vulva. Monilia makes the outer lips of the vagina bright red and swollen. If a woman is in the habit of wearing airtight panty hose or tight pants or jeans, the inflammation might spread from the vagina down and around to the anal area. The redness and swelling will also be inside the vagina, and a frothy white discharge, similar to curdled milk or cottage cheese, will be evident. A woman might see the discharge on her panties and then, when she looks at her vagina with a mirror, the lumpy white secretion will be easy to spot.

As the *Candida albicans* grow, the vaginal walls become more inflamed and a woman feels an incredible itch. When she scratches, she can break the skin and worsen the infection. Sometimes a Monilia infection can be so severe that a small ulceration on the vulva occurs and a woman finds it painful to walk.

Along with the redness, swelling, discharge, and itch, a woman might notice a disagreeable yeast smell emanating from her vagina.

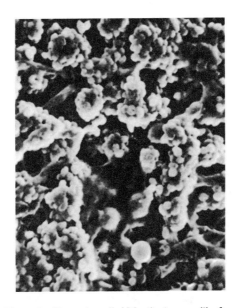

*15-1 **Candida albicans.** C. albicans,* also called Monilia, is a yeastlike fungus that commonly inhabits the mouth and gastrointestinal and genital tracts. Approximately 25 percent of asymptomatic carriers have been found to have *C. albicans* in their vaginas. When symptoms do occur, a woman experiences a cheeselike discharge and a vaginal itch. The monilia multiplies under various pathological conditions such as diabetes or during excessive sugar intake. When women take antibiotics, become pregnant, or use birth control pills, monilia might also proliferate. The picture illustrates the *C. albicans* as viewed under a scanning electron microscope. The fungus has been enlarged 700 times. *Reprinted by permission. From Breen, James L., M.D., and Smith, Charles I., M.D. "Sexually Transmitted Diseases—Part I,"* The Female Patient, *July 1981.*

The symptoms of Monilia/*Candida albicans* are uncomfortable and unpleasant, but this particular type of vaginitis remains in the outer portion of the vagina and proper treatment, although it requires knowledge, patience, and time, can cure it.

*How is Monilia/*Candida Albicans *Treated?* A woman who is suffering from what she thinks is moniliasis must visit her doctor immediately. The physician will take a culture to diagnose her condition, and once he confirms the spread of *Candida albicans,* his first reaction should be to recommend an antiyeast suppository or cream. Doctors used to prescribe these medications, but today products to fight yeast infections, such as Monistat, are sold over-the-counter. Other medications are Mycostatin, Vanobid, Gyne-Lotrimin, Myocel-G, and Terazol. Suppositories or creams must be inserted deep into the vagina once or twice a day to stop the spread of *C. albicans.* Diflucan (fluconazole) can be effective in a single 150-mg tablet, although sometimes Diflucan must be taken for a couple of days. Mycolog, a cream that combines antiyeast and cortisone medications, makes the outer lips of the vulva less sore. The goal is to restore the vagina to its natural environment, first with antiyeast medication, and then by taking healthful measures. A woman might be advised to avoid unventilated panty hose and tight jeans and slacks, which enclose the infected area and encourage the fungi to spread. When she is at home, in between the insertion of creams and suppositories, a woman might try to air her vagina by not wearing panties at all.

A woman might add yogurt to her diet, since yogurt contains lactobacillus, a healthy bacteria that helps return the pH balance to the vagina. Women who do not like yogurt might purchase acidophilus—yogurt culture—capsules at vitamin counters in quality drugstores or in health food stores. Since sweets, which elevate the blood sugar level, upset the vaginal acidity, a woman should also cut down on desserts, candies, sugary snacks, and sugar in general. A douche with vinegar and water (two tablespoons of white vinegar to a one-quart douche bag of lukewarm water), once a day every two or three days for one or two weeks, puts acid back into the vagina and aids in subduing the *Candida albicans.*

In addition, certain physical circumstances, if changed, can help to cure Monilia infections and stop them from returning. If a woman is prediabetic, she could probably eliminate her infection by controlling her diabetes. A pregnant woman will find that her vagina spontaneously improves after the birth of her child. If the birth control pill is the cause of a woman's problem, a different contraceptive might be in order.

The treatment of a Monilia infection aims at restoring the vagina to its natural environment, first with antiyeast medication, and then by eliminating conditions that might cause the vaginitis to recur. Sometimes a woman needs weeks of treatment before her moniliasis is under control.

During the treatment phase a woman should avoid sexual intercourse, because a yeast infection can sometimes be sexually transmitted. In fact, to avoid reinfecting her, the partner of a woman who has moniliasis should also be treated for a yeast infection.

Trichomoniasis

Trichomoniasis, the second most common vaginitis, is characterized by a greenish white or yellowish discharge that causes a foul smell. A woman might detect an odor when she sits down or crosses her legs. She might become upset and embarrassed when she realizes that the odor is hers, but she should be thankful that she has been given a sign of trichomoniasis, possibly before the condition becomes severe.

Unlike the *Candida albicans* fungi, which are naturally present in the vagina, the *Trichomoniasis vaginalis* protozoa are not harbored in a healthy body. *Trichomonas is always sexually transmitted.* The infection can be asymptomatic in men, who pass it on without realizing that they are carriers.

Sometimes a woman might be the recipient of a trichomoniasis infection that is discovered when it shows up on a routine Pap test.

More frequently, a few weeks after the trichomoniasis is transmitted, the protozoa proliferate to the extent that they cause discharge, odor, and itching that send a woman to her doctor. A woman's vagina becomes red and sore with trichomoniasis, and if the infection is not treated the itching can become almost intolerable. Irritation and pain can even spread into the abdomen, and a woman can feel fatigued and sick all over.

A doctor can confirm the presence of trichomoniasis by taking a sample of the vaginal discharge, placing it on a slide with a drop of saline solution, and examining it under a microscope. The trichomoniasis protozoa, or trichomonads, are pear-shaped microorganisms with tails called flagella that briskly move back and forth to propel the protozoa all over the medium. The trichomonads look like a bunch of amusement park bumper cars all constantly moving and bouncing off one another. They are easy to spot under a microscope, which is why they show up so readily when a Pap smear is evaluated.

How Is Trichomoniasis Treated? The most effective treatment for trichomoniasis is Flagyl (metronidazole), taken in a dose of 500-mg tablets twice a day for seven days, or 250 mg three times a day for 100 days, or a single 2-gram dose. The single-dose treatment requires a woman's sex partner or partners to be treated, too, even if they show no symptoms, or the woman can be reinfected. The drug clotrimazole can be used if a woman has an allergic reaction to Flagyl. Metrogel, vaginal gel, can also be used successfully.

Flagyl has a 90 percent cure rate; it is the prime treatment for trichomoniasis, but it is not without its detractions. Alcoholic beverages must be completely avoided when a woman or a man takes Flagyl because, when mixed, alcohol and Flagyl can make a person extremely dizzy, nauseated, and ill. Also, reports have shown that fetal abnormalities have occurred in the offspring of pregnant laboratory animals who were given Flagyl. There has never been any human birth defect directly related to Flagyl, but it is recommended that a woman not take the drug during the first three months of a pregnancy, and if possible, Flagyl should be avoided until pregnancy is over. Betadine, a povidone-iodine douche, is recommended for a pregnant woman with trichomoniasis, but if the douche does not bring relief, she might, as a last resort, used Flagyl vaginal suppositories to treat the infection.

Although reports have indicated that cancer has developed in laboratory animals who received high doses of Flagyl, there has been no evidence that Flagyl is carcinogenic in humans. Flagyl is still the best treatment for trichomoniasis. However, a woman should try to reduce her exposure to the drug by making sure that her sexual contacts seek treatment and do not reinfect her. Sometimes a man who has no sign of sickness does not want to take medicine. Whether trichomoniasis shows up in his semen analysis or not, he should willingly take the prescribed medicine.

Bacterial Vaginosis

Bacterial vaginosis (BV), used to be called *Hemophilus vaginalis* vaginitis and then *Gardnerella vaginalis* vaginitis (in deference to Dr. Herman Gardner, the gynecologist who described the symptoms of *Hemophilus vaginalis* vaginitis back in 1954). This particular bacterial infection has also been called *Corynebacterium vaginale*. Only the name, not the disease, has changed.

BV, or Gardnerella, is a bacterial infection that produces a grayish white discharge with an extremely unpleasant odor. The Gardnerella bacteria *do not* irritate the walls of the vagina, so there is no itching, swelling, or redness in the vaginal area—only a discharge less abundant than the discharge associated with trichomoniasis, and a smell.

Like the *Candida albicans* fungi, the Gardnerella bacteria can reside within the vagina without causing vaginitis. A study conducted among hundreds of college students found that young women with no sexual experience were harboring the Gardnerella bacteria. It is possible that in the close quarters of college dormitories, the microorganism could have been transferred through means other than sexual intercourse. Shared clothing and linens might be factors to consider. However, it is rare to find symptoms in women who have not been sexually active. *Bacterial vaginosis, or Gardnerella, is considered a sexually transmitted disease.* Usually, a woman and her partner both have the infection, although the man might not have symptoms.

A doctor can diagnose the vaginitis by taking a sample of a woman's vaginal secretion, examining it under a microscope, and identifying Gardnerella's characteristic "clue cells" (these cells sometimes show up in women who have no symptoms of infection). Studies have also shown that a whiff test leads to an exceptionally accurate diagnosis. A doctor adds potassium hydroxide (KOH) to his slide sample, and if a fishy odor emanates he can be close to 100 percent sure that his patient's vaginitis is Gardnerella.

How Is Bacterial Vaginosis Treated? Controversy exists over the treatment of bacterial vaginosis. Should an asymptomatic woman be treated? Does the male sexual partner have to be treated? Although there is evidence of sexual transmission, studies have not proven that there is a reduced rate of BV recurrence in women whose partners were treated. Also, half of the women with BV do not have symptoms. The main complaint from women who do have symptoms is an odorous vaginal discharge.

BV has often been treated with topical sulfa remedies, but many studies have shown that these are not very effective. There is a long list of remedies that do not work well: triple-sulfa creams, the antibiotics erythromycin and tetracycline, acetic acid gel, povidone-iodine douche—these are not the choice treatments for bacterial vaginosis.

The preferred treatment is Flagyl (metronidazole), 500 mg a day for seven days, or 250 mg three times a day for ten days, along with topical vaginal applications of clindamycin cream, 2 percent, at bedtime for seven days, or metronidazole gel (Metrogel), 0.75 percent, once a day for five days. As an alternate treatment, in tablets, a woman might also take 2 grams of Flagyl as a single dose in a single day, or clindamycin, 150 mg, two or three times daily for seven days.

A woman who has been diagnosed with BV might still be spreading the infection if her doctor is prescribing only topical sulfa creams to her. Some physicians believe in treating this condition with anti-biotics in combination with antiyeast or sulfa cures. This approach might work in some cases; however, studies have indicated that Flagyl, the same drug used to cure trichomoniasis, is the most effective treatment for BV.

Other Aspects of Bacterial Vaginosis. It used to be thought that if a woman's vaginal discharge did not reveal moniliasis, trichomoniasis, or gonorrhea (see page 486) when it was examined under a microscope, a woman had "nonspecific vaginitis." The 1954 reports of Gardner and Dukes showed that many women with this nonspecific vaginitis had a common bacillus that produced *Gardnerella vaginalis* vaginitis (now called bacterial vaginosis).

Recently it has appeared that some forms of vaginitis are related to the presence of other bacteria such as colibacilli, or *E. coli,* and possibly T-mycoplasma. These bacteria alone do not cause vaginitis symptoms, but physicians are beginning to link them with vaginitis and, in turn, connect them with problems of infertility and miscarriage. Vibramycin, a 10-mg tablet taken twice a day for ten to twenty days, is advised for a woman and a man who are having an infertility problem caused by T-mycoplasma.

If a woman who is diagnosed as having nonspecific vaginitis is emitting a grayish white, foul-smelling vaginal discharge and her vaginal pH is between 5 and 5.5, she most likely has Gardnerella, or BV. A doctor can confirm this by extracting a vaginal smear from a woman's discharge, placing the smear on a slide with a drop of saline solution, and examining his sample under the microscope. Gardnerella is identified by short motile rods and so-called "clue cells," which are easy to spot under microscopic magnification.

A woman who has been told that she has a vaginitis that is difficult to diagnose should ask her doctor to check her for BV/Gardnerella and examine her discharge for the bacteria. If a woman does not feel that her vaginitis has been thoroughly diagnosed, she might consult another physician.

QUESTIONS ABOUT VAGINITIS

How Can I Get Rid of My Vaginitis?

I have had a very heavy discharge ever since my son was born four years ago. I've been to five different doctors and none of them have been able to help me. In fact, one of them just said that I should consider myself lucky that I had more than enough wetness. "Just think if you had none," he said. "You'd be in big trouble." I can't stand it. I have to wear a pad all the time and the discharge has an offensive smell. It's embarrassing, uncomfortable, and every so often an itch comes over me, sometimes when I'm in public, and I feel like I'm going to die. I've been treated for the itch but it doesn't go away. Also, I am a borderline diabetic and I am overweight. I dread the thought of going to Doctor Number Six and not getting any satisfaction while I keep spending money. Will I ever be cured?
—A.R., Minford, Ohio

First, this woman must work on her prediabetic condition. Since she is prediabetic, her blood sugar level is probably higher than average, a situation that promotes vaginal infection. She might control her prediabetic state with the proper sugar-free diet, which might also help her to lose weight.

A weight gain or loss can affect the vaginal environment. Ms. R.'s vaginitis appears to have started after her pregnancy, when she had lost weight, but perhaps soon after childbirth she gained weight and her vaginal environment never had a chance to stabilize. If this woman can control her prediabetes with diet or diet and medication, she will also be helping herself to lose weight. She must, however, do both things—control the prediabetes and lose weight.

Ms. R.'s main goal should be to restore her vaginal environment to its natural balance. She most likely is suffering with a Monilia/ *Candida albicans* infection, and she might read the "How Is Monilia/ *Candida Albicans* Treated?" section of this chapter (pages 462 to

463). As mentioned there, the friendly bacilli in yogurt or acidophilus capsules help to change the composition of the vaginal milieu. Ms. R. might try the yogurt or acidophilus, and she might also douche with vinegar and water, as also described in the section on moniliasis, since this particular mixture introduces needed acidity into the vagina. While she is working on her vaginal situation, Ms. R. should avoid airtight panty hose, leotards, and tight jeans and slacks, all of which promote the spread of vaginitis.

While Ms. R. is doing everything she can to make her vagina healthy, a doctor might treat her with antifungal creams or suppositories, some of which are listed in the previously noted treatment section. Ms. R. might need prolonged medication, perhaps for two or three weeks at a time, to make sure that the abnormal fungi are subdued.

Ms. R. must understand the *cause* of her vaginitis and treat the cause, not the symptoms. When she does find that her vagina has become normal and healthy again, she should be very careful to keep her blood sugar low and her weight down. Becoming her own strict physician, she must try to prevent a recurrence of the vaginitis that has plagued her.

I'm Premenopausal; Could That Be the Cause of My Vaginitis?

I am fifty-two years old and for the past year I have been bothered by a cloudy white discharge. I do not have itching, burning, or pain, but when I get up in the morning, the discharge is there. I douche with white vinegar and water, and the discharge seems to clear up for the rest of the day, but it doesn't disappear. The next day, there it is, back again. I've also noticed that my periods are not as regular as they used to be and I think that the change might be coming. Could menopause be the reason for my discharge? Or do I have an incurable yeast infection? I've been to three doctors, I've used AVC cream and Monistat, but nothing seems to work.

—E.A., Vidor, Texas

It could be that the change-of-life has led to a lower estrogen level in Ms. A.'s body, and a drop in estrogen might cause a different type of vaginal discharge or irritation. Although myth has it that all vaginitis goes away during menopause, some menopausal and post-menopausal women do develop moniliasis or bacterial vaginosis.

As recommended in chapter 13, Ms. A. might take vitamins and exercise during this premenopausal period. She needs to get her body into good shape while her hormones are readjusting. If she is over-weight, she should reduce her sugar intake and lose a few pounds.

It is possible that Ms. A. might be suffering from moniliasis. If she is, she might be helped with an estrogen cream such as Premarin in combination with an antiyeast medication, which might stabilize her vaginal environment. Once again, by avoiding unventilated panty hose and clothing that clings to her genital areas, Ms. A. will prevent her infection from festering and spreading.

If this regime does not improve her condition, the possiblity that she has bacterial vaginosis, which might be appropriately treated with Flagyl, must be considered.

My Vaginal Infection Is Killing My Sex Life

I am twenty years old and I'm engaged to marry the only boy that I've ever been with sexually. We have been very frustrated lately because we cannot have relations. I've had a vaginal infection for the last two years and when we attempt it, sex just caused me too much pain. My doctor has tried all kinds of creams and vinegar-and-water douches. I am not diabetic and I've been off the pill for a while now. I had a miscarriage a couple of years ago and I wonder if that could have caused the infection. I don't know what to do. The wedding is getting closer all the time and I don't want to be like this on my honeymoon.

—E.Y., Windsor, New York

First, Ms. Y. should know that her miscarriage did not contribute to her vaginal infection. It is possible that the birth control pill she took a while ago might have initially contributed to the infection, but now the problem is eliminating the vaginitis.

She might prevent the spread of the infection by dressing in loose clothing and forgoing tight jeans and panty hose, if she wears them. As suggested in the Monilia/*Candida albicans* treatment section in this chapter (pages 462 to 463), Ms. Y. might add yogurt or acidophilus capsules to her diet in order to introduce friendly bacteria into her vagina. Vitamin B-complex, taken daily, might also help since it will promote the stability of the vaginal milieu.

Finally, Ms. Y. might benefit from gentian violet, a time-tested bactericide and fungicide. When other remedies have failed, women have been cured with gentian violet. A homeopathic pharmacy might be able to make a gentian violet vaginal insert.

To insure a healthful honeymoon, her boyfriend should also receive treatment, because Monilia/*Candida albicans* is sometimes sexually transmitted. A man might have no symptoms, mild symptoms, or might constantly be developing swelling, redness, and itching, in the penile area. Since the penis is an external organ, it does not retain moisture the way a vagina does. A yeast infection on the penis, in contact with drying air, might improve without treatment. However, Ms. Y.'s boyfriend should see a doctor. Her problem might be recurring because he is reinfecting her all the time. Since the yeast organism might have attacked his prostate gland, he should be treated with Mycostatin oral tablets, 500,000 units, three times a day for ten days or longer, in combination with an antiyeast cream such as Mycolog applied to the penile area.

Could My IUD Be Causing My Vaginal Infection?

I have been battling a yeast infection for four years. I had it before, during, and after my pregnancy. I have been to three doctors and I've tried everything—creams, suppositories, tablets, gentian violet, Betadine douche—and nothing has worked. I have to wear support panty hose because I have varicose veins, but I do use cotton underwear and I dry my vaginal area with a hair dryer after I bathe. I have an IUD, but I have never had a problem with it. My problem is this infection. It is interrupting my sex life with my husband. We used to enjoy all the sexual pleasures, but now I can barely stand for him to touch me in the vaginal area because I'm so sore and tender. Could my IUD be causing my infection after all? It is so discouraging to do everything I'm told and still have this condition.

—H.B., Pfofftown, North Carolina

When a woman has an intrauterine device she experiences a watery discharge that is more excessive than usual. In addition, the tail of an IUD might cause vaginal irritation. Therefore, it is possible that the IUD might be the source of Ms. B.'s problem.

A doctor should do a culture of her vaginal discharge to determine whether the infection is due to Monilia/*Candida albicans* or a mixture of bacteria. Ms. B. might, in the latter case, be treated with oral antibiotics such as tetracycline or ampicillin in combination with a vaginal cream. If Gardnerella vaginitis shows up in the culture, Flagyl, possibly 250-mg tablets three times a day for ten days, might relieve her symptoms. If there is only a Monilia infection evident in her vaginal culture, Ms. B. might take Mycostatin oral tablets, 500,000 units, three times a day for ten days, to cleanse her bloodstream and return her vaginal environment to stability. The tablets should be taken in combination with a vaginal cream, jelly, or suppository to ensure the most successful treatment.

If Ms. B. follows her doctor's instructions, based upon what he has observed in her culture, and she still finds no relief, she might need to have her IUD removed to see whether the absence of the device makes a difference. A few months later, after Ms. B. has healed, she might have a new IUD inserted.

Can Potassium Sorbate Help Get Rid of My Vaginal Odor?

I have had a yeast infection for three years and I've run the gamut of antiyeast medications. Right after I stop a medication the discharge and odor always return. I am constantly wearing tampons or pads and I've been embarrassed a couple of times by the smell. Needless to say, my sex life with my husband has been horrible because of this condition. Not only does intercourse cause me pain, but I'm self-conscious about the odor. The only thing I've heard about that I haven't tried is potassium sorbate. Do you think this would help me?

—J.L., Rahway, New Jersey

As I suggested to the woman with the IUD in the previous letter, a doctor should culture Ms. L.'s vaginal discharge and look for bacteria to tell him the kind of vaginitis she has. Then, she might ask her doctor to prescribe liquid potassium sorbate, which she would mix with lukewarm water for a vaginal douche. This treatment has been helpful in some cases.

Restoring the vaginal environment to stability is important, and Ms. L. can find suggestions for making her vagina healthy in this chapter's section on treatment of Monilia/*Candida albicans* (pages 462 to 463). Ms. L. might use vaginal creams or suppositories and, at the same time, she might take oral Mycostatin tablets, 100,000 units, three times a day for ten days or longer, to change her vaginal odor. Remember, though, that both body and vaginal odors react to diet. Certain spicy foods, for example, cause worse body smells than others. A woman should be her own diet detective and try to vary the foods she chooses to see if her vaginal odor varies with them.

Regular douching with Betadine or vinegar and water might also help Ms. L. reach her goal of vaginal stability. Also, by reducing her sugar intake she will be taking a big step toward maintaining body balance. Most important, however, Ms. L. must find a competent physician who will properly evaluate a culture of her vaginal discharge and find the cause of her problem.

If Ms. L.'s condition does not improve with treatment, her partner should be examined and, if necessary, also treated. If he has an infection, he might be the source of her troubles.

Can Stress Cause Vaginitis?

I had been worried about my job because there had been so many layoffs in my office, but then my mother, who had been sick with cancer, took a turn for the worse and died. All my problems seemed minor in comparison to her death. Being the oldest child, I helped my father make the funeral arrangements. Two days after my mother was buried, I got a terrible vaginal infection—itching, burning, and thick white discharge. My doctor said that my stress could have caused the infection. Is it true? Can stress cause vaginitis?

—C.O., Boston, Massachusetts

People who have suffered the loss of a loved one have talked about their bodies "going into shock" at the news. They say that they have felt "numb." This particularly stressful event can change the body's balance.

When a woman is under stress, her muscles, especially her vaginal muscles, tighten, and the steroids in her bloodstream increase. When steroids increase, the body's immune system cannot function properly. Resistance drops and germs flourish. A vaginal infection easily takes hold at this time, and with the muscles tightened, vaginal secretions are not released.

Ms. O., and any woman who is going through a stressful period, must learn how to relax the vaginal muscles to give the discharge a free flow. She should insert a finger into her vagina and tighten her vaginal muscles in a manner that would be squeezing the finger. After a few seconds, she should relax the muscles that would allow her finger to feel released. Using this technique, Ms. O. would learn how to control her vaginal muscles, and she could then perform the tensing-and-relaxing exercise any time—when she is sitting at a desk, driving a car, standing on line at the market. The exercise should be performed twenty to thirty times a day for the muscles to respond. Then in addition to vaginal relaxation, taking vitamin

B-complex with folic acid, as well as extra vitamin B_6, or yogurt or acidophilus capsules and reducing the amount of sugar in her diet will help her fight the physical problems caused by stress.

Creams and suppositories prescribed to cure an infection from the growth of Monilia/*Candida albicans* should be used while a woman under stress is trying to regain her peace of mind. Ms. O. might benefit from these medications as she builds up her resistance. Since stress can definitely cause vaginitis, a woman has a good chance to stay healthy if she can keep stress under control as much as possible.

A Hysterectomy Is Not the Cure for Vaginitis

I have had a yeast infection since my baby was born last year. I've used vaginal creams, Flagyl, ampicillin, and douches, but my infection has never cleared up. The last doctor I went to gave me more Flagyl and AVC cream and told me that if my infection did not go away in eight weeks, I would have to have a hysterectomy. I have had surgery for cysts in my uterus, but the doctors say I don't have cancer. I am scared that I might be going for surgery I do not need if I agree to a hysterectomy. I'm just praying that the medicine works this time.

—G.V., Virginia Beach, Virginia

A vaginal infection is a localized problem that cannot be cut out, scraped away, or burned off. It is impossible to remedy vaginitis through surgery. *A hysterectomy is not the cure.* Vaginitis can be healed only with medication and by restoring the natural balance of microorganisms in the vagina.

Any time a doctor suggests surgery as a cure for a problem, or says that the source of an infection must be surgically removed, a woman must seek a second opinion. Ms. V.'s fear and uncertainty are understandable and appropriate. No woman should agree to surgery without consulting more than one doctor.

I'm Allergic to All Cures; What Can I Do?

I have had chronic vaginal infections for the last five years. My infections have come from yeast, trichomoniasis, and Hemophilus. I have used so much medication that I have become allergic to the creams and douches. Still, my vagina constantly aches and swells and the doctor does not know how to treat me anymore. He says I have to "learn to live with it." What can I do now that I seem to be unable to use any cure?

—F.A., Jacksonville, Florida

Ms. A. might have to evaluate her lifestyle to see if there is anything she can do to inhibit her infections. Stress can cause vaginitis. If she is living under stressful circumstances, she might confront the source of her stress and try to diminish the pressures and tension in her life. Exercise and proper nutrition, especially a reduction in sugar, can help stabilize her vagina. Ms. A. does not mention whether her douches have been with vinegar and water or with yogurt. If she has not tried natural douches, she might see how they work. She must look into all possible causes and cures. Perhaps she has a sexual partner who continues to reinfect her.

It is difficult to eliminate the rampant spread of fungi, protozoa, or bacteria without prescribed medication. An astute doctor could study Ms. A.'s medical history, obtain a vaginal culture, and while she is trying to correct her body balance naturally, he might be able to suggest a cure that she has not previously tried.

My Pap Test Shows Trichomoniasis, But I Have Not Had Sex

I am a forty-five-year-old widow. My husband died a few years ago and I have not had sexual relations since his death. The other day, however, my doctor told me that my Pap test showed I had a trichomoniasis infection. I always thought trichomoniasis

came from sex, but I haven't had sex. My doctor wants me to take Flagyl, but I wonder if I really have the infection.
— D.B., San Angelo, Texas

A Pap test is one way that a trichomoniasis infection can be detected. Often a smear will show cells that indicate that trichomoniasis protozoa could have been in the vagina for a long time. Sometimes the results are not certain; maybe the infection was there, and maybe it was not. It is felt, however, that if Flagyl is not given, the cells might possibly lead to further abnormalities on Pap tests, and they might even become cancerous.

The recommended treatment for the appearance of trichomoniasis cells on a Pap test is Flagyl, 500-mg tablets twice a day for five days, or 2 grams in a single dose. Of course, in this case the condition is chronic and a partner does not have to be treated.

Do Women Have "Jock Itch"?

Since I've started running I've found that I'm itchy in my vaginal area. I went to my doctor and he says that there is no infection, but the itch hasn't gone away. My husband says I have "jock itch." I laughed when he said it, but now I'm wondering. Do women, like men, get some sort of "jock itch" from athletics?
— P.N., Washington, D.C.

Sweaty jogging outfits, tight tennis clothes, and wet bathing suits, especially if they're made of nylon, can cause itching and irritation because they trap moisture. Many women find that as they exercise they become itchy even though they are not infected. These itches can lead to vaginitis, however, if precautions are not taken.

Outfits made from cotton or any other kind of porous material are best for exercising. Cotton panties are recommended, but they should not be sealed in with tights or panty hose during physical exertion. A woman should keep her vaginal area aired as much as she can.

If a woman already has an itch like Ms. N.'s she should, after exercising, shower and gently towel-dry her vaginal area. After toweling, she can set her hair dryer on "warm," hold it at a safe distance, aim the warm air between her legs for a minute or two, and eliminate the moisture that provides germs with easy breeding.

A vaginal itch that becomes annoying can be treated with an over-the-counter hydrocortisone cream approved for vaginal use. If it doesn't go away, an itch should be checked by a doctor. Unless it is ruled out, the possibility of vaginitis or a sexually transmitted disease always exists when an itch persists. If a doctor does not find a pathogenic microorganism, he might suggest an excellent treatment for jock itch in both women and men, over-the-counter Mycolog, a cream applied three or four times a day to the sore area. It might be a good idea for a woman and her partner to purchase Mycolog, and then to keep a tube of the cream in the refrigerator just in case.

Could My Bathtub Give Me Vaginitis?

I'm a single twenty-five-year-old woman who loves to soak in the tub at the end of a day. I've never had any kind of itch or drip from my vagina until recently, when my doctor diagnosed Hemophilus vaginitis. He had read in one of his journals that this infection might come from my bathroom cleanser. That sounds pretty farfetched to me. Do you know anything about it?
—K.T., Chicago, Illinois

It has been found that antibacterial soaps and cleansers might stick to the surface of a bathtub after scrubbing. When a woman takes a bath, the bacteria fighters enter her vagina and kill microorganisms that keep the vaginal environment in balance, and then infection-causing bacteria begin to multiply. These same antibacterial agents can be found in swimming pools, whirlpools, and Jacuzzis. Women who swim when they're using tampons might even be more susceptible to infection because absorbent tampons might draw the bacteria fighters into the vagina.

Ms. T. should switch cleansers or simply wash out her tub with plain soap and water. Any woman who has recurring vaginitis might consider this antibacterial finding when she evaluates her lifestyle in an effort to learn the cause of her infection. This recent discovery also means that she should be vigilant about vaginal cleansing after she has been in chemically sanitized waters.

SEXUALLY TRANSMITTED DISEASES (STDS)

The all-encompassing category of sexually transmitted diseases contains everything that used to be called veneral disease (VD), plus a number of long-recognized enteric and other disorders that can be contracted in many ways and that in the past were not known to be transmitted sexually. The United States has the highest rate of STDs of any developed country in the world. Yet change is occurring among the most well-known of the diseases. Figures from 1996 show a decline in gonorrhea and syphilis, with syphilis rates the lowest in history. We are in a good news/bad news situation, however, because millions of people suffer with silent infections: chlamydia, the human papillomavirus (HPV) that causes genital warts, trichomoniasis, and hepatitis C—and their numbers are growing. Also, although fewer men have contracted the human immunodeficiency virus (HIV), which causes the deadly acquired immunodeficiency syndrome (AIDS), more women have become infected. Diseases such as amebiasis, giardiasis, salmonellosis, shigellosis, hepatitis B, and cytomegalovirus infection, which are severely debilitating, are now also considered sexually transmitted. These latter diseases, which can be transmitted by oral and anal sexual practices, are especially prevalent among male homosexuals.

Of course, sex is not the only way some of these diseases are transmitted. For instance, *moniliasis* (described earlier in this chapter) is not always considered an STD because it can be caused by stress or other environmental factors.

Acquired Immune Deficiency Syndrome/AIDS

In 1982 the fatal disease that took everyone by surprise was given a name: Acquired Immune Deficiency Syndrome, or AIDS. How the disease spread was a mystery that led to the discovery of the human immunodeficiency virus, or HIV, now better known as the AIDS virus, which traveled from one person to another through an exchange of body fluids, usually semen and blood.

HIV destroys the CD-4 blood cells of the body's immune system. The virus can live in the human body for ten years or more before it takes its toll and signs of AIDS appear. All the while, if a woman is unaware that she is infected, she can be passing the virus along to others. Eventually, HIV debilitates the immune system and stifles a woman's ability to stave off infection. As AIDS progresses, unusual infections such as pneumocystitis pneumonia and toxoplasmosis can prove fatal.

At first, AIDS was diagnosed predominantly among homosexual men and intravenous drug users. Today, the spread of the disease has slowed among these groups; however, the number of new infections remains at about 20,000 per year with a rise in heterosexual transmission of HIV among young minority women and men. New cases among young people thirteen to twenty-four years old are causing the figures to remain elevated. Of 7,200 people thirteen to twenty-four years old whose HIV infections were reported between 1994 and 1997, 44 percent were female, 63 percent were African-American, and 5 percent were Hispanic. There is a particular concern about the spread of HIV/AIDS among teenage girls, who could protect themselves from this life-threatening STD with the use of a spermicide-containing condom during sex. Pregnant women who harbor HIV can also pass the virus to their unborn children in the uterus and after childbirth, during breast-feeding.

How Do You Contract HIV, the AIDS Virus? HIV, the AIDS virus, is passed from one person to another through an exchange of body fluids, usually semen and blood, although it can also be spread through vaginal secretions. HIV has been detected in minute amounts in urine, feces, tears, and saliva, but there are no known cases of transmission through these fluids. French kissing, or deep kissing, is considered risky only because there could be an exchange of blood if either partner has a cut in or around the mouth.

Most of the time HIV is sexually transmitted through unprotected intercourse because the virus is in a man's semen and can be ejaculated into the vagina or anus—or, during oral sex, into a woman's throat. Since an infected woman would have HIV in vaginal moisture and menstrual blood, she can pass it on to a sexual partner during intercourse if he has a cut on his penis. Circumstances that make a woman more vulnerable to HIV during unprotected sexual intercourse are:

- An uncircumcised male; AIDS cases are usually lower among circumcised males.
- Harboring another STD such as venereal warts, chlamydia, trichomoniasis, or gonorrhea.
- Cervical ectopy, a condition in which abnormal tissue covers part of the vagina, more common in teens and young women in their twenties.
- Touching the penis of an infected male when a cut exists on your hand and semen penetrates the cut.

HIV is also spread through unclean, infected needles; a woman might be pricked by a needle used by an infected person and still tainted with blood. A woman can also be exposed to infected blood from shared toothbrushes, razors, and needles used for tattoos and ear piercing. With the screening of blood supplies, blood transfusions are unlikely sources of infection.

All pregnant women should have prenatal HIV counseling and testing. As mentioned earlier, a pregnant woman who has HIV/ AIDS can transmit the virus to her unborn baby in the uterus or later on, during breast-feeding. Studies have shown that the likelihood of transmission to a newborn can be significantly reduced if an expectant mother delivers by cesarean section and, at the end of her pregnancy, takes the drug zidovudine (Retrovir), formerly known as AZT.

A woman who thinks she might have been exposed to HIV can have a blood test for the presence of HIV antibodies, which is the only way to test for AIDS. The antibodies can take up to six months or longer to show up, so a negative test result within six months of suspected exposure should be followed by a second test.

What Is the Best Protection Against HIV/AIDS? The surest method of protection from HIV/AIDS is to not have sexual intercourse and to never use needles, whether for drugs, tattoos, or ear piercing, that have been used by anyone else. If a woman is sexually active, then:

- Every time she has sex with a partner who has not been recently tested for HIV antibodies, she should use a spermicide-containing condom. Even if a partner has never been an intravenous (IV) drug user, has never had sex with an IV drug user, and has never had sex with a man, he might have picked up HIV by having sex with someone who had sex with someone who has AIDS. The possibilities are endless and tragic.
- Sexual relations with only one partner also offers more protection.
- Any questions about AIDS might be answered by calling the National AIDS Hotline at 1-800-342-AIDS.

How AIDS Is Treated. There is no cure for AIDS, and this disease is spreading rapidly in Africa and other parts of the world. Due to safe sex methods of protection, however, AIDS cases and AIDS deaths in the United States have declined in recent years. With combination drug therapy, an increasing number of people infected with HIV are living longer. As of mid-1997, 612,078 AIDS cases had been reported to the Centers for Disease Control, and 379,258 people had died of AIDS. A woman living with HIV can receive a powerful three-drug combination to interrupt the life cycle of the virus and slow the disease. This "drug cocktail" includes three main classes of HIV-fighting drugs: nucleosides, nonnucleosides, and protease inhibitors. The drug combination a woman receives—which can be so complicated it involves taking fifteen to twenty pills a day, either alone or together, some on a full stomach, others on an empty stomach—will be based on her condition and her response to each drug's side effects. Included among the effects are diarrhea, fatigue, anemia, kidney stones, possible diabetes, high blood pressure, high cholesterol, and a strange redistribution of body fat. A typical drug cocktail includes zidovudine (Retrovir), lamividune (Epivir), and the protease inhibitor indinavir (Crixivan). One hopes that a vaccine against AIDS will become a reality and that this disease will one day be eliminated.

Hepatitis C

At least 4 million Americans, 2 percent of the U.S. population, are infected with the hepatitis C virus (HCV). That percentage means four times as many people have HCV as have HIV, the virus that causes AIDS. Each year as many as 180,000 people are diagnosed with HCV, and each year 10,000 to 12,000 people die from its effects. A person who has HCV may have no signs or symptoms for 10 to 40 years, but about 85 percent of those infected will develop chronic hepatitis C, and 20 percent of these chronic sufferers are likely to face serious liver damage. Chronic hepatitis C can lead to cirrhosis, a scarring of the liver that's severe enough to end the functioning of the liver, and life-threatening liver cancer. The fact that you can go on for years without knowing you harbor the virus makes hepatitis C a rampant, silent epidemic. Many people only learn they have HCV after they have blood tests for other reasons. When elevated liver enzymes are discovered, a follow-up blood test for the antibodies to HCV confirms the presence of the virus. Hepatitis C is conservatively reported to affect some 180 million people worldwide, and it is claiming more and more lives annually. By the year 2010, the death rate related to HCV is expected to triple.

HCV is mainly spread through exposure to infected human blood. You may have been infected with HCV if you received blood transfusions and blood products before 1992, before reliable tests were used to screen blood supplies. HCV appears in this chapter on STDs because unprotected sexual intercourse brings some risk of exposure, although health experts say they do not know how high or low that risk may be, or how effective condoms may be in preventing HCV infection. The American Liver Foundation reports that there have been "occasional documented cases of people with chronic hepatitis C transmitting the virus to their only, long-term sexual partner," but the majority of physicians do not recommend that partners in monogamous relationships change their sexual practices. At present, the risk of contracting HCV during sexual activity is viewed as slight for those who have only one sexual partner, but higher for those who have multiple partners. The bottom line is that there is a risk of becoming infected if you come into contact with an infected person's blood, so if your partner is diagnosed with HCV, you should be tested.

In addition to exposure through blood transfusions and blood products used before 1992, and through sexual transmission, you may also have been exposed to HCV-contaminated blood if you ever shared drug needles or sniffed drugs through communal straws. Shared razors and toothbrushes, and needles used for tattooing and body piercing can also spread the virus. A mother can transmit HCV to her baby during birth. Health care workers and people on long-term kidney dialysis are at high risk. Military personnel who had vaccinations with pneumatic jet injectors may be at risk, and so may anyone who received a gamma globulin injection in the 1960s and 1970s. One-fifth of the population of Egypt, at least 10 million people, were infected with HCV from nationwide vaccinations that began in the 1950s and went through the 1980s, to fight the parasitic illness schistosomiasis.

Hepatitis C is still an unsolved mystery. There was no way to identify HCV until a blood test for it was developed in 1989. At least six different genotypes of hepatitis C, and more than 30 subtypes, have been discovered, but the virus has defied efforts to grow it in a test tube. HCV mutates quickly to disguise itself from the body's immune defenses and is extremely hard to pin down.

How Hepatitis C Is Treated. There is no vaccine against hepatitis C, and the drugs used to fight HCV—interferon (interferon alpha-2b, interferon alpha-2a) and the antiviral compound ribavarin—are debilitating, costly, and not always effective (only 40 percent of sufferers experience a long-term remission of the disease). Treatment involves daily doses of ribavarin plus self-administered injections of interferon three times a week. Two new versions of interferon, called pegylated interferon, require only one weekly injection, and the drug companies Schering-Plough and Hoffman-LaRoche are separately working to get their versions approved. The side effects of treatment may include fatigue, headache, nausea, vomiting, fever, chills, diarrhea, partial balding, abdominal pain, depression, insomnia, dizziness, and anorexia. Only 40 percent of those being treated with the interferon/ribavarin combination will get some benefit. An alternative therapy, milk thistle herb, is purported to lower liver enzymes and make people feel better, but there is no scientific evidence that milk thistle has any real effect on the disease.

A woman who is diagnosed with HCV should seek care from a hepatologist or gastroenterologist who can perform blood tests to monitor her liver enzymes and perform biopsies to monitor her condition. An FDA-approved at-home blood test is available for about $70 from the Home Access Health Corporation, for anyone who wants the privacy and convenience of this type of testing. For more information about obtaining a test kit, Home Access health counselors are on call at 1-800-867-5655, or you can visit the Web site: www.homeaccess.com. Anyone who has HCV must avoid alcoholic beverages and should be vaccinated against hepatitis A and B. Depending on a woman's liver enzyme levels and the condition of her liver, her physician will recommend a course of treatment; if liver enzymes are consistently normal and no liver damage has been discovered, she may be able to avoid medication. That's one end of the

HCV spectrum; the other end may result in a liver transplant. Hepatitis C is the number one reason for a liver transplant since so many people suffer extensive liver damage from the disease.

For more information about hepatitis C, a woman can contact the American Liver Foundation at 1-800-GO-LIVER (1-800-465-4837) or visit the ALF Web site: www.liverfoundation.org.

Sexually Transmitted Hepatitis B

More clearly an STD than hepatitis C, hepatitis B is transmitted by oral and anal sex. The hepatitis B virus has been found in saliva, semen, and vaginal secretions, and can be passed on through kissing or oral/genital contact. The incidence of this disease is ten to twelve times higher for homosexuals, but heterosexuals are not immune. Unfortunately, the fluish symptoms that develop into jaundice have no definitive treatment, but they are usually overcome by bed rest and proper nutrition. A woman who is infected or has been exposed to hepatitis B might request a gamma globulin injection from her doctor. As the body builds antibodies to fight the virus, this hepatitis becomes self-limiting. This natural healing is still the only known cure, although scientists have stepped up the effort to find a way to combat this disease. A person should refrain from sexual activity until her or his doctor says that the hepatitis is no longer contagious. A vaccine against hepatitis B is now available, and the incidence of this disease should begin to fall.

Gonorrhea

Gonorrhea, which used to strike almost 3 million people annually, has declined to the point where an estimated 650,000 cases will be diagnosed in a year. The use of condoms has helped reduce its existence. When gonorrhea does surface, however, it can be in the form of a new drug-resistant strain.

Gonorrhea knows no social boundaries and has the ability to hide within a woman. A man usually knows he has gonorrhea because he experiences burning upon urination and a discharge from the penis, but 80 to 90 percent of the women with the disease do not have symptoms. Such a woman is completely unsuspecting but remarkably dangerous. *She might be a carrier without ever knowing she has the disease.*

Women become infected by contagious men with whom they have sexual intercourse. Men pass on *Neisseria gonorrhoeae,* a gramnegative, kidney-shaped bacteria that thrives in the mucosal tissue of the penis, vagina, anus, or throat. In these areas, the temperature and acidity are just right for breeding gonorrheal germs. It is almost impossible to propagate the bacteria outside the body, so the disease is usually not spread through toilet seats, although contamination has occurred this way. Sexual intercourse and oral or anal sex are the main means of transmitting gonorrhea.

A woman who realizes that she has gonorrhea can be easily treated, because the bacteria are very sensitive to antibiotics. When treatment is immediate, the disease is easily overcome. The maddening problem comes from gonorrhea's new strains. The old reliable medicines are not destroying the disease and doctors have to combine a number of new antibiotics to find a cure.

What Are the Symptoms of Gonorrhea? As mentioned before, 80 to 90 percent of the women with gonorrhea have no symptoms, which is why pregnant women are tested for the disease right away. The disease is known to cause blindness in newborns, and a pregnant woman who has gonorrhea can infect her baby during childbirth.

From two days to three weeks after a woman is exposed to gonorrhea, symptoms might develop. She might have a vaginal discharge and a minor irritation, but lower abdominal pain is a far more frequent indicator. Most likely, though, she will have no signs. If a woman has been exposed to the disease, it is hoped that the integrity of her partner will prevail and he will tell her to go to the doctor. A man with gonorrhea will usually have an obvious discharge from his penis and painful urination two to seven days after exposure. If a gonorrheal infection is in the throat, a woman or a man will feel only a slight soreness. If the gonorrheal infection is in the anus, which happens most often in homosexual men, it will be evidenced in painful bowel movements with blood and mucus in the stool.

Gonorrhea is usually diagnosed by a swab of the cervix, urethra, throat, or anus. The swabbed sample is put into a special transport medium and sent to a laboratory, where it is placed in a Thayer-Martin culture medium, which enhances the growth of gonorrhea. Within two or three days a lab can identify a diseased culture. Sometimes gonorrhea can also be detected with a Gram stain—a stained slide sample of the mucus from the infected area, viewed under the microscope. A blood test for this disease is just beginning to be used.

Once diagnosed, gonorrhea must be treated immediately. If a woman with gonorrhea is not treated, during her menstrual period uterine contractions might pull the disease into her uterus and Fallopian tubes. Once inside a woman's reproductive organs, gonorrhea can spread quickly and cause pelvic inflammatory disease (PID), an infection of the uterus, Fallopian tubes, and ovaries. PID can lead to damage of the Fallopian tubes that can make a woman infertile. The potent gonococci, even if they were asymptomatic in the beginning, are behind many tragic cases of PID and infertility.

How Is Gonorrhea Treated? Gonorrhea is usually cured fastest and easiest with penicillin. A woman receives a total of two injections of penicillin G, 2.4 million units each, one shot in each buttock, for a total of 4.8 million units. In addition, she swallows 1 gram of probenicid, a medication that helps prevent the excretion of the penicillin. (The longer the antibiotic stays in the body, the more time it has to kill the bacteria.) A man with gonorrhea gets half the dosage that a woman does—namely, one injection of 2.4 million units of penicillin G. A single oral dose of 3.5 grams of ampicillin in combination with 1 gram of probenicid is an alternative to a penicillin injection.

If a woman or a man is allergic to penicillin, the recommended treatment is 1.4 grams of tetracycline taken orally, followed by 500 mg of tetracycline, four times a day for four days, or one injection of spectinomycin, 2 grams. A pregnant woman with a penicillin allergy might take an oral dose of 1.5 grams of erythromycin, followed by 500 mg of erythromycin, four times a day for four days. Newer antibiotics being used to fight gonorrhea include cefixime, 400 mg in a single oral dose; ceftriaxone, 125 mg by injection; ciprofloxacin, 500 mg in a single oral dose; ofloxacin, 400 mg in a single oral dose combined with azithromycin, 1 gram in a single oral dose; or doxycycline, 100-mg tablets for seven days.

Any woman or man who has had gonorrhea must return to the doctor seven days after treatment for a follow-up examination. A new culture must be obtained to make sure that treatment has been successful.

QUESTIONS ABOUT GONORRHEA

Could an Old Case of Gonorrhea Have Made Me Infertile?

When I was in college eight years ago, I got gonorrhea from my boyfriend. After two shots of penicillin the disease went away (as did the boyfriend) and I didn't think about it until recently. My husband and I have been trying to have baby for a year, but I haven't conceived. Could my old case of gonorrhea have made me infertile?

—J.Q., Embarrass, Minnesota

Generally, if gonorrhea is properly treated it does not lead to sterility. It appears from Ms. Q.'s letter that she saw a doctor immediately, was treated, and was successfully cured; therefore, I doubt that her long-gone gonorrhea is the cause of her infertility.

Gonorrhea might make a woman infertile when it is not treated, because then it can easily spread to the Fallopian tubes, where it results in pelvic inflammatory disease (PID). If Ms. Q. had PID, she would have experienced abdominal pain and discomfort at some point during the disease. Since she does not mention any discomfort, she most likely has no reason to fear any aftereffects from her old bout with the disease.

How Can Gonorrhea Lead to Arthritis?

Recently my joints started swelling and becoming very painful. I thought I might have arthritis and I went to the doctor. He ran tests and stuck a needle into my joints. Later on he told me that the tests showed I had arthritis from gonorrhea. I never even knew I had an STD and I still don't understand how it causes the arthritis. What does arthritis have to do with sex?

—L.H., Valdosta, Georgia

Gonococci can enter the bloodstream and attack the joints, causing swelling, redness, and pain. Ms. H.'s doctor was right to insert a needle into a joint and withdraw a sample of the joint fluid to be cultured.

Since the culture showed positive for gonorrhea, Ms. H. should have received high doses of antibiotics. After treatment, she should have visited a doctor who specializes in sexually transmitted diseases. Such a specialist conducts a follow-up culture to make sure that gonorrhea has been wiped out. The arthritis, its symptoms and problems, will usually also disappear with the treatment.

Can I Get Gonorrhea from a Toilet Seat?

Is gonorrhea only sexually transmitted? I have a friend who has had it twice and I'm always afraid to use her bathroom or to let her use mine. I'm worried that she might get it again, and I'm scared I'll get it too.

—P.J., Springfield, Massachusetts

Two of the girls in my dorm have gonorrhea, but neither of them has had sexual intercourse recently. Could they have picked it up from a toilet seat?

—A.A., Ann Arbor, Michigan

Most gonorrhea is transmitted through sexual intercourse, but in one study the bacteria that causes gonorrhea stayed alive for up to twenty-four hours in a moist towel. Do the two young women in Ms. A.'s letter share towels? If so, the towels, theoretically, could have transmitted the disease.

If the temperature is right and a toilet seat is moist, gonorrhea bacteria contained in a discharge might survive for several hours. However, the chance that the bacteria would exist on a toilet seat at all is extremely slim since no gonococci were found in random samples taken from seventy-two toilets in public rest rooms. Also, researchers who have studied the likelihood of catching gonorrhea from a toilet seat have found that more than merely sitting on a seat would be needed to bring the disease to the genital area. A woman's hand would first have to touch the discharge, and then the vaginal area, before gonorrhea could be transmitted.

Nevertheless, I cannot say, absolutely, that the college women did not pick up the disease from a toilet. Even a slim chance is still a chance, and I would recommend that a woman always consider whether or not a toilet is sanitary before she touches it. If possible, it is always a good idea to line the seat of a public toilet with paper before use. In some countries there are often no seats in public toilets and women must squat to urinate—a little awkward, but the position prevents contact with a possible contaminant.

Besides being transmitted by sex and the remote toilet seat, gonorrhea can also be spread after it has contaminated the eyes and caused conjunctivitis, or infiltrated and abscessed the gums, or infected the throat to the point of pharyngitis.

It is probably wise for both Ms. J. and Ms. A., since they have been in close contact with people who have gonorrhea, to visit their doctors and request tests for the disease.

Can Gonorrhea Lead to Endometrial Cancer?

*I had undiagnosed gonorrhea for years. Finally, I was diagnosed
and cured, but I've been worried ever since. Could the disease have
predisposed me to endometrial cancer? I am too embarrassed to ask
my own gynecologist.*

—M.W., Truckee, California

Gonorrhea cannot lead to endometrial cancer. The disease might
cause pelvic inflammatory disease (PID) and infertility if it spreads
to the uterus and Fallopian tubes. Arthritis might arise if the gonorrhea bacteria enter the bloodstream and penetrate the joints. Cancer,
though, is not a possibility.

Since Ms. W. does not say that she is in ill health, she has probably conquered gonorrhea with no aftereffects.

Is There a New Kind of Gonorrhea?

*I am stationed at a military base in California where some of
the guys have been talking about STD that you can't cure with
penicillin. They say it's going around. What should I do if I get it?*
—L.S. Pfc., Fairfield, California

It is heartening to receive letters from men who are concerned. I
hope Private S. is thinking not only about himself but also about the
well-being of the woman, or women, in his life.

It is true that there have been new strains of penicillin-resistant
gonorrhea reported. One strain, which was brought to California by a
soldier who had been stationed in the Philippines, did not respond to
spectinomycin, a potent antibiotic used to treat gonorrhea. Only tetracycline, 500 mg every six hours for five days, brought relief. So,
although these new strains are difficult to treat, doctors are innovating
with antibiotics until they find drug regimens that do eventually work.

If Private S. does contract gonorrhea, before and after his treatment he should have a culture taken by a doctor who specializes in

sexually transmitted diseases. A shot of penicillin does not always mean that there has been a cure. A follow-up culture, which should be obtained two weeks after treatment, will show whether a case of gonorrhea has been overcome or has remained resistant.

Will Anal Sex Lead to Gonorrhea?

I hear that there is a lot of anal gonorrhea around these days. Does that mean that if you have anal sex you will always get gonorrhea if a man has it?
—C.K., New York, New York

The anal area is lined by a mucosa, a mucous membrane similar to vaginal lining, which is highly susceptible to the transmission of gonorrhea. The rising incidence of anal gonorrhea is seen more frequently among male homosexuals than heterosexuals, but a woman who indulges in anal intercourse might, of course, contract the disease. The symptoms include pain during bowel movements and an anal discharge with blood and mucus in the stool.

If a woman notices symptoms of anal gonorrhea, she should visit a doctor and request that a culture be made from her anal discharge. No matter which partner has the disease, the treatment, as explained earlier, is either penicillin or ampicillin. In the case of a penicillin allergy, tetracycline, spectinomycin, or erythromycin might be recommended.

How Do You Prevent Gonorrhea of the Throat?

A friend of mine thought she had a sore throat and she was taking aspirin, but she never got better. She went to the doctor, who discovered that she had gonorrhea of the throat. He said he was glad he got it in time, before the disease spread to other parts of the body. I have always liked oral sex, but now I'm worried. Should I stop it? Is there a way to prevent gonorrhea of the throat and still have oral sex?
—I.B., Philadelphia, Pennsylvania

Before a woman engages in any sexual activity she should, if possible, carefully inspect her partner. Examining a man's penis during foreplay might seem awkward, but in this world of HIV, AIDS, and other STDs, openness between sexual partners is needed. A man should willingly cooperate when a woman checks the state of his health, and he should use a condom.

This penile inspection, which might be a little worrisome for some women, has been successfully used by ladies of the night, who avoid STDs by gently squeezing a man's penis as if they were milking it. A sexually active woman might follow this technique. If a woman notices penile discharge from a man, she should suspect STD and refrain from sex. Oral sex is risky when a man has a penile discharge or an irritation. A woman might be exposed to HIV and AIDS or gonorrhea of the throat. The pharynx mucosa, like the mucosa of the vagina and anus, provides the right environment for the proliferation of the *N. gonorrhoeae.* The bacteria might move in and put a woman in a serious situation—she might not know she is infected. She might lack any signs of the disease, since 70 to 80 percent of all pharyngeal gonococcal infections are asymptomatic. A slight sore throat after oral sex should never be disregarded.

Before sex, if a woman does not know a man's health history, she should request that he wear a condom. Many STDs can only be stopped through assertiveness. If a woman hesitates, does not inspect a man, or is too shy to ask him to wear a condom for protection against STDs, she might be opening herself up to gonorrhea in her vagina, throat, or even her eyes. Oral sex can bring gonococci close to the eye's mucous membrane, where conjunctivitis can develop. She might also be turning herself into an unwitting carrier.

Ms. B. should take all the described precautions before oral sex. Afterward, if she has the least feeling that she is infected, she should ask her doctor to have a throat culture analyzed. Pharyngeal infections play a big part in the, so far, unmanageable spread of gonorrhea. It is essential that a woman who suspects gonorrhea in any area of her body act quickly to visit her doctor for diagnosis and treatment.

When Gonorrhea Leads to PID

My twenty-two-year-old daughter has been suffering with abdominal pain and heavy bleeding for two years. She has been to three doctors. One doctor operated and said that her tubes were infected and filled with pus. Then he didn't do anything but prescribe painkillers. Another doctor gave her a D & C and more painkillers. She got disgusted with gynecologists and went to an internist, who said that she had overactive bowels and an enlarged ovary. He gave her a diet and, you guessed it, painkillers. Now she has a discharge and she says she wishes she were dead. She is really suffering. Do you have any idea what's wrong with her? I'm her mother and I would do anything I could to help.

—W.H., Versailles, Indiana

Ms. H. doesn't say whether her daughter had STD tests. It seems to me that her daughter might have contracted a gonorrheal infection that went untreated, advanced into her uterus and Fallopian tubes, and developed into pelvic inflammatory disease (PID). When a woman has gonorrhea, disease-causing bacteria can be sucked into her reproductive organs during her menstrual period when the uterus is contracting. Once inside the uterus and tubes, the bacteria can generate PID.

Severe abdominal pain accompanied by a high fever could be a sign that PID exists. PID might be promoted by an intrauterine device, which can contribute to the spread of the disease. Since Ms. H. does not mention an IUD, such a device is probably not the source of infection in this case. With pus in her tubes, Ms. H.'s daughter probably has PID caused by gonococci or other bacteria. The exact bacteria can be identified only through a culture. In the past, PID was most frequently caused by gonorrhea, but today PID is often caused by a mixture of bacteria.

Painkillers will do nothing for PID, which is why Ms. H.'s daughter keeps getting worse. The complications continue to increase. Advanced PID can result in peritonitis, which might cause a woman to be admitted to the hospital for intensive care with high doses of antibiotics. Peritonitis—an infection of the peritoneum, the lining of the abdominal organs—is one offshoot of PID; infertility is another. As the bacteria multiply, pus continues to swell the young woman's Fallopian tubes and eventually closes them. Damaged tubes mean infertility.

Ms. H.'s daughter should consult a doctor who specializes in sexually transmitted diseases, preferably a physician associated with a teaching hospital or a large medical center. Doctors who are not familiar with PID have been known to suggest hysterectomies as cures for the disease. Ms. H.'s daughter must seek good care from a qualified physician. A hysterectomy will not cure PID, but antibiotics will. The young woman would probably respond to a triple antibiotic therapy—three different types of antibiotics combined to curb her condition. Then, when her infection is under control, she might need microsurgery to open her tubes and restore her fertility.

Ms. H.'s daughter needs another opinion. Pelvic inflammatory disease can be very dangerous and might lead to a fatal condition. She must be treated immediately. PID is yet another reason why today's STDs are so serious and tragic.

Is My Tubal Infection My Husband's Fault?

I've been suffering with a tubal infection for at least five years, but I didn't know it until recently. A pain on my right side was so bad I went to the doctor. He said he didn't know what was wrong with me and put me in the hospital for exploratory surgery. Afterward, he told me that I had such a bad tubal infection on my right side that I would have to have surgery with microscopes to patch it up. He also said that the left tube was blocked and would need surgery too. I want very much to have a baby. I have never used a contraceptive and I have never been pregnant. Five years ago I became afraid of doctors because I went to a gynecologist who told me that since my husband drives a tractor-trailer he had other women and had caused me the problem. Even then I had had an

*abdominal pain. If I can never have a baby, will it be my
husband's fault? Did he really give me a tubal infection?*
                              —T.D., Minneapolis, Minnesota

I don't see how driving a tractor-trailer gives a man more chance
to spread infection. The doctor who treated Ms. D. years ago was, of
course, implying that Ms. D.'s husband fooled around with other
women while he was on the road and picked up something that he
then gave to his wife. If an STD, specifically gonorrhea, remains
untreated, it can spread into the Fallopian tubes and cause PID.

STDs are occuring in epidemic proportions because so many
people have caught them and transmitted them. Married women
and men are not immune, especially if extramarital sex exists, but it
is totally off-the-wall for a doctor to say a woman has an STD
because her husband drives a truck. This woman knows her own
husband and his body. She would have noticed a penile discharge if
one had existed, and I venture to say that she would have known if
he had been having affairs. Women usually intuit those things.

Before Ms. D. agrees to surgery, she should consult an infertility specialist at a teaching hospital or a large medical center (see
chapter 8). It might be that she needs a combination of potent
antibiotics to curb the infection. After treatment, she should have a
blood test to make sure that the tubal infection is under control.
Then, a hysterosalpingogram, an X ray of her uterus and tubes, will
give an infertility expert a chance to evaluate any tubal damage and
decide whether microsurgery is in order. A tubal infection is a serious condition, and it is very sad that Ms. D. waited so long to seek
help. Her first doctor was certainly rash and unfeeling.

Syphilis

Syphilis in the United States is at its lowest level since the government started tracking it in 1941. Only 6,993 cases of syphilis
were reported to the Centers for Disease Control (CDC) in 1998.
Researchers attribute the drop, in part, to partner notification and

counseling. The disease is transmitted during sexual intercourse when a microorganism, a bacterium called *Treponema pallidum,* penetrates the site of intercourse, in women usually the vagina. The *T. pallidum* is a spirochete, a bacterium shaped like a spiral, which enters the mucosa, the sensitive mucous membrane of the vaginal area. During anal and oral sex the bacteria can invade either the anal mucosa or tissue in the mouth or on the lips. A lesion, a hard painless sore called a chancre, appears at the site of a *T. pallidum* infection. When it comes to syphilis, male homosexuals are a particularly high-risk group because an anal chancre often goes unnoticed and then the disease spreads rapidly within the homosexual community.

The syphilis chancre should not be confused with a herpes sore, which is very painful. The syphilitic sore is a sign of the primary stage of the disease. In total, syphilis has four stages—primary, secondary, latent, and tertiary. It is an insidious STD because it *seems* to disappear after the primary and secondary stages, even if it has never been treated. The sad truth is that while symptoms might abate, there is a 33 percent chance that the disease has not gone away. Syphilis slides into a latent stage, and decades later, when its victim is no longer thinking about it, syphilis has the power to reactivate itself and cause devastating complications.

Before the discovery of penicillin, syphilis was a major cause of insanity. If syphilis is not treated today, perhaps twenty or thirty years after a woman has contracted the disease she might succumb to cardiovascular problems and neurological disorders. The bacteria survive in the bloodstream and often progress to the vital organs. An undiscovered spirochete can pass through the placenta of a pregnant woman and might cause abortion, stillbirth, or infant death—or increase the chances that a baby might be born with syphilis and many physical complications. The worst is that, even in these modern times, doctors cannot eliminate the possibility of brain damage and even death if a person has untreated syphilis.

A woman can almost always prevent herself from catching a serious case of syphilis, however, if she knows her body and examines her partner's penis before sexual intercourse.

What Are the Symptoms of Syphilis? Within ten to ninety days after intercourse with a syphilitic partner, a woman has a 30 percent chance of developing the disease herself. At some point during those ten to ninety days a small elevation of the skin will appear at the site of sexual contact. The bump becomes a *chancre,* a hard painless sore usually located on the vaginal labia. Approximately 5 percent of syphilis chancres erupt on the lips, breasts, or in the mouth. A man will usually notice the sore on his penis. Chancres can also appear in the anal area. A sore is a sign of primary syphilis and at this stage a person is highly contagious.

Since there is no pain with a syphilitic chancre, a woman might not know she has it. The sore might be hidden in the folds of her vagina. A woman who notices a sore that she thinks might mean syphilis should consult her doctor immediately.

By squeezing or scraping the lesion, a doctor can get a sample of the content of the sore that he can place on a glass slide. Then, if he views the slide under a dark-field microscope, an instrument especially designed for diagnosing syphilis, he might be able to tell his patient right away if this STD exists. Very often the dark-field scopes are available only at public health clinics, in hospital labs, or in the offices of doctors who specialize in sexually transmitted diseases. A physician might, therefore, take a blood sample and send it to a lab for a VDRL (veneral disease research laboratories) blood test. The VDRL has replaced the old Wasserman test and might be required for couples applying for marriage licenses, and for newly pregnant women.

If a VDRL, which is considered a nonspecific test, is found to be positive, it might be followed by another, specific serological test called an FTA-ABS (fluorescent treponemal antibody-absorbed). This latter test pinpoints the specific antibodies that the body is producing to combat syphilis and helps doctors gauge their treatments.

If primary syphilis goes undetected, the chancre might heal itself and disappear in one to five weeks. The spirochete bacteria remain in the bloodstream, however, and about six weeks after the first appearance of the sore, now healed, syphilis shows itself in its secondary stage. A woman might develop a skin rash, possibly accompanied by enlarged lymph nodes, a mild fever, or hair loss. Lesions on the palms of the hands and soles of the feet are especially suspicious, as well as flat, wartlike growths called condylomata in the genital area. This secondary stage lasts about two to six weeks, as long as the rash does.

A sexually active woman who notices a long-lasting skin rash should ask her doctor for a VDRL blood test. If allowed to advance, syphilis is most dangerous.

Once a woman passes through the primary and secondary stages of syphilis without treatment, the disease enters the latent phase. A woman might have no symptoms. She might feel perfectly fine, but she has a 33 percent chance of being stricken with life-threatening complications from the disease. When she least expects it, maybe twenty or thirty years after her initial exposure to syphilis, she might begin to show signs of paralysis. In its last, or tertiary, stage, syphilis strikes the neurological and cardiovascular systems. The disease has been known to cause brain damage, psychosis, manic-depression, and schizophrenia. In England, there has long been a rumor that a royal duke turned into Jack the Ripper due to syphilis. King Henry VIII, the most royal syphiltic, died from the disease. Syphilis can eventually kill.

When it is diagnosed early, syphilis is easy to treat. A woman who is unafraid to examine her partner and is not shy about touching herself will always know when a sore, a sign of sickness, appears.

How Is Syphilis Treated? The most common treatment for primary or secondary syphilis is Benzathine penicillin-G, 2.4 million units given in two injections of 1.2 million units each, one shot in each buttock, as a one-time therapy.

If syphilis exists for more than a year, Benzathine penicillin-G, 2.4 million units (1.2 million in each buttock), is injected weekly for three weeks for a total of 7.2 million units.

Women who are allergic to penicillin might be treated with oral erythromycin, 2 grams a day for fifteen days for a total of 30 grams;

or oral tetracycline, 2 grams a day for fifteen days for a total of 39 grams.

Syphilis is an extremely dangerous, potentially fatal, disease that should always be treated by a doctor who specializes in sexually transmitted diseases.

Syphilis and Pregnancy. A pregnant woman should be tested for STDs at her first visit to the obstetrician. A positive result means further testing must be performed by a specialist in STD. If an expectant mother is known to have syphilis in the first trimester, some doctors would recommend pregnancy interruption. After the first three months of pregnancy, an expectant mother who has syphilis can pass on the disease to her unborn child. Early detection of the disease and prompt treatment can protect the developing fetus from harm.

If an infected pregnant woman is not treated during the first trimester she might have a miscarriage, a stillbirth, or her baby might be born with congenital syphilis. An infant with congenital syphilis might have problems with skin, bones, liver, and spleen at birth. Many babies infected with syphilis in the womb will not show any symptoms for two years or more. Sometimes the disease is latent until puberty. If allowed to progress, syphilis can lead to blindness, brain damage, and other serious problems in the child.

Genital Herpes

Herpes was once called "the new leprosy," "the virus of love," "the 'now' disease of the eighties." The word itself comes from the Greek word meaning "to creep," and herpes does just that. The disease moves from one person to another at a steady, undiminished pace. These days, disease-control experts estimate that about 30 percent of all sexually active Americans have been exposed to herpes, while less than ten years ago they were saying 5 percent came into contact with the disease. It is difficult to pin down the exact number of people who have herpes since, unlike gonorrhea, it does not have to be reported to the health authorities. Educated guessers feel that from 5 to 20 million people are harboring *herpes progenitallis*, better known as genital herpes.

Herpes took hold after the now-historic sexual revolution of the sixties encouraged sexual freedom. Women and men experienced many partners and inadvertently promoted STDs. All types of people found themselves with the highly contagious, often painful, itching, burning sores of genital herpes. Only protective use of a condom has slowed the silent outbreak.

Once a sore appears, the herpes virus has already entered the body, and that virus never leaves. The sore might disappear, but the disease has only retreated into a latent stage. When the disease is active and an open sore is festering, as it tends to do from time to time, herpes is very contagious and sexual intercourse hurts. Researchers at the University of Wisconsin have recently found that the virus might even be spread between flare-ups, when no symptoms exist. Their study found the herpes virus to be a constant prescence in genital secretions.

Herpes has strained marriages and postponed weddings. Sometimes a woman is so worried about being near a man with a history of herpes that she will not only refuse intimacy, she will barely shake his hand. People are gaining awareness that, like a fire in a windstorm, the disease spreads rapidly. Still, herpes might be considered only a mild illness if it were not for the severe consequences that women might suffer from it. Herpes can be a very painful disease, but unlike gonorrhea and syphilis, which have the potential to kill, it is not fatal.

A pregnant woman should know that, like gonorrhea and syphilis, herpes might attack a newborn during childbirth. The baby might die or suffer neurological disorders. (Newborns are damaged by herpes *only* during the birthing process. Herpes does not cause birth defects in utero.) But whether or not she is pregnant, studies have shown that a woman might be at a higher risk for cervical cancer if she has ever contracted herpes.

The most anxiety-provoking fact about this STD is that we can lessen severity of outbreaks but there is no cure. Many doctors have misinterpreted the disease, and they diagnose vaginal irritations from herpes as "yeast infections." Herpes has nevertheless been fully acknowledged as a serious problem. Its life-threatening effect on a newborn and possible cancer-causing presence in women have made it a disease with which to be reckoned. Researchers are now pushing for a way to combat the hardy herpes virus, and doctors are being encouraged to consider the possibility of herpes when they examine women for vaginal abnormalities.

What Are the Symptoms of Genital Herpes? Genital herpes comes from the DNA-based herpes simplex virus, types 1 and 2, or HSV-1 and HSV-2. The first type, HSV-1, is responsible for fever blisters or cold sores around the mouth. This type might also infect the eyes and, in the extreme, lead to blindness. The second type, HSV-2, accounts for most of the herpes that attacks the genitalia of women and men. In women, HSV-2 might show up on the cervix, vulva, perineum, and occasionally on the thighs and buttocks. It used to be thought that HSV-1 remained above the waist and HSV-2 was a below-the-waist condition, but researchers discovered that both types can be transmitted from mouth to genitals and vice versa during oral sex. (The difference between HSV-1 and HSV-2 is discussed at length in the next section.) However, most often genital herpes turns out to be HSV-2.

The beginning signs of a herpes sore usually appear about two to eight days after a woman has been invaded by the virus during sexual intercourse. Highly aware women might notice unusual vaginal discharges that send them to their doctors, but most women detect the disease only when they see or feel tiny, itchy red bumps on their vulvas. Very rapidly, the small bumps grow into ugly painful blisters that burst and spew forth millions of vital germs. A woman might have a slight fever and a general malaise at this time. She might also have a burning urination, especially if sores are festering near her urethra. On the other hand, if a herpes sore is located on her cervix, a woman might have no symptoms at all. Herpes might not be as pronounced on the cervix as it is on the vulva. On the cervix, a herpes sore might appear to be a small, often painless ulcer that is usually visible only to a physician. However, genital herpes hidden in the cervical area can be spread just as easily as when it is noticeably situated on the vulva.

When open sores are discovered, whether they are on the mouth or the genitals, a woman should avoid intimacies. The disease is in the active stage when open sores are festering. It is then that herpes spreads on contact. A woman should wait until the sores have disappeared, when herpes has retreated into the latent stage, before she engages in sex. However, the recent research suggests that there might be some level of contagion when sores disappear, since the virus has been found in genital secretions of herpes sufferers when they have no symptoms.

Still, the fact remains that a woman is mostly highly contagious after herpes sores erupt, a time when she is also susceptible to various kinds of disease-causing bacteria that might enter her body through the open wounds. So sexual intercourse is doubly dangerous at this time. Since there is no recognized cure for herpes, the body needs a quiet interval to build antibodies against the disease. Intimate contact during low resistance can easily spread the disease in her own body as well as transmit it to her partner.

In about ten or twelve days the sores heal, but the herpes virus stays in the body. The virus retreats into other cells, possibly near the lower spinal cord, where it remains until something happens to decrease the body's immune response. A stressful situation, menstruation, a poor diet, insomnia, anything that disrupts the body balance, can cause herpes to recur. About half of the people who get HSV-2 will have a recurrence within six months. Other herpes victims might live the rest of their lives without outbreaks of the disease or they might have attacks years later.

A woman must be alert to the signs of herpes to prevent herself from giving and getting the disease. On a man, herpes begins with the same itchy blisters that attack a woman. These blisters later break and cause painful open sores that are easy for a woman to spot before intercourse. By checking a man before sex, a woman can prevent herself from getting the disease. But since there is no real treatment for herpes, the only way a woman can be sure she will never get the disease is if her partners always wear condoms during sexual intercourse.

When a woman has vaginal pain or her instinct tells her that something is not right, she should visit her doctor. A gynecologist can rupture a sore and examine the fluid he extracts on a stained slide. Herpes viruses have giant, multicentered or multinucleated cells that are clearly recognizable under a microscope. A doctor can also send the sample fluid or a swab of the lesion to a lab for culture analysis. It will take a few days to get the answer. A blood test that determines a rise in herpes antibodies can also identify the disease.

A Pap smear is usually the best determinant for herpes on the cervix. A Pap test can tell a doctor about cervical herpes even before sores become visible. The viral cells stand out in the test.

But all these tests, in the end, should only confirm or deny a woman's suspicions. It is essential for a woman to examine herself when she bathes and showers, and if she finds any abnormality she must not be afraid to ask her doctor about the possibility of a sexually transmitted disease.

A woman who knows she has had herpes in the past should be open with her doctor about the condition. If she becomes pregnant, her baby could be affected during childbirth. Pregnant or not, she herself must be monitored for recurrence of the herpes, and also checked for early signs of cervical cancer, a disease that has been linked with herpes.

What Is the Difference Between Type 1 and Type 2 Herpes? Herpes simplex virus type 1 usually shows itself as a fever blister on the upper portion of the body, most frequently on the lips and mouth area, although on rare occasions it could infect the eyes. Herpes simplex virus type 2 usually affects the genital area and results in genital herpes. The sores involved in both types of herpes look exactly the same, but the viral strains are slightly different.

Originally it was thought that a cold sore on the lip was caused by a virus that was different from a genital herpes virus, but now it seems that the virus from a fever blister can be transferred to the genital area. During oral sex either a type 1 cold sore could be transmitted to the genitals or a type 2 genital sore could infect the mouth. Also, if a person touches an open sore on her or his lips and then handles a partner's genitals, herpes might be spread. *Herpes types 1 and 2 are not strictly confined to specific areas of the body.*

When a woman who has never had a cold sore gets an attack of genital herpes, HSV-2, she will have symptoms much more severe than a woman who has previously suffered through HSV-1. A woman who has had to deal with type 1 cold sores all her life has probably found them to be annoying and she has most likely wished they would just go away. Finally, she is being compensated for her suffering.

Having endured cold sores, a woman has had a chance to build antibodies against the herpes simplex virus. A woman who has been plagued by cold sores is less likely to succumb to the type 2 virus than a woman who has never experienced a cold sore or fever blister in her life. If a woman who gets type 1 does contract genital herpes, her symptoms will be milder than the fever and pain that can envelop a woman during her first bout with genital herpes, which might last from two to four weeks. If herpes starts on the cervix, a woman might have no symptoms or only mild symptoms, whether or not it is the first time the virus has ever entered her body.

HOW IS HERPES TREATED?

One of the main problems with herpes is that there is still no official cure. A reported one out of five Americans is infected with HSV and will carry the virus for life. However, sufferers now have a choice of medications for relief. Three antiviral oral drugs—acyclovir (brand name Zovirax), valacyclovir (Valtrex), and famciclovir (Famvir)—are effective at healing the sores of HSV-2 and calming flulike symptoms. Any of these medications may be taken whenever the itching that signals the onset of a herpes sore occurs. Any of these medications may also be taken daily for a year to prevent a recurring outbreak. More than 80 percent of people with genital herpes experience a recurrence after the initial outbreak, and most people average four recurrences a year.

While it is true that there is no effective cure for herpes, much can be done to relieve discomfort and prevent a recurrence of the disease. As it does against any other viral invader, the body will form antibodies to fight off herpes. The several weeks that it takes for antibodies to build up the body's defenses might be prolonged, however, if a woman becomes increasingly distressed by the disease. That is why *the first step in curing herpes is to try to eliminate stress* that might come from fear and worry over the disease itself. A woman should get plenty of bed rest, eat a proper diet, increase her vitamin intake, and generally strengthen her body to combat the virus. Then, her physician can combine her own experience with the latest information from researchers and can offer some form of treatment. If a doctor has no suggestions for relieving herpes, a woman should seek a new physician.

Considering the nature of the disease, it might be helpful, before the herpes blisters erupt, to apply cortisone ointment to the sores at frequent intervals. The cortisone should shrink the blisters before they burst. The disease will thereby be contained within cells and retreat into latency. (Remember, in the course of the disease the sores disappear but the herpes simplex virus is not destroyed. The disease has simply moved from its active stage into its latent phase.) With cortisone preventing open sores, there is little chance that a secondary infection will occur, which is often a problem with herpes.

There have been suggestions that herpes can be fought off naturally. Some scientists recommend megadoses of vitamin C, 1 gram

(1,000 mg) a day for every 20 pounds of body weight. A woman who weighs 120 pounds, for example, would need to take 6 grams a day. It has also been said that an increase in the amino acid lysine, 2 to 3 grams a day, might be helpful. This might be partly achieved by consuming milk products, fish, red meat, brewer's yeast, and potatoes—all foods that contain high amounts of lysine. At the same time that lysine is increased, arginine, an amino acid found in nuts, seeds, and grains, should be decreased, and no more than 100 units of vitamin E a day is recommended.

The most serious concern about an outbreak of HSV-2 is during pregnancy, especially around a woman's due date. A newborn exposed to the sores of herpes simplex virus during natural childbirth through the vaginal canal might be born blind. I recommend that a culture be taken two weeks before delivery to determine whether HSV-2 is active. If a woman tests positive, then a cesarean section should be scheduled. In her last trimester, an expectant mother might be treated with acyclovir, and sometimes her baby is treated after birth.

QUESTIONS ABOUT HERPES

Did I Get Herpes from Being Run-down?

> I got a herpes virus a few months ago and my doctor told me it was because I was so run-down. I have not had sex with anyone but my husband and he doesn't have herpes, so it seems that the doctor is right. Still, everything I read says herpes is sexually transmitted. Did I get herpes from being run-down?
> —M.F., Green Bay, Wisconsin

This woman might have been infected with the genital herpes type 2 virus years ago. The virus might have retreated into latency by settling into body cells. When she became run-down, the herpes might have surfaced because her immunity was diminished. When a woman's resistance is low the virus has just the opportunity it needs to become reactivated.

Ms. F.'s run-down condition should not have generated a first-time attack of herpes, but her fatigued state could have given rise to a recurrence. Ms. F. needed contact from fluid from an erupted herpes sore in order to get the disease in the first place. If it was not sexually transmitted, such fluid might have been present on a moist or unclean toilet seat. If her husband has never had the disease, she might have been exposed before her marriage and she might have been harboring herpes since then. Perhaps her first herpes invasion was in her cervical area, where it went unnoticed.

Ms. F.'s husband might have a built-in immunity to the disease and might never have been susceptible to herpes. Not everyone exposed to herpes gets it. Ms. F. should try to build herself up with rest, a proper diet, vitamin B-complex (which includes at least 50 to 100 mg of vitamin B$_6$), and a minimum of 1,000 mg of vitamin C daily to prevent the disease from returning again.

Herpes Led to Divorce

One day my husband came home with herpes type 2 and accused me of giving it to him. I have never been sick. I am full of energy, have no discharge, pain, or swelling, and have never seen a sore. Still, my husband charged me with his illness and even our minister backed him up and said my husband's herpes was my fault. I went to a doctor who confirmed that I did not have herpes, but then my husband said maybe I didn't have it now but I might have had it in the past. I was shocked! I firmly believe that it is my husband who has had sex since our marriage. I know it is not me. I have filed for divorce. I have moved out and I fully intend to remove this man from my life. The only thing is, I would like to prove that I have never had herpes. Is there any way I can do that?

—A.R., Alexandria, Virginia

Certainly, if Ms. R. has no symptoms and feels well, she should not be accused of having herpes, and her outraged reaction is understandable. There is no way of knowing whether her husband is suffering a first-time attack of herpes or a recurrence of herpes that invaded his body years ago, since he does not seem open to honest communication. He does not appear to be a loving, trusting husband, especially since he has even turned the minister against his wife. As the letter that follows this one shows, herpes does not have to break up marriages if both partners are sensitive to the patterns of the disease. I sympathize with Ms. R.

A blood test for herpes antibodies can show whether she has ever been in contact with the disease. If Ms. R. has antibodies, she might have had herpes at some point in her life. Any doctor can perform a blood test for her.

Living in Harmony with Herpes

My husband and I both have herpes. We don't care who gave it to whom, we're just real sorry that we have it. We've been married for three years and it seems that we have never had a time completely free from the awful sores. We have recently started taking vitamins C and B, and when we're not using ointments and creams, we powder the sores to keep them dry. Is there anything else we can do?

—D.Y., New Rochelle, New York

This couple has come to grips with the problems of herpes without blaming each other or seeking a divorce. They might be an example for other couples who must face the onset of this STD. The disease might recur after it has been latent in the body for a long time. An outbreak of herpes might be from a contamination that happened years before the couple married. Of course, there is always the possibility that herpes is showing up for the first time, but since herpes can occur in a woman without her being aware of its presence, it is often difficult to speak in absolutes. If a woman and a man love and trust each other, they should focus on overcoming the disease together.

There is no real cure for herpes, but in time, when a person has remained healthy and bolstered her or his resistance, the body builds defenses against the virus. By increasing their vitamins, using ointments and creams, and keeping the sores dry whenever possible, Ms. Y. and her husband are on the road to resistance. They might also follow antiviral drug measures suggested in the treatment section of this chapter until a breakthrough cure from science offers more relief.

My Baby Got Herpes During Delivery and Died

I found out that I had herpes when I was pregnant. My doctor told me that if I had no sores when it was time to deliver, the baby would not be in danger. If I had sores, he said he would do a cesarean section. When it was time to give birth I didn't have any sores, but the doctor did a cesarean anyway. My son was born with herpes and died one week later. I keep reading that herpes will not harm a baby born by cesarean. Then why isn't my son alive today? No one can give me any information, and the more I ask the more I'm told not to get pregnant again. I want to be a mother, but I can't live through the death and burial of another child. Is there anything I could have done to save my baby? Would I be killing another person if I tried to have a child again?
—J.S., St. Charles, Missouri

This letter is heartbreaking. And to add to the sadness, Ms. S. is still in the dark about how her baby contracted herpes.

It is known that the herpes simplex virus can travel into the amniotic fluid and attack an unborn. This viral invasion can occur in one of two ways: either a *transplacental passage* takes place and the virus penetrates an intact fetal membrane, or a woman goes into labor and her "water breaks," which means that the fetal membrane ruptures and the virus has easy access to the fetus.

An unborn child has no immunity to the disease since defenses against such a virus only begin to develop when a child is three weeks old. The fragile newborn who is exposed to herpes can do little to fight off the inevitable. About 50 to 100 percent of the newborns who are contaminated by HSV die, but safety measures can be taken.

A pregnant woman who has visible herpes sores should be delivered by cesarean section in order to prevent her baby from contact with the virus in the birth canal. Even if no sores exist and a vaginal culture has been negative for at least two weeks before a woman is due to deliver, there is concern about whether to recommend a cesarean section. Some obstetricians perform C-sections even though a woman tests negative and has no visible herpes sores; others permit natural childbirth. Sometimes acyclovir is given as a protective measure. A recent study has found that when a woman experiences a first-time outbreak of herpes during pregnancy, if she takes 400 mg of acyclovir at thirty-six weeks of gestation, she gains significant protection against a recurring outbreak and reduces her need for a C-section.

What unfortunately often happens if there is herpes contamination in the newborn is that the baby, not initially sick, is sent home, where she or he becomes ill and succumbs to the disease. If observation and treatment are provided in a neonatal unit, there is a greater chance that a baby can survive. In one case, doctors saved the life of a herpes-infected baby by giving the child a blood transfusion with serum from a woman who had had genital herpes and had built up antibodies against the disease. The newborn was also treated with an adenosine arabinoside ointment. In other cases, infants were treated with gamma globulin for their first ten days to build their immune systems. They fought off their infections nicely. The successful outcome of such cases offers hope for other newborns who might become infected by herpes, but the only way such therapies can be administered is if doctors suspect that babies are contaminated in the first place.

Ms. S. knows that she has a history of herpes, but I honestly think that she could try to become pregnant again. The chance that another child will succumb to the disease is practically nil, but as a precaution, she should have vaginal cultures tested for herpes at regular intervals during the pregnancy. Approximately a week before her due date, she should undergo an amniocentesis. If all her culture reports are negative and her amniotic fluid is negative, she should be permitted to give birth vaginally, even though she has previously had a cesarean section. If a vaginal culture is positive at any time, and if the amniotic fluid is negative, a repeat cesarean section should be recommended. After delivery, her baby should be observed in a neonatal unit.

My Herpes Disappeared Before Delivery; Why Did I Need a Cesarean?

I developed herpes three weeks before I went into labor with my son. A week before I delivered, the herpes had cleared up, but my doctor said that when any of his patients got herpes in the last trimester he delivered them by cesarean section. He also said that if my water broke there was a chance of the herpes traveling up the birth canal and infecting the baby. He wanted me to avoid labor, but as it turned out, I went into labor without knowing it and I was contracting every three minutes when I arrived at the hospital. Still, the doctor did a cesarean. I really didn't think he had to since the herpes had gone away. Now I want to get pregnant again, but my doctor and two other doctors I've talked to say that I would have to have a cesarean again. They believed that "Once a cesarean, always a cesarean." Why do I have to have a C-section again, especially when I think the first one was unnecessary?
—C.B., South Dennis, Massachusetts

As mentioned in the previous letter, a newborn with genital herpes faces between 50 and 100 percent mortality. It is important that everything be done to prevent a newborn from being contaminated by the virus—sometimes, even if a sore has disappeared, the virus might still be active. As explained in the previous letter, Ms. B.

should have had a vaginal culture to determine whether the herpes virus was still present. Then, she would have had no doubts about her cesarean. If a vaginal culture had been positive a cesarean birth would have been absolutely necessary. If a vaginal culture had tested negative, a vaginal delivery might have been permitted, but there is a small controversy on this point.

Certain scientists believe that if a woman like Ms. B. has been contaminated for less than three weeks prior to her delivery, she has not had enough time to produce antibodies against the disease. They feel that if an expectant mother has no herpes antibodies, her baby might be more susceptible to herpes and a cesarean section will offer the newborn better protection. There is little debate when a woman has suffered a herpes attack more than three weeks before her due date. She would have had more time to produce antibodies, and if a vaginal culture and amniocentesis are negative, a vaginal delivery should be safe.

Ms. B. should be able to find an obstetrician at a teaching hospital or a major medical center who does not feel that "Once a cesarean, always a cesarean," I keep hoping that physicians throughout the country will one day realize that women *can* have vaginal deliveries after cesarean sections. Recently I saw a woman who had traveled all the way from Houston to New York because no doctor in Houston would allow her a "normal" delivery after her cesarean. The woman, as expected, faced no problem. She enjoyed an easy, natural, vaginal delivery in spite of her past experience.

Every month, hundreds of babies are born vaginally to women who have had previous cesarean births. If aware women like Ms. B. refuse to become the patients of doctors who operate for the sake of convenience, these obstetricians will eventually change.

I've Had Herpes for Years; Will I Get Cervical Cancer?

I've had herpes that has come and gone for the last four years. I get very painful lesions around and inside my vagina every time I get an attack. When I learned that there was no vaccine or cure for

herpes, I became very upset. I've never had a disease that would last me the rest of my life and the more I hear about it, the more worried I become. Will I get cervical cancer? I'm so sure that cancer is going to be my fate now that herpes has set in. It seems my whole personality has changed because herpes and cancer are always preying on my mind. Is there anything I can do?
—V.L., Los Angeles, California

A woman who has herpes should not assume that she will get cervical cancer. Most experts believe that while HSV-2 and cervical cancer often co-exist, they are probably not cause-and-effect related. These two diseases tend to spring from the same circumstances, connected to a woman's sexual activity (see below). Research has shown that the human papillomavirus (HPV), which leads to genital warts, is more strongly linked to cervical cancer.

Cervical cancer is seen more when women begin engaging in sexual intercourse during their teens, have many sexual partners, and bear children early in life. These are almost the same conditions that promote herpes. Still, although the conditions of cervical cancer are known, the causes remain unknown. Perhaps something in male sperm causes cancer, or women who develop cervical cancer might have certain biological deficiencies that are still mysteries to medical experts.

A woman who has had herpes should not worry about cervical cancer any more than a woman who has never had herpes, but at least once a year she should have a Pap test, which will pick up cervical cancer before there are any clinical signs. If Ms. L. keeps her resistance high and gets her Pap smear at least once a year, she is doing all she can to stay in good health.

Chlamydia

Chlamydia, which is sometimes called nongonococcal urethritis (NGU), is a shockingly serious, sexually transmitted disease that infects 3 to 4 million people in the United States every year.

For 80 percent of women and 10 percent of men, chlamydia provides no symptoms, which is why it is considered a sinister
"silent infection." The chlamydia bacterium, *Chlamydia trachomatis*,
infects the mucus membranes in the penis, vagina, cervix, anus,
urethra (the tube that enables urine to pass from the bladder
through the penis in a man and opening near the vagina in a
woman), or eye.

A woman is usually infected on the cervix, and then chlamydia
travels. It moves into Fallopian tubes and ovaries, and through the
abdomen. Unless chlamydia is treated, it results in pelvic inflammatory disease (PID), an infection in the abdominal area that can
spread to the Fallopian tubes and ovaries. PID often can cause
chronic pain, internal scarring, and infertility. The scar tissue that
forms in the Fallopian tubes can prevent conception or cause an
ectopic pregnancy, which means that a conception grows outside the
uterus, usually in a tube. Ectopic pregnancy is a life-threatening
condition (see chapter 11).

Men who catch chlamydia might become sterile with epididy-
mitis, an infection of the testes and the epididymes, the ducts that
transport sperm from the testes to the vasa. Also, conjunctivitis, an
infection of the eyes, might be transmitted to anyone who swims in
a pool where the water is contaminated by *Chlamydia trachomatis.*

Another great danger, however, is contamination of newborns.
Each year, conjunctivitis is seen in about 75,000 and pneumonia in
about 30,000 babies born to infected mothers. Conjunctivitis usually
appears a week or two after delivery, when a baby's eyes become
swollen and runny. Untreated conjunctivitis might appear to heal by
itself, but it might recur as a child grows up, and she or he might
eventually suffer conjuctival scars and corneal damage. Chlamydia
is also a cause of infant pneumonia, which usually appears when
newborns are four to eight weeks old. Infants suffering middle ear,
genital, intestinal, and rectal infections might also have infected
mothers. Pregnant women might give birth prematurely or deliver
stillborn babies. In one study, stillbirth and sudden infant death

syndrome were shown to be ten times greater for the offspring of women with chlamydia.

What Causes Chlamydia? Although the *Chlamydia trachomatis* bacterium sometimes settles into healthy tissue, chlamydia finds its best growth environment within the ulcerated lesions of an inflamed cervix in a woman, or an irritated urethra in a man or a woman. The disease is spread through vaginal and anal sexual intercourse; also, it can spread from a woman to her fetus during birth. The only method of protection against chlamydia is the use of a male or female condom during intercourse.

Women who have multiple sex partners, who have sex without condoms, and who have a health history of other sexually transmitted diseases and infections, are more likely to be susceptible to chlamydia. Teenagers have the highest rates of chlamydia today.

Chlamydia can result in pelvic inflammatory disease (PID), which then could lead to miscarriage and ectopic pregnancy. Chlamydia is also linked to stillbirth and sudden infant death syndrome, and might be the reason why some newborns have low birth weight, eye infections, pneumonia, and other life-damaging diseases. Health professionals are deeply involved in fighting the spread of chlamydia through awareness.

Women must inform their sex partners of their infections and be sure that their partners are screened and treated at the same time they are. When being treated for chlamydia a woman should refrain from sexual intercourse, and when she returns to sexual activity she must use a condom every time.

What Are the Symptoms of Chlamydia? The bacterium *Chlamydia trachomatis* is sexually transmitted by both sexes. In men, urethritis usually begins two to three weeks after exposure to the disease. A man will have burning urination, maybe some pain and tingling, and a urethral discharge. Many men think they have gonorrhea, but gonorrhea occurs two to three *days* after exposure; chlamydia shows up two to three *weeks* later. Often with chlamydia, the discharge is min-imal—it might be clear white, like mucus, and appear only at the first urination of the day.

Women are at a disadvantage because they usually have no symp-toms. The rare woman might notice a slight urethral discharge. Sometimes a woman has one or some of these symptoms: bleeding between menstrual periods or after intercourse, abdominal pain, painful intercourse, low-grade fever, painful urination or the urge to urinate more than usual, a vaginal discharge, or mucopurulent cer-vicitis (a yellowish, odorous discharge from her cervix). Most often chlamydia is detected by a doctor who spots an inflamed or irritated cervix during an examination. A cervical inflammation does not usually cause a woman pain.

Every sexually active woman, even a woman who has only had one sexual partner, should be tested at least once for chlamydia. A woman who is under age twenty, or a woman who has more than one sexual partner, or a new sexual partner, or who engages in sexual intercourse without the protection of a condom, should ask her doc-tor for a chlamydia test every year. It can be done at the same time she has her Pap test.

The Chlamydia/PID Link. Chlamydia is the leading cause of pelvic inflammatory disease (PID), which is sometimes a woman's first sign of chlamydia. PID is an infection that causes abdominal pain with fever, and sometimes pain with intercourse. It starts in the abdominal area and spreads to the Fallopian tubes, ovaries, and often leads to infertility. In the tubes it can form scar tissue that blocks conception or leads to a life-threatening ectopic pregnancy. As explained in chapter 11, a doctor must remove an ectopic pregnancy either surgically or through medication. The longer an ectopic pregnancy grows before it is removed, the greater a woman's chance of losing the use of her tube. The chlamydia/PID link is known to be a cause of infertility.

Chlamydia and Pregnancy. Every year almost 200,000 newborns suffer eye infections, ear infections, and pneumonia as a result of being born to mothers infected with chlamydia. An infant's symptoms usually appear about four weeks after birth. A baby who is sick with chlamydia can be difficult to treat. If chlamydia is diagnosed when a woman is pregnant, however, it is usually treated easily and successfully. Chlamydia infections that go undetected have been associated with miscarriage, stillbirth, low infant birth weight, and premature delivery.

How Is Chlamydia Diagnosed? Usually a doctor detects chlamydia during a gynecological examination when he notices an irritated cervix or a cervical discharge. A doctor might also do chlamydia testing as part of a woman's biannual checkup or an infertility workup. It can be done at the same time as a Pap test. Traditionally, a doctor takes a swabbed sample from a woman's cervix and sends it to a laboratory for cell-culture test.

As mentioned above, every sexually active woman and infertility patient, even a woman who has had only one sexual partner, should have a chlamydia test at least once. Women under age twenty, and women with multiple partners, should have annual chlamydia tests. I urge teens who have sexual intercourse without condoms to be tested every six months. A young woman's cervix is more open to infection at this time of her life, which is one reason why chlamydia is so common among teenagers.

It is important that a woman's sexual partner be tested when a woman's chlamydia is confirmed. Until recently, testing for a man involved obtaining a swabbed sample of his urethral discharge, an unpleasant process. Now a new chlamydia test has been developed that requires only a urine sample. It is available to women and men. This latest test is a high-tech DNA amplification that is proving to be much more accurate, but also more expensive, than the chlamydia culture test.

What Is the Treatment for Chlamydia? Once it is found, chlamydia can be cured easily with an antibiotic. A woman and her partner must take the antibiotic at the same time so that they do not risk passing the disease back and forth. Tetracycline or erythromycin have been given in the past, but recently other antibiotics have been recommended for treatment. Doxycycline or Vibramycin, 100 mg orally twice a day for seven days, is one course of treatment; another is azithromycin, 1 gram orally in a single dose. It is astounding that a single, inexpensive dose of an antibiotic can permanently cure a disease that, when left untreated, can devastate a woman's ability to reproduce.

Lymphogranuloma Venereum

Lymphogranuloma venereum comes from a sexually transmitted chlamydia infection that causes lymph nodes in the groin area to become swollen and tender. The chlamydia causing this disease is a different strain than the one described earlier. In the highly contagious lymphogranuloma venereum, a single painless blisterlike lesion on the perineum appears three to twenty-one days after a woman has been exposed to the disease. The chlamydia then travels to the neighboring lymph nodes, causing them to become painfully swollen about three weeks after the initial lesion appeared. At this point, the primary sore has already healed. The infection, though, begins to spread upward to the vagina. Swollen lymph nodes form a hard mass, and the overlying skin turns dusky, stretches, and eventually breaks open into painful sores that take a long time to heal and leave linear scars when they do. A woman might have headaches and fever during the course of the disease. If swelling and lesions spread into the vagina and the anus, both canals might subsequently become fibrous and close, and severe complications can result.

If a woman has a suspicious groin lesion when she visits a doctor, he should be able to biopsy the sore and have a lab determine whether a specific chlamydia pattern exists. Most often, though, a woman goes to the doctor for the swollen lymph nodes. Then, lymphogranuloma venereum can be diagnosed by a Frei test, an injection into the forearm that causes a red bump to appear in forty-eight to seventy-two hours if the test is positive. A doctor might also choose to conduct a complement fixation (CF) test to see if chlamydia antibodies are present in the patient's blood. Such a test can be performed only at a lab that specializes in VD analyses.

Even though the two STDs are caused by chlamydia, lymphogranuloma venereum is much less common than NGU. If a woman is diagnosed as having lymphogranuloma venereum, she and her partner should be treated with oral tetracycline or oral erythromycin, 500 mg every six hours, or four times a day, for at least three weeks.

Genital Warts

Genital warts (*Condylomata acuminata*) are very different than warts that appear on the fingers. Caused by the human papillomavirus (HPV), genital warts are uneven growths that might be round or long; pink, white, or gray; small or enlarged into clusters. They are usually seen on the penis or in the vaginal area because the warmth and moisture of the genitals is especially conducive to wart development. Often the warts on a woman travel to her perineum and anus because fluid from the growths carries the virus downward (see figure 15-2, page 561).

The wart-causing HPV initially invades the genital area because the vaginal environment, often unbalanced by yeast infections or other types of vaginitis, birth control pills, pregnancy, or stress offers good breeding grounds for germs. The moist vaginal enclosure becomes a prime target for a viral invasion, as does the moist area of a penis, particularly of an uncircumcised man. In fact, although the virus attacks every type of penis, men who are not circumcised more often have venereal warts than men who are circumcised. Of the over 100 types of HPV, about twenty-three infect the human genital area. A woman diagnosed with HPV can sometimes have a follow-up Digene Hybrid Capture test to determine whether her strain of HPV is linked to cervical cancer. Ninety-five percent of cervical cancers contain genetic material from HPV.

The genital warts are spread during sexual intercourse, but they might not appear until six weeks to six months after exposure. Usually a woman feels a small protusion of the skin on the vulva or the outer portion of her vagina. Most of the time the growth is painless. Using a mirror, a woman should perform a self-examination of her genital area to confirm her finding of an abnormal growth. She might investigate the inner wall of her vagina to see whether the warts have spread. If her doctor diagnoses genital warts, she should tell her sexual partner or partners that they should also be examined and treated for warts. The only way to curb this, and every, STD is to prevent infection and reinfection with the use of a condom and honesty between partners.

While the link between HPV and cervical cancer is clear, the good news is that the HPV types responsible for most of the visible genital warts do not cause cancer. Also, cervical cancer is still relatively rare. As long as a woman has biannual Pap smears and any abnormal results are followed up by her doctor with colposcopy and biopsy, she can be successfully treated.

Most of the time genital warts are detected by an abnormal Pap smear and a colposcopy, essentially a doctor's magnified well-lit look at a woman's cervix. A doctor can also apply acetic acid to a suspicious area; HPV-affected spots will whiten. A cervical biopsy can be done to find out whether any cells are precancerous or cancerous. Genital warts can also be a problem for a pregnant woman (see page 524).

How Are Genital Warts Treated? Available antibiotics do not affect a virus. Eventually genital warts might become self-limiting because the body, once exposed to the HPV, begins to produce natural antibodies. A physician might treat genital warts either with podofilox (Condylox), imiquimod (Aldara), or podophyllin, all wart-killing medications.

- Condylox is a liquid; Aldara is a cream. Both are available by prescription for home use. A woman's physician should instruct her on how to apply these medications.

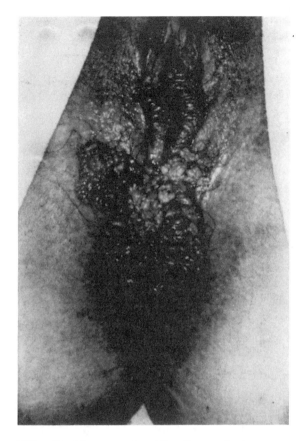

15-2 **Venereal Warts** *(Condylomata acuminata).* Sexually transmitted warts are caused by the papova virus. The warts spread during sexual intercourse and usually begin as small pink, white, or gray growths. If not treated, the growths multiply to such an extent that they might cover the entire vaginal opening. The photograph illustrates how the venereal warts have spread from the bottom of the vulva to the perineum and the anus. Venereal warts are very contagious, and a sexual partner should be examined and treated if he or she has evidence of warts.

- Podophyllin is a medication the doctor applies directly on the heads of the warts during an office visit. A woman remains on the examining table ten to fifteen minutes after a podophyllin application to give the medication time to penetrate and destroy the warts. A woman might need several treatments before all the warts are gone, and in some cases warts have to be removed through electrosurgery or laser surgery.

At the same time that a woman is treated with podophyllin, she should receive antiyeast medication to restore the balance of microorganisms in her vagina. The presence of yeast makes the warts multiply, and the growths will not disappear unless the natural environment of the vagina is restored through aggressive therapy.

Until all the warts are gone, a woman should return to her doctor every two weeks for an internal examination and reapplication of podophyllin. Some warts do not disappear right away, and small warts are often hidden. Only constant treatment will truly eliminate the growths.

If podophyllin treatments do not remove the warts, they can be electrocauterized, or burned away. This procedure is performed after a doctor injects Novocain around the warts, which he then burns to their stems with the aid of a fine probe. If there are only a few warts, a doctor can complete the electrocauterization in his office. A doctor might also offer a woman the option of burning away her warts through electro- or laser surgery, or by destroying them through cryosurgery, which involves freezing them off with liquid nitrogen. If warts have spread extensively, a woman might have to be admitted to the hospital to have the growths destroyed while she is under anesthesia.

A NOTE ABOUT PREGANCY: Genital warts can become large enough to obstruct the birth canal and prevent a vaginal delivery. A cesarean section is then necessary. Even if a woman has small warts that do not prevent vaginal delivery, the warts could affect the newborn. Sometimes the baby aspirates the virus as she or he passes through the birth canal, and warts are subsequently found on the baby's vocal cords. Therefore, it might be best for a woman afflicted with genital warts of any size to be delivered by cesarean section. *Important: A pregnant woman should never be treated with podophyllin since the medication can cross the placenta and lead to birth defects or fetal death.*

What Can I Do If My Warts Won't Go Away?

Six months ago my doctor told me I had venereal warts and he applied some kind of solution to the bumps which burned like fire. I had to stay on the table with a light shining on the area for fifteen minutes afterward. I've had this treatment once or twice a month for the last six months and the warts still keep coming back. I tried not to have sex for a while, but the warts still don't disappear completely. When I get treated I can barely wear clothes because my vaginal area is so tender and sore. What can I do if the warts won't go away? I'd like to get married someday, but how can I if I have this problem?

—D.G., Union City, Tennessee

As mentioned above, genital warts are usually carefully inspected and diagnosed by a physician, who then applies podophyllin, the acidic, wart-killing medication. After treatment, especially if a woman has felt a burning sensation, Mycolog cream can be used to salve irritated vaginal lips. Intravaginal application of antiyeast medication should be prescribed at the same time as the podophyllin treatment is undertaken. Warts are often accompanied by a yeast infection, and if both ailments are not treated simultaneously, the warts can stubbornly persist. (See "How Is Monilia/*Candida Albicans* Treated?" pages 462 to 463.) Remember, a wart cure is not complete without an effort to stabilize the vaginal milieu.

A woman should be treated with podophyllin every two weeks until her warts completely disappear. If recurrence continues, as it has with Ms. G., a careful wart removal through electrocauterization should be attempted. Electrocautery produces only minor discomfort. It seems that Ms. G. would be a candidate for this procedure, but still she might become reinfected if her partner or partners are not also treated for warts. She should inform her sexual contacts about her condition and ask them to be evaluated by their own physicians. Then, with luck, her wart misery will be over.

Molluscum Contagiosum

Molluscum contagiosum is a sexually transmitted disease that shows itself as small, dimpled pimples, often mistaken for venereal warts, appearing on the vulva. The molluscum contagiosum growths are smaller than warts and contain foreign tissue known as molluscum bodies. Sometimes they appear when a woman is being treated for gonorrhea or NGU because when bacteria are killed the molluscum contagiosum virus has an opportunity to breed.

The growths are not harmful in that they will not lead to debilitating illnesses. Usually if a woman tries to stabilize her vaginal environment with proper diet and rest and keeps her genital area as clean and dry as possible, her body will work to produce antibodies to fight the virus causing molluscum contagiosum. If the growths do not disappear by themselves after a few weeks, the recommended treatment for venereal warts might be advised for this disease. Treatment with podophyllin might be attempted, but it is usually not successful. To overcome molluscum contagiosum, electrocauterization might be necessary.

Granuloma Inguinale, or Donovanosis

Granuloma inguinale, an STD usually confined to people who live in the tropics, is caused by the bacterium *Donovania granulomatis*, currently referred to as *Calymmatobacterium granulomatis*. The bacteria proliferate during instances of poor personal hygiene, are harbored in the gastrointestinal tract, and are transmitted during anal sex. With the rare case of granuloma inguinale, painful red bumps might appear on a woman's cervix, vagina, perineum, or anal and groin areas. The bumps turn into inflamed, itchy, ulcerated sores that cause the pain to escalate. A doctor can have scrapings of the sores cultured for a diagnosis. Tetracycline, erythromycin, or ampicillin, 500 mg four times a day for two or three weeks, is the usual treatment.

Chancroid

Chancroid is another infrequently seen STD that involves genital sores. About three to five days after exposure to the *Hemophilus ducreyi* bacteria, which cause chancroid, a woman might notice one or several pustules—pus-filled blisters—near her clitoris or on her vulva. The sores erupt rather quickly into foul-smelling, shallow, soft, painful ulcerations. The disease can be diagnosed by a culture and treated with Gantrisin (sulfisoxazole), 1 gram four times a day for two weeks, or tetracycline, 500 mg four times a day for two weeks. If a woman is pregnant or allergic to sulfa drugs and tetracycline, she might be treated with erthyromycin, 500 mg four times a day for two weeks.

Enteric Sexually Transmitted Diseases

There is a new rash of enteric, or intestinal, sexually transmitted diseases that never used to be considered sexually related. Shigellosis, amebiasis, giardiasis, and salmonellosis have moved into the category of sexually transmitted disease with the rise in oral and anal sex. These diseases have become more prevalent among homosexuals than heterosexuals. The symptoms include abdominal pain, diarrhea, nausea, vomiting, fever, and chills. Diagnoses are made from stool cultures, but treatments vary depending on the disease. Shigellosis, caused by bacteria, can be treated with antibiotics, preferably ampicillin or tetracycline. Amebiasis, giardiasis, and salmonellosis are protozoan invasions. For giardiasis, the first-choice treatment is Atabrine (quinacrine), but Flagyl (metronidazole) is also effective. Salmonellosis is often self-limiting, but in severe cases chloramphenicol or Terramycin have been used successfully. With amebiasis, Diodoquin (diidohydroxyquin) is often the drug of choice, given in combination with Flagyl or tetracycline.

Crabs, or Pubic Lice

"Crabs" are responsible for a sexually transmitted condition officially known as pediculosis or phthirius pubis. They are tiny bloodsucking lice (*Phthirius pubis*) that breed in the pubic hairs, although they are sometimes also found on underarm hair, eyelashes, and mustaches—but never in head hair. These hungry parasites bury their mouth parts into the skin and hold on to the pubic hairs with their hind legs. Disturbed by the heat of lovemaking, crabs loosen their grips and travel from one partner to another. Crabs do not live long away from their human feeding grounds, but sometimes they can be found in recently infested clothing, towels, and bedding, and even on toilet seats, which all can be sources of contamination.

A woman might not notice that she has crabs at first. The insects lay their eggs, which are called nits, at the bases of pubic hairs. In two weeks the nits become adults and then an overwhelming symptomatic itch begins. A woman might see small dark spots on her underwear. When she looks at her itchy genital area, she might discover what appear to be moving dots or traveling freckles. These are the crabs. Lice are often carriers of such epidemic diseases as typhus and trench fever, so crabs should be eliminated quickly.

A doctor might prescribe Kwell lotion or shampoo, to be rubbed into the infested areas and washed off in twelve to twenty-four hours. Usually Kwell lotion is left on overnight. Without a prescription, a woman can purchase over-the-counter pediculicides such as A-200 Pyrinate, RID, Triple X, and Vonce, which are also effective crab killers. As a woman washes off a medicated solution, she should try to pick away the dead crabs and nits with her fingers. All of her clothing, towels, and bedding should be washed in very hot or boiling water to prevent reinfection. A week or two later, the lotion or shampoo should be repeated and a woman should examine herself with a magnifying mirror to make sure all crabs are dead and gone.

Should I Shave My Pubic Hair If I Have Crabs?

*I just turned nineteen and I've only had sex with one man in
my life. I knew him a long time and I trusted him, but I didn't
know what to do when he called and told me he had crabs. At first
I thought he was talking about seafood. I never heard of crabs on
your body before and I was shocked to discover that he was actually
discussing a venereal disease. He told me to shave off all my pubic
hair and go to the drugstore for a bottle of A-200. I was never more
embarrassed than when I went into that store and asked for A-200
in front of a whole bunch of customers. I didn't dare question the
pharmacist, but when I got home I realized that I had a bottle with
instructions in Spanish. I was so scared that live things would be
crawling all over me I washed my entire body in the medicine for
three days. I shaved my pubic hair too. Now I'm worried because I
don't know how I can tell if I really had crabs. I've also heard they
could crawl inside your body and make you sterile. Is there
anything else I should do? Should I shave again?*

—P.L., Albuquerque, New Mexico

Crabs are usually sexually transmitted; however, they could be
passed on through infested clothing, towels, or bedding. Ms. L.'s
boyfriend might have caught them from any of these media if he
had no other sexual relationship prior to his discovery.

The lice look just like saltwater crabs under a microscope, so Ms.
L.'s "seafood" assumption was perfectly reasonable. These crabs, however, will be seen only in the pubic hair, eyelashes, armpit hairs, or
mustache. They will never appear on head hair and they are easily
treated with Kwell, the prescription lotion or shampoo, or over-the-
counter remedies such as A-200 Pyrinate or Triple X. These medications should be smeared onto the pubic hair, armpit area, or on the
mustache, in two applications one to two weeks apart. A woman or a
man with crabs does not have to shave her or his pubic hair in order
to treat the condition. The medication is usually sufficient. Although

crab lice could crawl into the vagina or the nostrils (if a man has them in his mustache), they cannot enter the internal organs. Crabs will not cause infertility or brain damage by entering orifices. Whether or not Ms. L. had crab lice, if she does not have any sign of them now she need not worry about unforeseen complications.

Scabies

Scabies occurs when a tiny mite (*Sarcoptes scabiei*) burrows under the skin and lays eggs. In ten days the eggs become adults and the infestation continues. The scabies mite is barely visible, but sometimes when a woman realizes that she is itchy, she might notice a small opening in the skin where a mite has invaded. Scabies attack in the genital folds; between fingers and toes; inside wrists or elbows; around the waistline, nipples, or navel; and in the creases of the buttocks—but never above the neck. The mites are easy to diagnose from the burrows, the short wavy lines they make in the skin.

The big problem with scabies is that it does not have to be sexually transmitted. Scabies can spread through an entire family and leave everyone itching and scratching. The infected person and everyone who lives with her or him should be treated with an application of Kwell lotion from the neck down. The Kwell should be left on for twenty-four hours and then washed off. A second application is not usually necessary, but the Kwell treatment might be repeated a week later if a woman feels she would like double protection. As soon as scabies is diagnosed, a woman should wash her clothing, towels, and bedding in very hot water to prevent reinfection.

Tinea Cruris

Tinea cruris, or ringworm of the thigh, is a fungal infection. Since it has recently been discovered that the fungus can travel from the skin of one person to another during the close contact of sexual intercourse, tinea cruris has become another sexually transmitted disease.

Actually, there are no worms involved in a "ringworm" condition. Tinea cruris appears in the form of round or irregular spots that grow into widening rings on the inner upper thighs. The disease might restrict itself to just a few lesions, or it might spread to a woman's perineum, vulva, and labia. On a man, tinea cruris will often attack the area between the thighs and behind the testicles. The brownish red spots are itchy and they can become very painful if scratching causes a secondary skin infection to develop.

Tinea cruris has often been thought to be a "jock itch" by its victims. Usually the heat rash from jock itch spontaneously disappears within a few days, but tinea cruris, without medication, persists. A woman who itches on her inner upper thighs should hold a mirror to the area and see if she notices the spots of tinea cruris. If she sees anything that looks suspicious, she should visit her doctor for diagnosis and be ready to suggest the possibility of tinea cruris to him. Since the infection has only been considered an STD for a short time, a doctor might not yet be familiar with its symptoms.

A doctor might diagnose tinea cruris either by recognizing its unique appearance or by sending a scraping of a lesion to be cultured. Once positively diagnosed, tinea cruris can be effectively treated with antifungal antibiotics such as Grifulvin V or Fulvicin, taken orally in tablets. In addition, local application of medicated creams such as Mycolog or Tinactin might help to speed recovery.

Cytomegalovirus Infection

One of the oldest viruses known to man, cytomegalovirus infection is considered an STD because it can be spread through intimate contact with saliva, vaginal secretions, cervical mucus, and urine. (Occasionally, the disease has also been found in semen.) A woman who gets cytomegalovirus will experience symptoms similar to those of mononucleosis—malaise, lethargy, a rapidly ascending and descending fever for as long as three weeks. The disease is distinguished from mononucleosis because it is not accompanied by tonsillitis, pharyngitis, or enlarged lymph glands. As with any other viral ailment, there is no effective treatment for cytomegalovirus infection, although antibiotics have been used to curtail secondary infection. The biggest problem comes when the disease attacks a woman during pregnancy, and 3 to 4 percent of all pregnancies are affected by it.

If cytomegalovirus infection occurs in the first trimester, there is a strong chance that the disease will have a teratogenic (cell-changing) effect on the fetus since the virus attacks growing cells most rapidly. Congenital malformation of the newborn, with brain damage, might result, but most often the disease ends a pregnancy in miscarriage or fetal death in utero. For the damage it can do during pregnancy, cytomegalovirus has often been compared to rubella (German measles), but since women can now be vaccinated against rubella, cytomegalovirus is the most severe and harmful viral infection an expectant mother might contract.

Cystitis—Honeymoon Cystitis

Cystitis, a bladder infection, is not technically a sexually transmitted disease, but it can be related to a surge in sexual activity (which is why we use the term "honeymoon cystitis"). During frequent sexual intercourse, bacteria can be pushed up into a woman's urethra. After the bacteria travel from the urethra into the bladder, a woman feels a pressure to urinate. When she tries to void, she might have either a burning sensation, burning urination, or bloody urine. Women who use diaphragms are more commonly afflicted with cystitis because the diaphragm presses against the urethra and distorts the passage. A woman who uses a diaphragm should urinate before and after intercourse to relieve the pressure on her bladder. If cystitis develops, it can easily be treated with Macrodantin, Negram, or sulfa medications. If a woman with cystitis increases her intake of vitamin C and drinks a lot of cranberry juice—both also good for *preventing* cystitis—she will be making her urine more acidic and hastening her cure.

15.

Fibroid Tumors and Ovarian Cysts— Do They Mean Hysterectomy?

"CUT IT OUT!"

The twenty-eight-year-old woman dangled her legs from the edge of the examining table as she waited for the gynecologist. She automatically pulled the tissue paper gown more tightly around her body as she thought about how much she hated this appointment. Maybe she would like this new doctor, but the prospect of a medical checkup made her cringe. Feeling that she was too busy with work to take time out, she had not seen a doctor in three years. She had always been in good health and this was probably going to be a needless ordeal. She gathered the force of her conviction and stared directly in front of her. Suddenly the door she was facing abruptly opened and the doctor walked toward her, followed by his officious nurse.

"Okay, dear, you can lie down and put your feet in the stirrups," said the redheaded nurse. "Come a little farther down. That's fine. The doctor will be right with you."

"How are you?" asked the doctor as he pulled a chair closer and positioned himself between her legs. Without further conversation, he began his internal examination.

"Hmm" he said as he furrowed his brow. Then he squinted slightly. "Have you ever been told you have a tumor?"

"A tumor?" she repeated in disbelief. She pushed her heels into the stirrups, propped herself up on her elbows, and stared down at him. All she could see was the top of his head between her legs.

"Yes, you have a uterine tumor the size of my fist," he said as he raised his clenched hand to illustrate.

"Oh my God," she gasped with her eyes on his fist. It looked tremendous. "My God, is it . . . is it cancer?"

"I'm not sure. We'll have to cut it out and take a look."

"Cut it out?"

"I'll have my nurse book you for surgery."

"Wait, this is all happening too fast. Are you sure it's that serious? Maybe you should check it again."

"I've done all I can right now. There's nothing more we can know before we take it out and send it to the lab."

The nurse was already on the phone to the hospital as the doctor prepared to leave the examining room. At the door, he looked back, nodded to his patient, and smiled. "See you in the OR," he said, and closed the door behind him.

Luckily, this woman did not fall for the doctor's scary, insensitive approach. Her intuition told her that she felt too good to require surgery. She phoned a girl friend to ask for the name and number of the physician her friend had always praised as kind and competent. This second-opinion doctor confirmed a small fibroid tumor in her uterus.

"Your fibroid is not as large as a fist," he told her. "It's only about two inches in diameter." He went on to explain fibroids in detail and ended by saying, "A tumor is not synonymous with cancer. *Tumor* is a Latin word that simply means 'swelling.' You don't need surgery. We only need to see you in the office every four to six months to monitor the growth of the fibroid."

The second doctor was an exemplary physician. *A tumor does not necessarily mean cancer,* but doctors like the first gynecologist might say *tumor* knowing that the word alone might panic their patients into agreeing to surgery. The discovery of a tumor often puts a woman in the frame of mind to accept whatever a doctor suggests, even if his advice is hysterectomy. An important aim of this chapter is to help every woman understand that in the great majority of fibroid tumor cases, *there is no need for alarm* as long as there is no hemorrhaging or severe pain.

Fibroids, common uterine growths in women, sprout from the muscle wall of the uterus. In more than 99.5 percent of diagnosed cases, fibroid tumors are benign. During the rare occasion when a fibroid might become cancerous, it will begin to grow very rapidly. This sudden expansion can be found on pelvic examination and can be documented by X ray or ultrasonography.

A woman should alleviate any fear by becoming fully aware of her condition. She should ask the doctor to explain the size of her fibroids and learn what symptoms might mean trouble.

If her doctor finds a growth that is not in the uterus but on the ovary, then an ovarian *cyst,* another usually benign tumor, exists. During a woman's childbearing years, many ovarian tumors are referred to as "cysts." A *simple cyst* is a fluid-filled sac that can form on an ovary any time during the menstrual cycle. A *dermoid cyst* (from *derma,* meaning "skin") is a unique growth that contains all types of skin tissue and is a more solid, less typical, ovarian enlargement.

Most simple ovarian cysts that appear during a woman's fertile years are benign; they will often disappear spontaneously after one or two menstrual cycles. A dermoid cyst does not dissolve naturally, but the surgery required to remove it is easily performed. The real need for medical concern occurs if an ovarian growth is caused by endometriosis or if ovarian tumors are found in a woman who is over fifty. In older women, ovarian cysts often become dense growths that are much more likely to become malignant. No matter what a woman's age, however, her condition should be carefully evaluated, and transvaginal as well as abdominal ultrasound can help a doctor's assessment. By and large, fibroid tumors and ovarian cysts are not serious health hazards, but a doctor must carefully follow their growth. The rapid growth of a fibroid or cyst might be a sign of malignancy.

FIBROID TUMORS

There is scientific disagreement over the origin of the fibroid tumor since it is not a true fibrous growth. A uterine fibroid tumor (referred to medically as a leiomyoma, fibroma, fibromyoma, or myoma) contains mostly muscle cells bound together by varying degrees of fibrous connective tissue.

It has been suggested that a primitive cell within the uterus, a cell that normally would develop into muscle, connective tissue, or blood vessel, undergoes a mutation and forms the nucleus of a fibroid tumor. Various researchers have theorized that fibroids might spring from adult muscle cells, connective tissue cells, cells from the outer covering of blood vessels, or from the muscle cells inside blood vessels. Scientists only agree that fibroid tumors are probably hereditary.

Approximately 20 percent of women over twenty have fibroid tumors, and about 30 percent of the hysterectomies performed are blamed on fibroids. The convoluted masses are most often discovered when women enter their late thirties, and it has been estimated that approximately 40 percent of women over thirty-five have fibroid tumors in their uteri even though many of them might never have noticed any signs of discomfort. The tumors occur three to nine times more frequently among black women than white or Asian women, and are more prevalent among white women of Eastern European or Jewish descent than among women of other origins. For an unknown reason, Asian women rarely experience fibroids.

It is believed that a woman who has a fibroid tumor was born with its seed in her uterus. That seed might have remained dormant for years, but then something triggered its growth, perhaps pregnancy or the taking of the birth control pill, both of which increase the body's level of estrogen. The seed was activated by the estrogen jolt and began to emerge into a tumor, which, like an onion, slowly added layer after layer until one day it was felt to be quite large.

Female Hormones and Fibroid Tumors

There is a definite correlation between fibroids and estrogen. Fibroid tumors are rarely seen before menarche, when the amount of estrogen in the body is low. The tumors burst forth and multiply during the childbearing years, when the estrogen level rises. After menopause, when the estrogen level drops, fibroids begin to shrink and disappear. Whenever a woman is in a situation in which her estrogen increases, such as during pregnancy or when she is taking birth control pills, previously inactive fibroid tumors might enlarge to palpable levels.

Often fibroids are associated with certain disorders that are themselves related to boosts in estrogen:

- Estrogen-producing ovarian tumors will spurt the growth of fibroids.
- Women suffering from polycystic ovarian syndrome (PCOS) have high estrogen levels and might be the bearers of fibroid tumors. (See "What Is Polycystic Ovarian Syndrome?" in chapter 8, pages 219 to 221.)
- Women are also more susceptible to fibroids when they are overweight because fatty tissue converts into estrogen and increases the likelihood of developing tumors. (See "Menopause in the Overweight Woman" in chapter 14, pages 435 to 436.)
- Fibroid tumors might be found in association with hyperplasia, an enlargement or thickening of the uterine lining also caused by an overstimulation of estrogen (see pages 663 and 667).

Any one of these conditions could put a woman at high risk for fibroid tumors. By keeping a close check on her health and by learning all about fibroids, a woman can prepare herself for their possible appearance within her womb.

Are There Different Kinds of Fibroid Tumors?

There are three different types of fibroid tumors (see figure 15-1), defined according to their locations within the uterus:

A *submucosal* fibroid grows just below the surface of the uterine lining, making the lining bulge out into the uterine cavity. There might be bleeding and cramping as the tumor invades the uterus. A submucous fibroid can get so big that it breaks the endometrium, the uterine lining, and results in such heavy bleeding that a woman might have to be rushed to the hospital for emergency surgery to save her life. If a woman with a submucous fibroid becomes pregnant, she might miscarry. The fibroid might prevent the placenta from properly attaching itself to the womb and block the nourishing blood supply that is supposed to reach the developing fetus. Sometimes a submucous fibroid can swell out and break through the uterine lining into the uterine cavity but still be attached to the uterus by a broad- or narrow-based stalk. At this point it is called a *pedunculated* tumor, which the uterus might consider a foreign body and attempt to abort through the cervix. This is a very painful condition. No matter how much the uterus contracts, the fibroid will always remain attached, but it might become infected by the process and require surgical removal.

An *intramural* fibroid is located within the muscle wall of the uterus. This type of tumor is unobtrusive and creates a problem only if it is growing within a portion of the uterus that might expand, block a Fallopian tube, and cause infertility.

The third type of fibroid, the *subserous* tumor, grows in the outer layer of the uterus, actually outside the womb. A subserous fibroid can occasionally become so large that it fills the pelvic cavity and blocks the birth canal. Also, like a submucous fibroid, the subserous kind might become pedunculated, twist on its stalk, and cause severe abdominal pain.

In general, fibroid tumors, as long as they are monitored by a doctor and do not show sudden growth, should not give rise to concern. A woman usually has more than one fibroid if she has any, and she

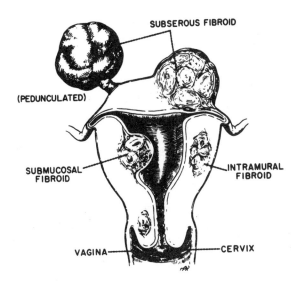

15-1 **Fibroid Tumors.** There are three types of uterine fibroid tumors: the *submucous*, the *intramural*, and the *subserous*. All three types are composed of fibrous muscle tissue and are named according to their locations in or on the uterus. The submucous fibroid might cause the most serious problems since it protrudes into the uterine cavity and can break through the uterine wall. A submucous fibroid is often associated with heavy vaginal bleeding, and it can lead to miscarriage after conception. The intramural fibroid is located in the muscle wall of the uterus. This fibroid is rarely associated with any difficulties, although it occasionally can obstruct the Fallopian tube. The subserous fibroid can grow very large but it is generally not associated with any serious problems. Sometimes a subserous fibroid can become pedunculated and twist on its own stalk; then it will cause severe abdominal pain that might necessitate surgery. (Note the fibroid at the upper left-hand corner of the drawing.) Fibroids are benign tumors and surgery is needed only if they lead to excessive bleeding or pain. In such cases an operation called a myomectomy, in which only the fibroids are removed and the uterus is left untouched, should be considered. A hysterectomy is required only when fibroids are extremely large or if they cause excessive and uncontrollable bleeding.

should ask her doctor how many fibroid tumors he can feel and what size they are. Of them all, the submucous fibroid, as a possible source of cramps and bleeding, is the most troublesome.

What Are the Symptoms of Fibroid Tumors? Fibroid tumors usually are asymptomatic, without symptoms. A fibroid might be so small that one doctor misses it during an internal examination while another physician, blessed with a responsive sense of touch, discovers it. A woman's experience will depend on her doctor's skill. By the time some doctors detect fibroids, the tumors are already growing. Then, suddenly, a slight increase in size might make a tumor seem enormous to the touch and a doctor might rush a woman into a hysterectomy by telling her that the fibroids are overtaking her uterus. In the operating room these "enormous" tumors usually turn out to be smaller than originally perceived.

Before agreeing to an operation, a woman should ask her doctor to show her the exact size of her fibroids with the aid of ultrasonography. A woman should not worry about cancer if she hears the word *tumor* because, as mentioned earlier, more than 99.5 percent of all fibroids are benign. After a woman and her doctor review the ultrasound image of the tumors, they can then talk about the necessity of removal, and as discussed next in the treatment section, hysterectomy is *not* the only method.

Sometimes a woman can attune herself to signs that might indicate a fibroid or two (even though the condition has no specific symptoms) and avoid the shock of surgery through early detection. By being alert to periods that are heavier than normal, a woman might be helping her doctor find that a submucous fibroid is disturbing her uterine lining. A woman who is bleeding heavily should be evaluated by a D & C. A doctor can use the curette, an instrument designed for the procedure, to feel whether the uterine cavity contains any swelling or abnormality. A doctor might also suggest that a woman have a hysterosalpingogram, an X ray of her uterus, to determine whether she has submucous fibroids.

Fibroids might also be suspected when a woman notices frequency of urination, which might mean that tumors are pressing against her bladder. In another instance a woman might feel abdominal pain if a pedunculated tumor is starting to twist. Fibroids that are disintegrating can also be painful. Infertility might be due to the particular position of a fibroid tumor. Depending on where and how large tumors are, fibroids might be considered the reason for a miscarriage, a premature delivery, or an obstructed birth canal.

A woman can live with fibroid tumors for her entire life with no problems. Still, she should expect to have her suspicions investigated if she thinks undetected fibroids are causing discomfort. She might know something her doctor has yet to discover.

How Are Fibroids Treated? Fibroids should never cause a woman to feel unhealthy. They must be monitored by a doctor at regular six-month checkups, when he might use transvaginal or abdominal ultrasound. However, unless they create problems, fibroids might remain untouched.

If fibroid tumors cause a woman to have prolonged, heavy bleeding, her increased flow might be controlled by progesterone in the form of Provera tablets, 10 mg two to three times a day for five to ten days, depending on the length of the flow. Or, a doctor might prescribe ergotrate or Methergine, medications that will contract the uterus and help lessen the flow. Recent studies have indicated that to enhance *hemostasis* (control of bleeding) even further, these drugs could be given in combination with prescription NSAIDs, such as Motrin or Anaprox, which are also antiprostaglandins (see chapter 3). Also, drugs called GnRH agonists (see chapter 7) can halt estrogen production, reduce menstrual bleeding, and temporarily shrink fibroids while the drugs are being taken. Danocrine tablets and injectable Lupron, a GnRH agonist, are most frequently used to treat fibroids. A woman should also take iron and vitamins (particularly vitamin C) and eat a high-protein diet to strengthen a body that may be weakened from the blood loss.

If different kinds of medication fail to bring relief, conservative management—a *myomectomy,* removal of the fibroids without hysterectomy—should be a doctor's next consideration. Also, he might have no choice but surgery if fibroids are the reason for miscarriage or if they are pressing on the Fallopian tubes and causing infertility. A fibroid tumor that is pedunculated, twists, and presses on the bladder or rectum makes another case for surgery. But in all these cases a *myomectomy, not a hysterectomy,* should be the operation under discussion.

There are only a few instances when a hysterectomy should be the treatment of choice. For example, if fibroids grow very large, bleeding becomes uncontrollable, the tumors become malignant, or pain seems unbearable, a hysterectomy might be unavoidable. Sometimes with an unskilled physician, bleeding is absolutely uncontrollable during a myomectomy and a hysterectomy is the final recourse. A hysterectomy might also be indicated when a woman in her mid-forties has decided not to bear any more children and fibroid tumors are adding pain to other physical difficulties. As a rule, however, *a hysterectomy is not the first-choice treatment for fibroid tumors.*

A growing number of health insurance companies and doctors are working to preserve a woman's womb by making myomectomy the first-choice surgery for fibroids. A myomectomy is usually undertaken as an abdominal laparotomy (described below), but if fibroids are small, a less invasive laparoscopy might be elected. Tiny submucosal fibroids can be removed during vaginal hysteroscopy.

Myomectomy Versus Hysterectomy

Removal of a uterus, a hysterectomy, should not be viewed as a minor, trouble-free event. A uterus does more than give a woman the capability of carrying a child. It aids in providing an adequate blood supply to the ovaries to keep them healthy and producing hormones. When a uterus is removed through hysterectomy, which entails major surgery, a woman's menopausal symptoms become much more severe because a hormone imbalance is likely to follow the loss. When confronted with surgery for fibroid tumors, a woman should make every attempt to have her doctor perform a myomectomy rather than a hysterectomy. In a myomectomy, the myoma, the fibroid tumor, is removed but a woman's uterus remains intact.

A woman who is going to have a myomectomy is given general anesthesia, and a doctor conducts an exploratory laparotomy in which he opens a woman's abdomen and examines her uterus. An appropriate incision for this kind of operation is a Pfannenstiel incision, a horizontal bikini cut below the pubic hairline. Unless tumors are extremely large, there is no need for a doctor to do a vertical incision, which can leave a woman looking like a "divided highway."

After exposing the uterus, the surgeon can cut into the womb and excise the fibroids, which shell out almost like oranges being pulled away from their skins. During a myomectomy it is important for a physician to command a good hemostasis, a good control of bleeding. A skillful surgeon should place a tourniquet around the lower portion of the uterus to create hemostasis and prevent excessive blood loss. More important, he should inject pitressin, a hormone normally released from the posterior lobe of the pituitary gland, into the *myometrium*, the muscular layer of the uterine wall. Pitressin will constrict the blood vessels in the uterus, further decrease the blood loss, and make surgery much easier.

A number of leading gynecological surgeons have found that during a myomectomy if a tourniquet is placed around the uterus and pitressin is injected, a woman will experience very little blood loss and she will have a much better chance for successful, uncomplicated surgery. A woman who learns about the use of the tourniquet and pitressin during myomectomy might tell her doctor that she has read about these techniques and that she would feel safer if they were used during her operation. A woman should also be aware that if her fibroids are small, a skillful doctor might be able to remove them during a laparoscopy; a tiny incision is made in or near her navel, a viewing instrument is inserted through a slim tube, and fibroids are either cut, vaporized by laser, or electrocauterized. As another alternative, a competent physician might have the ability to remove small submucosal fibroids through the vagina during a vaginal hysteroscopy.

During surgery, if there is a submucous fibroid, a tumor inside the uterine cavity, a surgeon will have to cut into the cavity, remove the fibroid, and close the uterus. Once the uterine cavity has been opened, due to the type of incision required for fibroid removal, in subsequent childbirth a woman can deliver only by cesarean section.

If a myomectomy can be performed without invading the uterine cavity, then a vaginal delivery would be possible if pregnancy occurred.

A *doctor should attempt to remove every single fibroid in the uterus,* even very small ones that could grow later on. He must place a lot of sutures around his excisions to make sure that bleeding continues to be managed. When he is sure all tumor sites are properly sutured, he can close the outer portion, the serosa, of the uterus with fine dissolvable sutures, which should be placed underneath the skin tissue to avoid adhesion. When the inner suturing is finished he might infuse hydro-cortisone solution and Dextran-70, a thick, viscous solution, into the abdominal cavity to smooth the uterus and keep the bowel, uterus, and other internal organs free from damaging adhesions. Before the operation is concluded, a doctor gives a woman the best chance to maintain her reproductive health if he performs a *uterine suspension,* pulls the uterus forward to decrease the formation of adhesions and scar tissue.

After surgery, a physician might elect to give a woman intra-venous Pitocin (oxytocin) for twenty-four hours to aid in uterine contraction. If this procedure is carried out and if a woman is given antibiotic treatment at the start of surgery and during her postoper-ative period, she will usually have few problems. On the third and fourth days after surgery she might experience a fever for a few days, but this is a common occurrence caused by blood and damaged tis-sue inside the uterine wall.

Approximately 40 percent of the women who have had myomec-tomies have become pregnant after their operations. It is amazing to see how completely a uterus heals a few months after surgery. I per-sonally removed thirty-two fibroid tumors from one woman's uterus and alterations in her womb were imperceptible.

Every woman should realize that fibroid tumors can be removed without her uterus having to go, too. No matter how old she is, and even if she feels her childbearing is over, a woman can seek out a myomec-tomy before she agrees to a hysterectomy. One doctor might not care about a woman's uterus, but another doctor might want to save every organ. When a woman's womb is at stake, a second opinion is crucial.

A hysterectomy should be performed only if fibroid tumors are so large that they are impossible to remove through myomectomy, if bleeding cannot be controlled, if there is a suspicion of malignancy, or if a myomectomy has failed. As mentioned in the previous section, sometimes a doctor who is not experienced in performing myomectomies will encounter such heavy bleeding during his surgery that he will have to perform a hysterectomy to save his patient. Many women who think they are going into hospitals for myomectomies are asked to sign consent forms allowing associated hysterectomies, should they be necessary. A woman must do her best to investigate her doctor's experience and competency in the operating room. However, she might never have to reach the point of surgery if she always keeps her six-month appointments with her doctor, fully understands this benign condition, and knows that her doctor is not knife-happy. By monitoring the size of her fibroids, a woman will be safeguarding her uterus. If fibroids begin to grow rapidly and unexpectedly, a woman can elect to have a myomectomy before the tumors grow so large her doctor can no longer perform this type of surgery.

QUESTIONS ABOUT FIBROID TUMORS

Is There Any Alternative to a Hysterectomy Advised for Fibroid Tumors?

I am forty-two years old and I have fibroid tumors. During the last two years I have had very heavy bleeding and my doctor performed two D & Cs. The blood loss has given me anemia. The D & Cs were supposed to help, but they haven't. Now the doctor says that the only way to solve my problem is to remove my uterus. He is one of the best doctors around here, but if there is any way to remove the fibroids and save my uterus I would like to know.

—M.H., Soldotna, Alaska

I am one of many women who has a fibroid tumor the size of a grapefruit. My doctor says the tumor is very hard and he advises an immediate hysterectomy. I am forty-six years old, so child-bearing does not enter into the picture. Still, I am very wary of this operation. Do I have an alternative?

—F.C., Coram, New York

My fibroid tumors have never given me any problems but my doctor has recommended a hysterectomy. I am twenty-eight years old and the thought of losing my uterus terrifies me. Is there any other way of treating fibroids?

—H.V., Brawley, California

Each case of fibroid tumors is always individual. A young woman who wants to have children in the future can usually benefit from a myomectomy, an operation that removes the fibroid tumors while it leaves the uterus intact. Technically, it is agreed that a doctor has cause to remove a uterus when it is the size of a twelve-week pregnancy, but even if a uterus is as large as a twenty-week pregnancy, a myomectomy can still be performed. Sometimes it is even easier to remove one huge tumor than a lot of small ones.

The story is different for an older woman who has completed her family and is contending with uncontrollable heavy periods caused by fibroid tumors. If she has submucous fibroids and her doctor has tried to no avail to relieve her condition with medication and D & Cs, then she might best be served with a hysterectomy.

Sometimes fibroids grow and press on other organs or make the uterus so big that it presses on other organs. A woman of any age might then suffer pain or urinary ailments that might be eased with a myomectomy. If a woman is older and she has no desire to bear a child, a hysterectomy might be the treatment of choice, but even so, she should be fully informed of all possibilities.

A hysterectomy is major surgery with ramifications. The uterus is more than just a childbearing organ. When the uterus is removed, the blood supply to the ovaries is diminished and the ovaries do not function optimally. A hormonal imbalance often ensues, and a woman might become physically and emotionally unsettled. If the ovaries are also removed during a hysterectomy, a woman might experience the severe menopausal symptoms described in chapter 13. Although there are certainly times when a hysterectomy is necessary, a woman should educate herself to her options and question her doctor about the myomectomy procedure. Above all, it is important to remember that if fibroid tumors are *not* causing any problems and have *not* suddenly grown, there is no reason to remove them.

Do I Need My Ovaries Removed During a Hysterectomy for Fibroids?

My fibroid tumors are causing heavy bleeding that cannot be controlled by D & Cs. I am forty-two years old, have four children, and I do not want any more babies. My doctor has recommended a hysterectomy. When he operates, I would like my ovaries to remain. Is this possible? Do I need my ovaries removed during a hysterectomy?

—A.M., Utica, Kentucky

This woman's symptoms indicate that she has submucous fibroids that cause bleeding. She does not want future offspring, and if she has a hysterectomy she will end her bleeding problem and she can forget about contraception. A hysterectomy might be right for Ms. M., but she should retain her ovaries.

There is no need to remove the ovaries when doing a hysterectomy as a treatment for fibroid tumors. Fibroid tumors represent a benign condition, and if Ms. M.'s ovaries are healthy, her doctor should leave them alone. If he takes out her ovaries, Ms. M. will be thrown into surgical menopause as described in chapter 13. Then her life will never be the same.

Women undergoing hysterectomies to relieve problems caused by fibroid tumors must understand that removal of their ovaries is often unnecessary. A woman with fibroids who is scheduled for a hysterectomy should discuss the retention of her ovaries with her doctor. If he insists on removing the ovaries, she should cancel the surgery and seek a second opinion.

I Have Adenomyosis; Do I Need a Hysterectomy?

A few years ago I had a myomectomy and uterine suspension and then gave birth to my third and last child. I am thirty-nine years old and I do not intend to become pregnant again. About six months ago my gynecologist performed a D & C to alleviate my heavy bleeding. At that time he told me I had adenomyosis. My periods did not get any better after the D & C. I've had severe clotting and my menstrual flow has been like a hemorrhage. I have daily headaches and pain two weeks before menstruation, and my nerves are shot. My doctor recently suggested a hysterectomy, but I'm worried about saying yes. I am fearful of this surgery and I wonder if there isn't a better way.

—B.C., Newland, North Carolina

Adenomyosis, a condition most often seen in women after child-bearing, is technically called *endometriosis interna*. The endometrium, the uterine lining, infiltrates the uterine wall and makes it thick and spongy. Adenomyosis can lead to infertility because the resultant uterine lining prevents the placenta from adhering properly to the uterus. Adenomyosis might also cause uncontrollable heavy bleeding and pain.

Ms. C. might need a hysterectomy, but she might try alternative medication first. Danocrine or one of the GnRH agonists such as Lupron, both drugs used to treat endometriosis, might also relieve endometriosis interna. For example, if Ms. C. takes Danocrine, 200-mg tablets two to three times a day for six to nine months, her menstrual flow might stop and her uterus might decrease in size. I have treated several women suffering from adenomyosis with Danocrine. After a successful Danocrine cure, a woman's uterus should remain healthy as long as she keeps her weight down.

If Danocrine is ineffective and bleeding continues unabated, a woman might be treated with progesterone in the form of Provera tablets, 10 mg twice a day for five to ten days. An antiprostaglandin NSAID such as Motrin or Anaprox should be taken simultaneously with the Provera.

If Danocrine does not work and progesterone in combination with an antiprostaglandin does not work, then a hysterectomy might be in order. However, if Ms. C. does need a hysterectomy, her ovaries should remain unscathed after surgery. She is still a young woman and her ovaries should be allowed to provide her with the hormonal fluctuation she needs for continued equilibrium and good health.

I Have No Trouble with My Fibroids; Do I Really Need a Hysterectomy?

I have fibroid tumors that give me no trouble except that they make my stomach protrude. My periods are normal and I have no pain. My problem is that I do not want surgery and I'm confused. The doctor who discovered the fibroids wants to do a hysterectomy. I am almost afraid to get a second opinion because I do not want another doctor to tell me the same thing. Do you know alternative treatments? Are there medications that can shrink the tumors? Why do I need a hysterectomy?

—H.C., Raytown, Missouri

Since this woman has no troubling symptoms from her fibroid tumors, on the surface there seems to be no need for surgery. However, a judgment cannot really be made without knowing Ms. C.'s age. If she is in her mid-forties, has been checked twice a year by her doctor, and her fibroid tumors have shown no rapid sign of growth, then she probably does not require surgery. A problem sometimes occurs in the late forties when fibroids start to grow rapidly, because this is the time when they might become cancerous. Generally, as a woman approaches menopause her estrogen level is dropping and her fibroid tumors should be starting to shrink. If her fibroids begin to swell, she could be experiencing rapid cell division that might be a sign of cancer. A hysterectomy is then indicated.

If Ms. C. is in a time of life when she wants to conceive children and her fibroids seem to be the problem, she might be advised to have a myomectomy to aid her in conception. No matter what her age, if she does not desire children and her fibroids are not causing many problems, she can probably do without surgery.

Ms. C. writes that her stomach is protruding, which means that her uterus is expanding. After the uterus has reached the size of a three-month pregnancy, the American College of Obstetricians and Gynecologists has decreed that a hysterectomy would be permissible. Ironically, if two doctors examine the same uterus, each physician can have an opinion as to the size of the womb, and the opinions need not necessarily match. Different physicians have different sensitivities, and doctors are sometimes surprised during surgery when they see uteri much smaller than they had anticipated. If Ms. C. is told she needs a hysterectomy because her uterus resembles a three-month pregnancy, she should request ultrasonography to see, in actuality, the size of her uterus. She might also seek the opinion of a second physician with a different sense of touch. If her uterus exactly equals the size of a three-month pregnancy, but she has no complaints, there should be no need for hysterectomy.

If Ms. C. is overweight, she will have an overproduction of estrogen in her fatty tissue and the hormone will subsequently stimulate the growth of her fibroids. Ms. C. might help to inhibit the expanding fibroids by keeping her weight down and staying fit.

Depending on her age and her condition, a woman might be able to avoid surgery if she does not take estrogen hormones, keeps herself fit, educates herself to the condition, and is cared for by a competent, sensitive, conservative physician who believes that surgery is only a last resort and that myomectomy should be attempted before hysterectomy.

There is medication that can shrink fibroids, but only temporarily. The drugs are Danocrine, or one of the GnRH agonists, such as Lupron. They are mainly used to dissolve endometrial growths, and can be taken for a few months. Their inhibiting of the brain hormones FSH and LH stops estrogen/progesterone production. These drugs are generally used to halt menstruation and shrink fibroids when a woman has heavy bleeding, which is not the case for Ms. C. When the drugs are stopped, fibroids grow back to their larger sizes.

Can I Be Pregnant with Fibroid Tumors?

I have fibroid tumors. My doctor has suggested surgery, but I want to have a baby. I went for a second opinion about the surgery and the second-opinion doctor said that I should get pregnant before the operation. Six months ago I miscarried when I was three months pregnant and now my regular doctor doesn't think I can hold a fetus. He wants to operate. I would hate to lose another baby, but I don't know what to do. Do you think I could refuse the operation and carry to term with fibroid tumors?
—E.D., Arvada, Colorado

Miscarriage is more common when a woman has fibroid tumors, particularly if they are the submucous kind that can protrude into the uterine cavity. The smooth uterine lining will swell out at the site of a submucous fibroid and the placenta will not be able to adhere properly to the uterus. As a result of this placental defect, a developing fetus will not receive the nourishment it needs, and it might spontaneously abort in a miscarriage. An abdominal ultrasound or hysterosalpingogram, an X ray of the uterus, will show whether there is an abnormality in Ms. D.'s uterine lining that could be a submucous fibroid.

If she does have submucous fibroids, Ms. D. might need a myomectomy to remove them. The uterine cavity will have to be entered, and remember, due to the type of incision a surgeon will have to make to penetrate the cavity, a woman will have to deliver by cesarean section in subsequent pregnancies. If a myomectomy is performed to remove subserous fibroids outside the uterus or intramural fibroids within the uterine wall, then surgery will not mean cesarean births for Ms. D.'s future pregnancies. As long as the uterine cavity is not touched, a vaginal delivery is still possible after a myomectomy.

If Ms. D. has submucous fibroid tumors or large fibroid tumors of any kind, she might be advised to have a myomectomy before pregnancy, She will be lessening her chance of miscarriage or premature labor.

A pregnant woman with fibroid tumors must take it easy at least during the last half of her pregnancy. She should not exert herself by lifting heavy objects and for the last three months she should refrain from sexual intercourse, which might stimulate the uterus into premature labor. A doctor might prescribe a beta-mimetic drug to relax the uterus and prevent premature birth. He might also place a cervical cerclace suture around the cervix to prevent dilation.

Ms. D. does not specify what type of surgery her doctors are suggesting. Assuming that she is a candidate for myomectomy, she should still be cautioned that due to uterine scarring she still runs a risk of giving birth prematurely. Whenever Ms. D. decides to become pregnant, she must treat herself gently.

Can the Birth Control Pill Cure Fibroids?

For six months my doctor has treated my fibroid tumors by giving me birth control pills. I have had continuous trouble with a heavy flow and spotting during the month. The doctor gave me a D & C, but neither that nor the pills have helped. Now he has recommended a hysterectomy. Do I really need major surgery? Why hasn't the birth control pill cured my fibroids?
—J.I., Mohnton, Pennsylvania

No, this woman does not need a hysterectomy, and she might have a reason to sue for malpractice. A birth control pill contains doses of estrogen, a hormone that spurts the growth of fibroid tumors, Her doctor, by giving her something that enlarges fibroids, is behaving unethically.

Sometimes a doctor will prescribe birth control pills to a woman he knows has fibroids in order to make the tumors grow fast. Then once the fibroids are big, he will have a reason to do a hysterectomy. This is exactly what Ms. I.'s doctor appears to be trying to do to her. She took the birth control pills, bled more, had a D & C, and now the doctor is beginning to scare her by saying she needs a hysterectomy soon.

Ms. I. has every right to file suit. She was given the wrong treatment. Any woman who has fibroid tumors must avoid estrogen tablets and must never take birth control pills. Estrogen stimulates the growth of fibroids. A woman with fibroids must use other forms of contraception such as an IUD or a diaphragm. She might even consider becoming pregnant early in life, before her fibroids have a chance to grow and interfere with gestation. If a woman only wants children later in life, she might undergo a myomectomy to remove the fibroids since they might become obstacles when she is older. But it must be repeated that *under no circumstances should a woman with fibroids take birth control pills.*

Can Fibroids Cause Severe Pain?

I am twenty-three years old and for two years I have had extreme pain in the lower left side of my pelvis. At first the pain was so great I vomited every half hour and lost fifteen pounds. I went to several doctors and had a laparoscopy and a hysteroscopy. Usually the doctors said they couldn't find anything, but one doctor told me that I had fibroid tumors that were shrinking and causing me to suffer. My current doctor, like all the rest, says there is nothing he can do for me, but the pain has not let up. Why do fibroid tumors hurt so much? I have never heard of something like this that can't be cured.

—W.F., Aiken, South Carolina

It seems unlikely that a twenty-three-year old-woman would be suffering from shrinking fibroid tumors. Degeneration of fibroid tumors occurs when they are very large and their centers, due to decreased blood supply, begin to rot. Then the tumors shrink and cause pain. This usually does not happen until a woman is over thirty-five.

Ms. F.'s symptoms of nausea and vomiting seem more like signs of menstrual cramps or even endometriosis (see chapter 7). In fact, I would suspect that this woman has endrometriosis rather than shrinking fibroid tumors. Unless they are very large or twisted, fibroid tumors are rarely painful.

Ms. F. might be helped by taking Danocrine or a GnRH agonist such as Lupron, drugs used to treat endometrial growths. Danocrine, administered in 200-mg tablets two or three times a day for six months or longer, will stop her menstrual flow and stabilize her hormonal fluctuation. If she has endometriosis, Danocrine will shrink it away and at the same time rest her organs.

If Ms. F. does have fibroid tumors, she might consider childbearing early in life rather than later. When she is older, her fibroids might be more problematic.

I Have Heavy Periods with My Fibroid Tumors; Is There Any Treatment?

For more than a year now I have been suffering with a heavy menstrual flow. I am forty years old and I have fibroid tumors. My gynecologist has already given me a D & C and he wants to do another. In fact, he says he would want to do them regularly. At least he is better than the family doctor, who advised a hysterectomy. I would like to find an alternative to either a constant D & C routine or a hysterectomy. I am taking iron pills to keep up my strength with the blood loss. I thought that perhaps I might find someone who would give me a myomectomy. What is the best way to treat heavy periods when you have fibroids?
                                        —C.L., Cleveland, Tennessee

As explained in the "How Are Fibroid Tumors Treated?" section of this chapter, when fibroids cause prolonged, heavy bleeding, progesterone in the form of Provera tablets might help control the flow. Also, uterine-contracting medications such as ergotrate or Methergine might reduce the bleeding. If these drugs are given in combination with an antiprostaglandin NSAID such as Motrin or Anaprox, the effort to reduce the flow might be even more successful. This woman's cycle might also be regulated by extra vitamin B and C.

If Ms. L.'s flow does not respond to medication, she might need a hysterosalpingogram, an X ray of her uterus, to see if she has submucous fibroids. The X ray might be unnecessary, however, if her doctor was able to detect uterine abnormality when he performed the D & C.

If Ms. L.'s tumors are located, she might benefit from a myomectomy, a removal of all the fibroid tumors. Not every physician performs myomectomies, but Ms. L. most surely will find doctors who use the latest surgical techniques at teaching hospitals or major medical centers. Informed physicians at reputable hospitals should be conducting myomectomies with the tourniquet technique and pitressin injection method, as detailed in the "Myomectomy Versus Hysterectomy" section of this chapter. Ms. L. should seek out a knowledgeable doctor who is an experienced surgeon.

I recently met a woman who was determined to have a myomectomy even though her doctor had suggested a hysterectomy for her fibroids. She traveled all the way from St. Louis to New York to find a doctor who would help her. Soon after her arrival in New York she underwent a successful myomectomy, and shortly thereafter she became pregnant. Had she submitted to the advised hysterectomy she would never have borne her son. Sometimes a woman must go miles out of her way for up-to-date care, but the trip is usually worth the effort.

Is There Any Way to Shrink Fibroid Tumors?

My gynecologist tells me that I have a fibroid tumor the size of a grapefruit and that the removal of my uterus is inevitable. I am thirty-five years old and I would not like to lose my womb at this

age. Is there any way I might be able to take a drug that would
shrink my fibroid? I heard there might be something but I'm not
sure of the name of it.

—T.D., Auburn, New York

At present, medications can only shrink fibroid tumors *temporarily*. Danocrine, and the GnRH agonists, such as Lupron, treatments for endometriosis (see chapter 7), can arrest estrogen production and shrink fibroids. Tumors will return to their original sizes, however, when medication is stopped.

Although fibroids cannot be permanently reduced through medication, there are steps that can be taken to prevent them from becoming larger. Estrogen is known to stimulate the growth of fibroid tumors. By avoiding estrogen tablets or birth control pills containing estrogen, a woman will be staying away from a hormone that could expand her tumors. Also, the slimmer a woman is the less likely that she is producing high amounts of estrogen in her body. An overweight woman will be converting estrogen from her fatty tissue and boosting the level of that hormone to the point where it might instigate fibroid development. By keeping her weight down with exercises such as swimming or jogging, a woman will be safeguarding the size of her tumors.

There was a study in which testosterone, the male hormone, was given to women to prevent the growth of their fibroids later in life. The results were such that the administering of testosterone is not recommended.

Danocrine (danazol), the drug that dissolves endometrial growths, has sometimes been used to treat fibroid tumors, but only in connection with endometriosis or other ailments that cause pelvic pain. Sometimes, when women have heavy bleeding with fibroid tumors, a GnRH agonist is given because it arrests the menstrual flow and allows other treatments to be administered. At this time, vitamins B with B_6 should be taken to regulate the menstrual cycle.

The bottom line here is that Ms. D. cannot make her fibroid tumor smaller but she might be able to stop it from getting bigger.

In the meantime, if the tumor is so large that it requires surgery, she should read the "Myomectomy Versus Hysterectomy" section of this chapter and attempt to find an informed gynecological surgeon who is associated with a metropolitan teaching hospital.

Can Fibroid Tumors Turn into Cancer?

I am forty-four years old and I am already having signs of menopause. I have fibroid tumors and I am worried that as my body changes the fibroids will go into cancer. Should I have a hysterectomy now?

—K.B., Chatham, Ontario, Canada

The chance that a fibroid tumor will become cancerous is very slim. A fibroid tumor is a benign growth composed of muscle cells and fibrous tissue that show a very low incidence of carcinoma.

A woman who has fibroid tumors must be examined twice a year by her doctor. If her uterus begins to expand due to rapid growth of fibroid tumors or if a doctor can feel the enlargement of the tumors themselves, myomectomy—surgery to remove the fibroid tumors alone—might be needed. A doctor can confirm the size of the tumors through ultrasonography.

If fibroid tumors always remain the same and a woman has no pain or heavy bleeding, she has no need to worry. Ms. B is forty-four and in the next few years, as her estrogen level drops, there will be even less chance of stimulating the tumors to grow. As long as Ms. B. keeps her weight down to prevent the possibility of estrogen conversion from fatty tissue, it is unlikely that her fibroid tumors will be activated, and even more unlikely that she will need surgery of any kind.

My Eighteen-Year-Old Daughter Has Fibroids; Should She Get Pregnant?

The doctors thought that my daughter was pregnant, but then they found out that she has fibroid tumors. They say she is going to

need a hysterectomy, but since she is only eighteen years old, they
want her to try to get pregnant first. After the operation they say
she won't be able to have children anymore. I don't think it is right
for her to have to get pregnant at such a young age, but does she
have any choice?

—I.A., Mt. Morris, Illinois

This woman's daughter is only eighteen, and from this letter, it does not sound as if she is ready to have a child. No one has the right to say, "Rx: Have a baby," as part of the treatment for fibroid tumors.

If the fibroid tumors are large enough to be causing heavy bleeding and pain, Ms. A.'s daughter might require surgery, but a myomectomy, removal of only the tumors, should do the job. A physician associated with an accredited teaching hospital or a major medical center should be well versed in the myomectomy procedure. Ms. A. might help her daughter find such a surgeon. After her fibroid tumors are excised, the young woman should then have no problem bearing children.

The reason doctors suggest early pregnancy is because they do not think "myomectomy" first. They know that there is a high incidence of hysterectomy among women with fibroid tumors. Feeling that a hysterectomy awaits a woman who has fibroids, doctors promote early pregnancy instead of myomectomy. Too often, doctors have no experience performing myomectomies, and they do not learn how to do these operations. They rely on hysterectomies instead.

A woman who has fibroids must investigate her doctor's experience with myomectomies and choose a physician who is skilled in the latest techniques.

Shrinking Fibroids Through Embolization

Fibroid embolization is a new, nonsurgical method for shrinking fibroid tumors, although still somewhat experimental, and may be quite risky. One woman who had a grapefruit-sized fibroid removed developed a blood infection from the withering fibroid and she died two weeks after surgery. Embolization must be performed by a radiologist and is recommended only for women who have completed their childbearing. The approach is so new that its safety and long-term effect on fertility are not yet known.

A woman receives local anesthesia and mild sedation to undergo a fibroid embolization. A radiologist (preferably one recommended by a knowledgeable gynecologist) inserts a fine catheter into a woman's femoral artery through a tiny incision in her thigh. He then threads the catheter into her uterine artery. He employs angiography, an injection of special dye into the artery, to help him track the blood flow to the uterus. Then he is able to inject, through the catheter, tiny plastic or sponge particles that travel through the uterine artery and block the smaller arteries feeding the fibroids. Once the blood supply to the fibroids is blocked, the growths shrink. A woman can go home the same day or stay overnight in the hospital.

Larger fibroids shrink more slowly, but most shrink by half in about three months. It is too soon to know whether plugged blood vessels might reopen or nearby vessels might start feeding a fibroid.

OVARIAN CYSTS

The ovaries are a woman's gonads. When a baby girl is born, her ovaries contain a lifetime supply of eggs (more than half a million) and tissue that produces estrogen and progesterone, the female hormones responsible for secondary sexual characteristics, menstrual regularity, and maintenance of pregnancy. As a woman matures, the responsive ovaries react to her hormonal highs and lows and ovulation results each month. (See chapter 3 for a complete description of the menstrual cycle.)

The monthly cycle is a delicately balanced process based on precise interaction between the brain and the reproductive organs. If something such as stress disrupts the normal flow of hormones, the cycle might become obstructed and an ovarian cyst might form during the ovulatory phase.

When a cyst forms due to a disturbed menstrual cycle, it is called a *functional cyst* because it is related to the way an ovary functions. A functional cyst, also called a *simple cyst*, is a fluid-filled sac that usually disappears and is almost always benign. However, a woman might become confused when she learns she has an ovarian cyst because the words *cyst* and *tumor* are often used interchangeably by doctors describing enlargements of the ovaries. Also, there are types of ovarian cysts that are *semisolid masses*, more like traditional tumors, and not fluid-filled sacs at all.

The ovarian cysts that are diagnosed after menopause are usually the dense type, which have a high incidence of becoming malignant. Rarely do these tumors form during a woman's fertile years. After the change-of-life, an ovarian abnormality should be carefully evaluated by a doctor because a new growth is not going to be a slowly disappearing functional cyst but is a suspicious tumor. A woman's age is a big factor in the type of cyst she has.

Functional Ovarian Cysts

The four most common types of fluid-filled, mostly benign, functional cysts are: follicular cysts, corpus luteum (or lutein) cysts, polycystic ovarian cysts, and endometriotic cysts.

Follicular Cysts. At the time of ovulation the Graafian follicle will burst, release the egg-of-the-month into the Fallopian tube, and allow the menstrual cycle to continue in its synchronized fashion. A follicular cyst emerges only when a Graafian follicle does not develop properly. When something such as stress or weight fluctuation alters the hormonal flow and interrupts normal ovulation, the Graafian follicle might turn into a follicular cyst with a very thin shell.

The follicular cyst might grow to the size of a peach or a small apple. Since only a thin membrane forms the cyst wall, after existing through one or two menstrual cycles the vulnerable cyst responds to hormonal surges and usually disappears by itself. Most often its fluid is painlessly absorbed into the body, but there are times, before a cyst has a chance to dissolve, that it might accidentally rupture.

A woman should be forewarned. After a follicular cyst is diagnosed, a blow to the abdominal area or vigorous sexual intercourse might break the cyst. Sometimes a cyst ruptures spontaneously. No matter how a break occurs, ovarian fluid spilling into the abdomen will be very irritating to the peritoneum, the lining of the abdominal cavity, and a woman might have severe pain. No surgery is necessary, though, since the pain will ease as the fluid is absorbed by the body.

At the start, a follicular cyst develops painlessly. It can be confirmed through ultrasonography. If a follicular cyst does not shrink after one or two menstrual cycles, a doctor might elect to place a woman on birth control pills. Oral contraceptives will stop a woman's hormonal fluctuation and aid in the disintegration of the cyst.

OVARIAN CYSTS

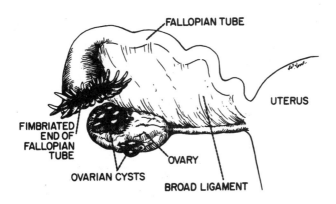

FALLOPIAN TUBE

UTERUS

FIMBRIATED
END OF
FALLOPIAN
TUBE

OVARY

OVARIAN CYSTS

BROAD LIGAMENT

15-2 **Ovarian Cysts.** A cyst is a fluid-filled sac. Ovarian cysts commonly occur in menstruating women. Most ovarian cysts are called functional cysts because they are related to the way an ovary functions. These cysts often develop from an area of the ovary in which ovulation has recently taken place. All functional cysts are benign. A functional cyst might be as small as a grape or as large as a grapefruit. In one or two months it will usually disappear by itself without the need for surgery. If a functional cyst does not disappear, it should be further evaluated through ultrasonography, or possibly with laparoscopy. Since most ovarian cysts are benign, a woman should always seek a second opinion if her doctor suggests surgery as a means of treatment.

If a woman takes the pill and the cyst does not disappear, a laparoscopy might be indicated to allow a doctor to scrutinize the cyst and possibly perform a biopsy. The cyst that appears suspicious should be surgically removed.

Corpus Luteum Cysts. After ovulation, the cells of the Graafian follicle transform into the corpus luteum, which produces progesterone and estrogen. These hormones relax the uterus and prevent menstruation until the egg has a chance to be fertilized. If the ovulated egg is not fertilized, the corpus luteum disintegrates in two weeks and triggers menstruation.

During this luteal phase of the menstrual cycle, if blood seeps into the corpus luteum, a *corpus luteum hematoma* is likely to form. Gradually, in a biological transference, the blood is replaced by clear fluid and the hematoma becomes a corpus luteum cyst. This is a completely benign occurrence that can happen to a woman at any time during her reproductive years.

Ultrasonography will confirm a corpus luteum cyst, which, like a follicular cyst, develops without any symptoms and usually disintegrates after one or two menstrual cycles. A corpus luteum cyst will not easily rupture, so a woman need not be as cautious as she might be with a follicular cyst. (The occasional rupture of a corpus luteum cyst could be associated with severe abdominal pain, which should subside within a few days.)

If a corpus luteum cyst does not disappear spontaneously, birth control pills may be prescribed. Should oral contraceptives prove ineffective, a laparoscopy might be indicated.

Polycystic Ovarian Cysts. Polycystic ovarian syndrome (PCOS) is detailed in chapter 8 (see pages 219 to 221), but it is appropriate to include within this chapter a description of the ovarian cysts marking the condition. During PCOS the ovaries become hard and glistening. The follicles that should release the eggs for ovulation cannot break through the tough outer shell of the ovary, and these entrapped eggs form cysts within the ovaries. A doctor can usually feel the cysts, which eventually cause the ovaries to swell. Usually, the cysts are benign and they will disappear on their own, but sometimes they become so large that they damage ovarian function. A woman might then become infertile.

When a doctor notices the PCOS cysts are not shrinking, he might prescribe Clomid, a fertility drug, to help the eggs escape the ovaries (see chapter 8). Sometimes, surgery with a so-called wedge resection, removal of a portion of the ovary, is necessary to restore normal ovarian function.

Endometriotic Cysts. Another type of benign growth a doctor encounters all too frequently is the cyst caused by endometriosis, the hidden disease described in chapter 7. During endometriosis, the menstrual flow—the endometrium, or uterine lining, with all its glands—is pushed backward into the abdomen, where it might spray out and adhere to the reproductive organs. Sometimes when the trapped endometrial tissue and glands attach to the ovaries, endometriotic cysts evolve. These blood-filled "chocolate cysts," so named because the encased blood gives them a deep, dark chocolate appearance, might overtake the ovaries by themselves or they might mix with existing follicular cysts to form combination cysts.

In their unbridled spread, endometriotic cysts change the shape and affect the functioning of the ovaries. These growths can interfere with ovulation and lead to infertility. Endometriosis itself is a painful disease that might be treated with GnRH agonists, medications that work to dissolve the cysts and restore a woman's fertility (see chapter 7).

A doctor can confirm an ovarian cyst through ultrasonography. After a time, if the observed cyst does not disappear and infertility cannot be overcome, a doctor might decide to perform a laparoscopy. During the laparoscopy, he can insert a special needle into the cyst and aspirate fluid. Lab analysis of the aspirated fluid can tell a physician what type of cyst he is treating and whether there is any suspicion of malignancy in the growth. When a diagnosis of endometriosis is made, a doctor should immediately begin drug treatments with Danocrine or one of the GnRH agonists, which should be continued for at least six months (see chapter 7).

Semisolid Ovarian Cysts

If a woman's ovarian cyst does not disappear spontaneously, her doctor will probably begin to suspect a semisolid cyst. The *dermoid cyst*, a regularly diagnosed semisolid ovarian cyst, is frequently seen during a woman's fertile years. Surgery is usually needed to excise the dermoid, but this cyst is rarely malignant. The most common of the suspicious semisolid ovarian cysts are the *serous cyst adenomas* and the *mucinous cyst adenomas*, the latter type being the largest cysts ever seen in the body.

All cysts develop so painlessly that a woman might be surprised when her doctor tells her she has one. To determine the type of cyst he has discovered, a doctor will observe a woman through one or two menstrual cycles. A functional cyst often disappears after one or two months, but a semisolid cyst remains. When a woman is under fifty, most ovarian cysts will usually be benign and immediate surgery will rarely be recommended.

As it becomes evident that a cyst is not going to disappear, a doctor might prescribe birth control pills or Danocrine in an attempt to shrink a stubborn growth, since they will stop the hormonal fluctuation. A persistent ovarian cyst might indicate a precancerous or cancerous condition, but a doctor will have to perform further testing and evaluation to make a diagnosis. He might want to view the cyst on an X ray (which can sometimes picture teeth inside a dermoid cyst), or, more likely, he will try to evaluate the cyst through ultrasonography. A doctor will then make a decision to perform either a laparoscopy for identification of the cyst or an exploratory laparotomy for cyst removal and analysis. He might also order a CA125 blood test to rule out the presence of ovarian cancer.

Dermoid Cysts. The dermoid cyst, named for its kinship with the dermis layer of the skin, contains all elements normally found in skin—fatty tissue, hair, sweat glands, and other skinlike tissue. A dermoid even occasionally incorporates cartilage, bone, intestine, and thyroid tissue. Sometimes the presence of a dermoid cyst can produce hyperthyroidism.

The origin of the dermoid cyst is not known. A woman might be born with the makings of this cyst, but the growth might appear only if a sudden hormonal stimulation causes its development to spurt. As a dermoid cyst grows, it might come to be known as a woman's "twin," because it will have many of the same biological elements that make a woman unique.

During an examination, a dermoid cyst might float up in front of the uterus rather than stay lodged in one place. Dermoids are light, mobile growths attached to the ovaries by stalks, or pedicles. Sometimes there is a danger that dermoids might twist on their stems and cause severe pain that can be alleviated only by a rush operation.

The diagnosis of a dermoid can be confirmed by either ultrasonography or X ray, and then a doctor will suggest a date for surgical removal of the cyst. Under normal circumstances a dermoid cyst does not require immediate surgery because it has only a *1 percent* chance of malignancy. However, a dermoid must eventually be excised because if it remains on the ovary there is a chance that it might rupture and spill irritating fatty fluid into the abdomen. Peritonitis, an inflammation of the abdominal lining, might ensue if a dermoid ruptures. A laparoscopy or barely noticeable bikini incision below the pubic hairline can provide a surgeon with access to this cyst.

Serous Cyst Adenomas. A serous cyst adenoma is often called "the 50 percent tumor" because half the time it is malignant and half the time it grows on both ovaries. After menarche, any woman can develop this cyst. Sometimes a serous cyst adenoma is so small it cannot be felt by a doctor during a pelvic examination, or it can be so large that it completely occupies the abdominal cavity.

If a doctor feels a cyst that does not disappear, he should suspect a serous cyst adenoma and perform a laparoscopy and a possible laparotomy to excise the growth. Before concluding surgery, a doctor should examine both ovaries for abnormalities. If lab analysis of an extracted tumor confirms a serous cyst adenoma, a doctor should check a patient regularly for a few years to make sure another cyst does not form. The appearance of serous cyst adenomas after menopause means that both ovaries should be immediately removed—the chance of malignancy multiplies after change-of-life.

Mucinous Cyst Adenomas. The biggest mucinous cyst adenoma ever reported was 328 pounds! I have personally removed a mucinous cyst adenoma that was the size of a newborn baby. Yet merely 10 to 15 percent of the suspicious ovarian cysts turn out to be mucinous cyst adenomas, and only 12 to 15 percent of these growths become malignant.

While functional cysts are usually filled with thin fluid, the fluid inside a mucinous cyst adenoma is thick. It normally appears on only one ovary, but it can grow very large. When a mucinous cyst adenoma is clearly visible through ultrasonography, a doctor should perform a laparoscopy followed by an exploratory laparotomy to remove the cyst for lab analysis. If the cyst is benign, the ovary can be saved in a young woman. After change-of-life the ovary should be removed even if the cyst is benign because the chance of malignancy increases dramatically.

How Are Ovarian Cysts Treated?

After a doctor discovers an ovarian cyst during an internal examination, he will want to determine what type of cyst it is. If a woman is in her fertile years, there is a good chance that she has a functional cyst, especially if the growth is accompanied by menstrual irregularity or prolonged bleeding. A woman should undergo ultrasonography to aid the doctor in his diagnosis. An ultrasound image will show whether or not a cyst contains fluid.

If a clear-fluid cyst is visible, it is probably a benign functional ovarian cyst. A doctor should monitor the cyst for one or two menstrual cycles to see if the cyst disintegrates by itself. Usually a spontaneous remission occurs and the cyst disappears. On the rarest of occasions a cyst might rupture and spill pain-causing fluid into the abdominal cavity, so a physician must be watchful. If a cyst stubbornly remains, a woman might be placed on birth control pills to help reduce the growth. Or, a woman might be treated with a GnRH medication such as Lupron, or the drug Danocrine, to overcome endometriosis by melting away its cyst. Certainly in the case of an endometriotic cyst, a GnRH drug is the first-choice treatment.

If ultrasonography shows a semisolid cyst, or if a fluid-filled cyst lingers without change, a doctor might perform a laparoscopy to get a closer look at the growth and to take a biopsy or remove it. A cyst that appears suspicious during a laparoscopy might warrant an exploratory laparotomy to remove the cyst for lab analysis. If during the laparoscopy the cyst looks benign, it could be punctured and its fluid aspirated and sent for cystologic lab analysis. Until the report is in, the benign-looking cyst is allowed to remain in a woman's body.

The major cause for concern occurs when a woman develops an ovarian cyst after menopause. This is the time when a cyst is at high risk for malignancy. A postmenopausal woman should not waste a minute in having her ovarian cyst evaluated and removed. The sooner ovarian cysts are detected and treated, the better are a woman's chances of avoiding extensive chemotherapy.

QUESTIONS ABOUT OVARIAN CYSTS

How Did My Ovarian Cyst Disappear by Itself?

I had been having sharp pains in my left side so I went to my doctor. He ordered a pelvic ultrasound and told me I had an ovarian cyst the size of an orange. He advised surgery. I would not agree to the operation and I waited five months. Then I went to another gynecologist who said that I didn't have an ovarian cyst. I

had some pain, which is why I went to the second doctor. I thought
the cyst might be causing me big trouble. You can't imagine how
shocked I was to hear that the cyst was gone! How did it disappear
by itself? And if it is gone, why do I still have pain?
                                        —A.Y., Turlock, California

This woman clearly had a benign functional ovarian cyst, probably a follicular cyst. It might have been as large as an orange and still it would have been capable of disappearing spontaneously after a few menstrual cycles. Benign cysts respond to hormonal fluctuations, and this is exactly what her cyst did. As her estrogen and progesterone increased and decreased, her cyst, which might have grown due to a sudden hormonal shift, lost its stimulation and shrank away to nothing.

Her current pain might exist because the cyst might have ruptured and irritating follicular fluid might have leaked into the abdominal cavity. This pain will disappear as the fluid becomes reabsorbed into her body.

I am so pleased to hear from a woman who listened to her body. Ms. Y. refused surgery and eventually sought a second opinion. She waited, and without birth control pills or other medication her cyst vanished. Her body healed itself.

Why Did My Cysts Come Back When I Went off the Pill?

I am having problems with ovarian cysts. My doctor put me on
birth control pills to keep the cysts under control. Recently I went
off the pill because I didn't want to take it anymore, but the cysts
came back. The pill seems to eliminate my cysts only temporarily. I
want to get rid of my cysts for good. I asked my doctor about
removing them, but he said my ovary would have to go too. Is there
any way I can eliminate the cysts but keep my ovaries? If I go back
on the pill, will the cysts return if I stop the pill again?
                                        —B.N., Rochester, New York

Birth control pills inhibit the release of the brain hormones FSH and LH, relax the ovaries, and help to speed the disintegration of benign functional ovarian cysts. When a woman's cysts have been controlled by birth control pills, they might re-emerge when the pills are stopped. After a few menstrual cycles, however, the female hormones readjust and the new cysts usually disappear by themselves. A doctor should be monitoring the cysts for changes in size. And in the aftermath of the pill, a woman might enhance her hormonal balance by taking vitamin B-complex with extra vitamin B_6.

If several months elapse and the returned cysts do not disappear, Ms. N. might be placed on birth control pills once more. After a time she might try to stop the pills again to see if the cysts stay away. At some point in her life her hormones will alter and the cysts will not reappear.

There is no need to panic. The growths are benign and Ms. N. does not need surgery. I have seen women rushed into the operating room to remove cysts that have grown back two months later. It appears to me that sometimes surgery seems to stimulate functional ovarian cysts. An operation is definitely inappropriate, and the idea of removing an ovary to cure a functional cyst is something like chopping off a foot to prevent a broken toe. This is unintelligent medicine. Under no circumstance should Ms. N. permit her doctor to excise her ovary as treatment for this condition.

What Can Be Done with a Hemorrhaging Cyst?

Five years ago I lost my left ovary and tube during surgery to remove an ovarian cyst. The cyst was hemorrhaging and gangrenous and the doctor could not save my organs. I was fine while I was on the birth control pill after surgery, but when I went off the pill I started having pains in my right side. I had a hemorrhagic ovarian cyst removed on my right side and I still have my right tube and ovary. Once again, I was fine for a while, but then I developed pain in my right side. The doctor said "Have a baby," so I did. My son is now a year old and I am still in pain. I

*do not want to lose my remaining tube and ovary. I would like to
have another child, but I do not know what to do. I was diagnosed
as having a pelvic infection and adhesions. After antibiotic therapy
in the hospital, I went home with my pain not cured. Could it be
that I have another hemorrhagic cyst? What can be done?*

—L.S., Montgomery, Alabama

Usually a hemorrhaging cyst is referred to as a *hemorrhagic corpus
luteum cyst.* It is a functional cyst that will generally disappear by
itself. A cyst becomes gangrenous when it grows very large and
twists on its stalk, cutting off the blood supply to the cyst tissue. The
decaying, gangrenous tissue causes tremendous pain and must be
surgically removed with the ovary.

It is not quite clear what is at the root of Ms. S.'s problem. She
should seek a second opinion from a doctor who can skillfully review
her pathology report from the hospital where she was treated. Her
pathology slides should be studied by this physician to determine
whether the pathologist misinterpreted her case. She might be suffering from endometriosis, which produces dark "chocolate cysts" on
the ovaries. With this disease she would be experiencing pain at
ovulation and before and during her menstrual period. If there is a
chance that she might have endometriosis, she should be placed on a
GnRH agonist for at least six months to rest her pelvic organs and
dissolve her endometriotic cysts.

Should the second-opinion doctor decide that her condition is
being caused by a hemorrhagic corpus luteum cyst, she might be
placed on birth control pills for several months. Oral contraceptives
might shrink her ovarian cyst, regulate her period, and make future
conception easier. After going off the pill she might have a pelvic
ultrasound or a hysterosalpingogram, an X ray of her uterus, to allow
her doctor to check the healthiness of her organs.

A diagnosis of Ms. S.'s condition might be extremely difficult, but
with her pain and history of abnormal cysts, I would, even with an
uncertain diagnosis, place her on Lupron or Danocrine to inhibit

her hormonal fluctuation. With Danocrine or a GnRH agonist treatment, her reproductive organs might heal themselves, and after, the rate of conception usually increases.

I Had a Dermoid Cyst; Did I Have to Lose My Ovary?

My doctor told me that my dermoid cyst had twisted around my ovary and during surgery he had to remove my ovary and tube with the cyst. He said that I had a 15 to 20 percent chance of getting a dermoid on the other ovary and I am beside myself with worry. I want a sibling for my daughter and I'm scared that if I get a dermoid I will lose the rest of my organs. What do you think is likely to happen to me if they find another cyst?
—E.T., Houma, Louisiana

As mentioned earlier, a dermoid often contains fatty tissue, hair, skinlike tissue, teeth, cartilage, bone, intestines, and thyroid tissues. It is humorously called a woman's "twin" because it retains her biological characteristics.

A dermoid cyst is a benign ovarian growth that can be excised without harming the ovary itself. As long as there is adequate blood supply to the ovarian tissue, even a dermoid that is twisted on its stem can be removed without damaging the ovary.

It appears that Ms. T. was not being cared for by a skillful surgeon. In the past, when doctors found an ovarian cyst, they would just carve out the ovary and the cyst together, without much thought to the possibility that at some point a woman might have a problem with the other ovary. Today, most doctors are trying to save ovarian tissue, to think ahead to a woman's future childbearing. Recently, I examined a twenty-two-year-old woman whose hysterectomy had been blamed on a twisted ovarian cyst that had grown on the only ovary she had after prior surgery. I hope I do not see any more women in her position, and I know that concerned physicians are trying to prevent other young women from losing their capability to conceive.

About 25 percent of the time, dermoid cysts occur bilaterally, on both ovaries. When a surgeon operates for one dermoid cyst, he should carefully examine the other ovary to make sure that he is not missing a second dermoid. Sometimes he must cut into the other ovary to assure himself that a dermoid is not developing on the inside of the organ. Only one-time surgery is necessary in most cases of dermoid cysts.

If Ms. T. ever learns that she has a dermoid cyst on her healthy ovary, she should seek out a doctor associated with a teaching hospital or a reputable medical center. A skillful surgeon will be able to remove the cyst—or, if it is unavoidable, a portion of the ovary with the cyst. He will know how to leave as much of the ovary as possible untouched. Remember, a woman has a quarter of a million eggs in each ovary. A doctor could remove even half of an ovary and there would still be plenty of good ovarian tissue to produce an egg for fertilization.

Can an Ovarian Cyst Make My Periods Irregular?

I am nineteen years old. My family doctor tells me that I have an ovarian cyst, but I have not been checked by a gynecologist. I am wondering if my painful cramps and heavy flow are from the ovarian cyst. About a year ago I had a heavy period with clots and then my flow went back to normal. Could I have had a cyst then too? My doctor tells me that I don't have to go to a gynecologist, but maybe a gynecologist could give me medicine for the cyst.
                                                    —M.B., St. Paul, Minnesota

When a woman has an ovarian cyst, the ovary becomes enlarged and the ovary does not function properly. Often the cyst develops during a month when ovulation might have gone awry and a follicle that was meant to contain the egg-of-the-month turns into a cyst. The hormonal imbalance that results from inadequate ovulation might bring on pain and prolonged bleeding.

The progesterone that is produced in the corpus luteum after ovulation relaxes the uterus to stop the bleeding. As long as a cyst remains, however, progesterone secretion will be thrown off balance. Without progesterone regulating the flow, bleeding will be irregular and unrestrained. Spotting can also occur, but for another reason. As a cyst disintegrates, the hormones inside it often spill into the abdomen and cause spotting. Thus, Ms. B.'s pain, prolonged bleeding, and spotting, if she has it, might be due to her ovarian cyst.

She should consult a gynecologist, who will want to monitor the cyst through the next few menstrual cycles. If the cyst does not disappear by itself and bleeding continues to be irregular, this woman, assuming she has a benign functional ovarian cyst, might be placed on the birth control pill. The pill will inhibit the release of the brain hormones FSH and LH, relax the uterus, and stabilize her estrogen and progesterone. Eventually, the action of the pill might help to shrink the cyst.

What Problems Will I Encounter with Polycystic Ovarian Cysts?

I have been told that I have Stein-Leventhal cysts and polycystic ovarian syndrome. I am worried that this syndrome could result in cancer. Also, will I suffer hair loss, weight gain, and dry skin? Is the fertility drug Clomid the only solution to this problem? I would like to get my body back to normal and have a child. Will I ever be the same again? I'm sorry to ask so many questions, but my doctor never seems to have the time to talk to me.

—O.C., Rome, Georgia

Polycystic ovarian syndrome might be inherited, or at least some abnormality in the ovary might be inherited. Ovulation does not occur every month. The ovaries enlarge and their surfaces develop hard shells. The egg-of-the-month, unable to break through the shell of the ovary, becomes a fluid-filled sac, a cyst trapped inside the ovary. As more and more eggs are locked within the ovaries, more and more cysts develop and the ovaries swell.

Since the ovaries produce male and female hormones, a woman will have an abundance of both. She will experience a higher estrogen level, which might mean heavier periods and bigger breasts. She will also experience an increase in testosterone, the male hormone, which usually means excessive male-characteristic hair growth. A woman might develop hair on her chin and around her nipples, and her pubic hairs might grow upward toward her navel. A woman with PCOS cysts is often overweight, but the cysts should have no effect on the condition of her skin.

The good news is that polycystic ovarian syndrome is a benign condition. It is not ovarian cancer. However, pregnancy might become elusive because the off/on ovulation pattern of the disease makes conception difficult. A woman with polycystic ovarian syndrome is often helped by Clomid, a medication that is specifically designed to induce ovulation. The chance of having twins is a little higher with Clomid, but generally it is a safe drug successfully used by women with this condition.

Ms. C. should refer to chapter 8, the sections "What Is Polycystic Ovarian Syndrome?" (pages 219 to 221) and "Could All the Hair I Have on My Body Be Connected to My Infertility?" (pages 221 to 223), which specifically detail the facets of polycystic ovarian syndrome.

A woman should not be worried about PCOS cysts, because they usually do not rupture. As for the excessive hair growth that accompanies this syndrome, hair does not disappear with hormonal treatment. The time-honored methods of hair removal—depilatories, electrolysis, waxing, and shaving—are still the best suggestions a doctor can give.

Ms. C. can get her body back in good condition, but she will never be exactly as she was when she was young.

I Have Cysts on Both Ovaries; Can I Still Have Children?

I have a cyst on each ovary. My doctor says there is no need to remove the cysts, but I have excruciating pain during my period.

Is my doctor right in not removing the cysts? I am also concerned because I would like to become pregnant, and my question is: Can I still have children with the cysts?

—K.J., Aurora, Illinois

It is difficult from this letter to know what type of cysts Ms. J. has. A follicular or corpus luteum cyst will usually occur in one ovary at a time. Polycystic ovarian cysts might appear on both ovaries at once and cause difficulty in conception (see previous letter). Also, considering Ms. J.'s menstrual pain, the possibility of endometrial cysts on both ovaries should not be excluded.

If Ms. J.'s cysts do not disappear after a few menstrual cycles, and if a diagnosis cannot be made through ultrasonography, she might be advised to undergo a laparoscopy. During a laparoscopy, a doctor will be able to view and aspirate the cysts. Lab analysis of the cyst fluid should then provide an identification of the cyst type so that they can be appropriately treated.

There appears to be no reason why she shouldn't be able to conceive and have a child.

Does an Ovarian Cyst Mean Hysterectomy?

I have an ovarian cyst sandwiched between my ovary and my bladder. My doctor says there is no way he can remove the cyst without taking my ovary and tube. He also informs me that if he finds a cyst on the other ovary, he will have to perform a hysterectomy. So far, I have refused to submit to surgery because I don't feel that a cyst should lead to hysterectomy. Will my delay make my condition worse, or should I agree to surgery?

—H.T., Easton, Pennsylvania

Most ovarian cysts are benign, so a woman should not be panicked by her doctor and rushed into surgery. If Ms. T. has a functional ovarian cyst, as it appears she has, there is no need for surgery, least of all a hysterectomy. If she is carefully evaluated and a fluid-filled cyst is viewed through ultrasonography, her doctor should not be pushing for surgery. Ms.T. should seek a second opinion.

As explained in the "How Are Ovarian Cysts Treated?" section of this chapter, if a clear-fluid cyst is diagnosed, a doctor need only monitor the cyst through one or two menstrual cycles to see whether it disappears spontaneously. A functional ovarian cyst that does not go away might possibly be reduced through birth control pills if a woman is under thirty-five. A GnRH agonist recommended for endometrial cysts might be given to women who cannot tolerate birth control pills in an effort to shrink their ovarian cysts.

Ms. T. need have cause for concern only if ultrasonography reveals a semisolid cyst. A semisolid cyst in a woman who is beyond menopause could be an indication of ovarian cancer. After a woman's change-of-life, if a suspicious semisolid cyst is found most physicians would recommend a hysterectomy to avoid development of another potential malignant ovarian cyst. However, if ovarian cysts are completely benign, a woman should find a doctor who is willing to remove the cysts alone.

I would suggest that Ms. T. be evaluated by a second-opinion doctor who will take the time to define her cyst and describe exactly how he plans to treat her condition.

I Had Adenomyosis and an Ovarian Tumor; Did I Need a Hysterectomy?

I am a twenty-one-year-old woman who has had a total hysterectomy. I had been in severe pain all the time. My doctor scheduled an operation and told me before the surgery that he would do a hysterectomy only if he found something. He said when he got in there he couldn't believe the mess. I had a tumor the size of a baseball on my ovary and my organs were full of adenomyosis. He did a total hysterectomy including my ovaries. I have a daughter, but I will never be able to have a baby again. The surgery was an extremely difficult decision for my husband

*and me. I am happy to be living without the pain, but now I
am on hormones and I worry about breast cancer. I try not to
think about that. Once before when you answered a letter of mine
you told me I was too young to have my female organs removed.
Yes, I know that you advised me against hysterectomy. I wanted
another child, but what could I have done? Maybe I don't want
to know.*

—S.F., Nashville, Tennessee

Without a pathology report, it is difficult to respond to Ms. F.
However, it is unlikely that such a young woman would have had
adenomyosis. Usually adenomyosis, a thickening of the uterine wall
that is described in the "I Have Adenomyosis, Do I Need a
Hysterectomy?" section of this chapter, is seen in older women who
have suffered severe menstrual cramps for years. It seems more
probable that Ms. F. might have had endometriosis. She might
have benefited from treatment with Lupron or Danocrine, which
would have stopped her menstrual flow and dissolved her ovarian
cyst.

She does not say whether she sought more than one opinion on
her condition. When a young woman is told she needs surgery, she
should consult two or three doctors before making her decision. If
she absolutely requires a hysterectomy, perhaps her ovaries can be
saved. Ms. F. obviously is saddened by this experience and her emotional adjustment will probably be more difficult than her physical
recovery. Now she will be taking female hormones for the rest of
her life.

I would encourage every woman who is faced with the possibility of
hysterectomy to learn all she can about the condition the doctor
tells her is making the surgery necessary. Certainly an ovarian tumor
does not warrant a hysterectomy. And Ms. F.'s adenomyosis is questionable. A woman must educate herself to the workings of her body
and always consult a second-opinion doctor when the subject is
surgery.

My Ovary Is Out of Place; Must It Be Removed?

My doctor says that my ovary is out of place and there is nothing he can do unless he removes it. He does not want to do that since I am twenty-five years old, but in the meantime the ovary is making sexual intercourse very painful. Is there anything to be done that my doctor might not know about?

—V.M., Gladstone, Missouri

Ovaries can be located anyplace. Sometimes adhesions can cause them to be below or above the uterus. Since Ms. M. does not mention that she has cysts or other ovarian abnormalities, her doctor is right to refrain from surgery.

The fact that she has severe pain during intercourse could indicate that she has pelvic endometriosis or pelvic inflammatory disease (PID). A doctor should keep checking for these conditions.

OTHER GYNECOLOGICAL CYSTS

How Did I Get a Vaginal Cyst?

I recently learned that I have a cyst growing on the outer portion of my vagina. Where did it come from? Do I need surgery? I want to have children and I'm worried that this cyst will make it impossible.

—G.N., Amarillo, Texas

Since Ms. N.'s cyst is located on the outer portion of her vagina, it is most likely a Bartholin's duct cyst. There is a Bartholin's gland on each of the two outer lips on the lowest part of the vulva. The Bartholin's glands secrete the mucus that lubricates the vagina and facilitates sexual intercourse. Sometimes, for no special reason, the duct of a gland clogs, swells up, and evolves into a cyst that looks and feels like a lump between a woman's legs. The cyst, however, is painless and does not interfere with childbearing. Generally, the enlargement drains by itself during sitz baths.

There is only a problem if the cyst becomes inflamed and abscessed. Then the lump can hurt so much that a woman can barely walk. A doctor will prescribe antibiotic therapy in combination with the sitz baths for a Bartholin's gland abscess. If the infection cannot be cured with medication, then a surgical drainage of the gland, a *marupialization,* might be necessary.

Ms. N. does not say she is in pain, so her cyst is not likely to be inflamed. Her Bartholin's duct cyst will not at all hinder her ability to conceive a child.

Is a Gartner's Cyst Dangerous?

My gynecologist told me that I have a Gartner's duct cyst in my cervical area. I can feel the pain when I withdraw a tampon. I wish the cyst would go away, but it has grown recently and caused me to have a D & C. The doctor said it was not necessary to remove the cyst at the time. I'm beginning to wonder, though, if this cyst is harmless. Should I press to have it removed?
—F. C., Walla Walla, Washington

A Gartner's duct cyst develops in the Gartner's gland, which secretes fluid to moisten the vagina. The Gartner's gland is located high in the vagina close to the urethra. Sometimes the Gartner's duct can become irritated, blow up like a cyst, and cause pain during sexual intercourse or with the use of tampons.

The Gartner's cyst, however, is a benign condition. The enlargement can be removed through surgery, but Ms. C.'s doctor is correct in not pressing for it. Surgery is not strictly necessary. Since the duct is inside the vagina, not on the ovary or in the uterus, it does not interfere with childbearing.

16.

Fibrocystic Breast Disease
and Other Breast Problems

Why Doesn't My Doctor Tell Me Anything?

*I am twenty-five years old and I have already had two
operations to remove breast cysts. I had two cysts removed from my
left breast and one from my right breast. My doctor says I have
fibrocystic breast disease, that I will have it the rest of my life, and
that I should just forget about it. He tells me that my cysts are not
malignant and there is nothing to worry about unless I find a
hard, painless lump. Then I'm supposed to come back to him,
because I might have cancer. Since I'm on my own to take care of
myself, I would like more information. My doctor isn't very
talkative when it comes to telling me about my breast, and
anyway, every time I find a lump, he sends me to a breast surgeon.
Like my doctor, the surgeon only communicates facts he considers
essential. Are breasts so mysterious that no one can explain them?*
—C.S., Cedar Rapids, Iowa

Many doctors still hesitate to explain the difference between
benign and malignant breast conditions. They even disagree among
themselves about when to proceed with further examination and

how to determine malignancy. The bottom line is that women are expected to discover their own breast lumps.

Generally, a cancerous lump is hard, fixed in the breast tissue, and painless, although on rare occasions it might be associated with minimal pain. Breast cancers are more likely to be found when women are between the ages of forty and seventy-one. The median age of women who develop breast cancer is fifty-four. Benign fibrocystic breast disease, also called fibrocystic change, appears most often during a woman's reproductive years, from age sixteen to fifty. A benign lump is softer than a cancerous growth, easier to move, and when it is a symptom of fibrocystic breast disease, it is usually painful. The median age for this condition is thirty, although it is seen more frequently in women over thirty-five.

Often women who are checking themselves for breast abnormalities panic when they feel a lump because they have never been told about fibrocystic breast disease or any other benign breast problem. One of the reasons so little attention has been paid to breast conditions is that when gynecology became a specialty a few decades ago, a gentleman's agreement was made between the surgeon and the gynecologist. The surgeon promised to stay away from pelvic disorders if the gynecologist kept "hands off" the breast. For years many gynecologists honored the pact and refrained from examining women's breasts. Those days are over now.

The American College of Obstetricians and Gynecologists has encouraged gynecologists to recognize the fact that for most women, gynecologists are primary physicians. As such, they should examine women completely, which means the breast as well as the pelvis. With gynecological interest in the breast increasing, endocrinologists and scientists have begun to conduct more investigations into breast conditions.

Until tests for the early detection of breast diseases are refined, a woman will probably still discover her breast problems before her physician does. When it comes to her breasts, which, as this chapter will show, are neither mysterious nor inexplicable, a woman should expect to become an expert.

BREAST ANATOMY AND FUNCTION

Breast Structure

Size, shape, and elevation of the breast, nipple position, and color of the nipple and the areola (the area surrounding the nipple) are inherited characteristics that vary from woman to woman. For most females it is quite normal to have one breast slightly larger than the other. Some women are naturally "high-breasted," while others are "low-breasted." The nipple might be located directly in the middle of the breast or below the center. Nipples might also be inverted or protruding.

Inside the breast, the mammary glands extend from about the second or third rib to the sixth or seventh rib, and from the breastbone into the armpit region, the axilla. Fasciae, bands of fibrous tissue, support the breasts on the chest wall, while a highly developed network of nerves and nerve endings connects the glandular activity of the breasts with the normal fluctuations of the brain and the ovaries.

The breast is a glandular mass interlaced with ducts and supported by a blood supply, a lymph system, and fat. There are twenty or more lobes of functional tissue in each breast. Each lobe encompasses a system of milk glands to the nipple. There are also several clusters of between ten to one hundred acini, glandular sacs grouped around the ducts. The Latin word *acini* means "grapes," which are what the acini resemble. These saclike acini are the basic structural unit of the mammary glands. Their numbers vary from woman to woman, but they are in greatest abundance in women between seventeen and twenty-two years old.

Surrounding each of the acini is tissue made up of *myoepithelial cells*, which give the tissue the ability to contract. Myoepithelial contraction enables the acini and the duct network to expel the milk from the breast when a woman breast-feeds. Actually, the ducts store milk in the *ampullae*, the enlarged duct terminals at the base of the nipple. In Latin, *ampullae* means "jugs," but if the ducts and ampullae are given the more simplified name "milk sinuses" the slang term is certainly avoided. To aid the squeezing and emptying of the ampullae, smooth muscle fibers contract and make the nipple erect and firm during breast-feeding.

The breast gets its main supply of blood from the internal *mammary artery*, which enters from underneath the rib cage through the chest wall near the sternum—the breastbone—and then branches into the breast tissue. The lymph system in the breast closely follows the pathways of the veins and is connected to the lymph glands in the armpit. During a breast examination the lymph glands in the armpit should be checked, since their enlargement could indicate that disease, infection, or even cancer, could be present in breast tissue.

In addition to everything else, the breast contains fatty tissue. Fatty cells vary from woman to woman. An overweight woman has more fat in her breast tissue, making her breasts look larger. A slim woman usually has less fat and smaller, firmer breasts.

Feeding: The Breast's Primary Function

In the female, the mammary glands provide nourishment for the newborn baby. The first milk, the *colostrum*, is highly recommended for an infant since it contains more immunological substances—bacteria fighters and antibodies—than subsequent breast milk.

It is now believed that breast-feeding will help a child have a healthier life since breast milk appears to protect against serious illnesses such as gastroenteritis and respiratory disorders. According to recent research, breast milk might also inhibit obesity in a child, promote brain development, and guard against adult disorders such as heart disease. For the mother, breast-feeding might also reduce the risk of fibrocystic breast disease and possibly breast cancer.

The Breast As a Sexual Organ

The female breast is structurally designed to serve as an erotic organ. Nerve endings located in the nipple send and receive erotic sensations to and from the brain. Like the male penis, the nipple of the female breast is an erogenous zone. Smooth muscle fibers cause the nipple to become erect on sexual manipulation and stimulation. Not only does the breast become responsive, but kissing and caressing of the breast can cause a higher pulse rate and increased respiration in a woman. In addition, the glands in the genital area secrete vaginal fluid more heavily when the breast is sexually stimulated.

Sexual sensitivity of the breast varies, not with the size or shape of the breast, but with the woman. For some women, stimulation of the breast is a necessary prelude to orgasm and sexual intercourse. In most women, stimulation of the breast increases desire for sexual intercourse, and in that way the breast is directly connected to reproduction.

HOW HORMONES INFLUENCE THE BREAST

The endocrine hormones that affect the reproductive cycle of a woman and bring on breast changes are produced by the pituitary gland (in the base of the brain), the adrenal glands (above the kidneys), and the ovaries. As explained in chapter 3's description of the menstrual cycle, the brain hormones FSH and LH stimulate the production of estrogen and progesterone in the ovary. As the estrogen increases after ovulation, in the last two weeks of the menstrual cycle, it influences the breasts.

There are cells within the acini called *estrogen receptors*. These estrogen receptors can be likened to keyholes waiting for their estrogen "keys" to be inserted. Estrogen activates these receptors and the breast glands grow. A woman will have breast enlargement at the end of the menstrual cycle.

If a woman is pregnant, there will be increased stimulation to the breasts by both estrogen and progesterone. The breasts will continue to increase in size. The pituitary gland also secretes *prolactin*, a hormone that stimulates the secretion of milk. By the time a woman begins to breast-feed, prolactin will have prepared the breast for milk production. When a baby sucks on a woman's nipple, nerve impulses then go to the brain, where the pituitary gland will release another hormone, *oxytocin.* The oxytocin will trigger myoepithelial—smooth muscle—contractions within the breast tissue and milk will be expelled. This is called the "milk ejection reflex" or the "letdown reflex." When a woman who is not pregnant experiences a normal menstrual cycle, the levels of estrogen and progesterone inhibit the release of prolactin.

Sometimes, when a woman has amenorrhea, an absence of regular periods, there might be insufficient estrogen in her body and overproduction of prolactin. She might notice a leakage of fluid from her breasts. This is not a cancerous condition, but a disorder called galactorrhea (see chapter 3, page 126). A new medication called Parlodel (bromocriptine mesylate) can block the prolactin, stimulate estrogen, lead to menstruation, and enhance fertility.

If hormones fluctuate normally, a woman might not experience breast problems. However, a hormonal imbalance, which women often experience during their teens and in their late thirties and forties, might abnormally stimulate breast tissue and lead to fibrocystic breast disease or other breast conditions.

BREAST SELF-EXAMINATION (BSE)

Since breast disorders are most successfully treated when discovered in early stages, it is important that a woman practice regular breast self-examination.

A woman should check her breasts at least once every month. Immediately after menstruation the breasts are in their least tender stage because hormones are at their lowest levels. This is the best time to perform a breast self-examination.

Before starting the self-examination, a woman should stand in front of a mirror with her arms at her sides and inspect her breasts. Is there any dimpling of the breast skin? Any new puckering or inversion of the nipples? Any changes in breast size or shape?

Discoloration of the breast? A woman should remain focused on her breasts as she presses her hands on her hips and then raises her arms above her head. If she notices abnormalities when she is in any of these positions, she should arrange a visit with her doctor.

A breast self-examination is best done when a woman is lying flat on her back in bed. To examine her left breast, she should place a folded towel under her left shoulder and her left hand should be underneath her neck. The right hand will be used to examine the left breast, and vice versa. The fingers should be flat together with the thumb extended, and the underside of the fingers, not the fingertips, should be used to "feel" the breast structure.

A woman should imagine her breast as being the face of a clock. She should start by pressing the top edge of the left breast where the breast meets the chest wall at a twelve o'clock point. While pressing, a woman should move her hand in a small circle about the size of a quarter in order to disturb the skin and move it over the internal tissue. A woman should then proceed clockwise around the face of the clock, making small circles as she presses at the point of each new hour. When she reaches twelve o'clock again, she should move her hand a little toward the nipple and go around the clock once more in the same fashion. Every time a woman reaches twelve o'clock she should proceed on another clockwise path closer to the nipple, until she finally reaches the nipple. This route to the nipple requires about four trips around the breast. Then she might examine the lymph nodes in her left armpit with her right hand.

After she finishes examining her armpit, a woman should lower her arm to her side and *repeat the entire breast examination* with her arm in this relaxed position. When she reaches the nipple this time, she should squeeze the nipple between her thumb and index finger to see if there is any discharge or bleeding. If so, she should inform her doctor right away.

Having completed the examination of her left breast, a woman should move the towel to a position underneath her right shoulder. With her left hand she should examine her right breast in the same way that she examined her left breast with her right hand. When she

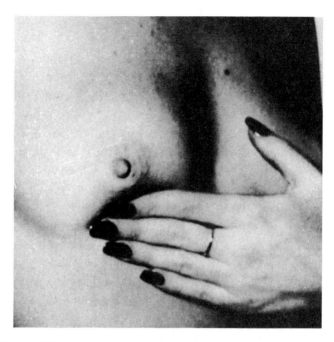

16-1 **Breast Self-Examination.** Ninety-five percent of breast lumps treated by doctors are discovered by women themselves. Breast self-examination is an extremely important procedure since early detection increases the chance for effective treatment. A woman examines her breast when she is either lying down or standing up. The woman in the photo is examining her right breast with her left hand. With the flat of her fingers, she firmly presses the breast tissue against her chest wall. She moves her fingers in small circles. She starts away from the nipple and carefully covers her entire breast by moving the hand clockwise toward the nipple. This pattern for a successful breast self-examination is detailed in the text. If any unusual lump is found, a woman should immediately call her doctor.

has finished, a woman should sit up and examine her left and right breasts again because the breasts often feel different when body positions are switched.

Sometimes the perfect moment for a breast self-examination is when a woman is standing in the shower and her skin is wet and soapy. She can keep one hand behind her head and examine her breast in the clockwise pattern with the other hand. If she has large, pendulous breasts, she might prefer to support a breast with one hand while examining it with the other. Her slippery skin might make it easier for her to feel lumps.

When she performs a regular breast self-examination, a woman becomes familiar with the contour of her own breasts and abnormalities become more apparent. It is important for every woman to know that she is looking for something that is new or unusual in her breasts. A lump, a thickening, a hardening under the skin, discharge from the nipple, any unusual appearance of the skin or nipple, could be a trouble signal. A doctor should be called immediately.

NOTE: *All women should be examined at least once a year by their doctors.* A gynecologist should perform a pelvic examination, a Pap smear, and a thorough breast examination when a woman appears for her annual checkup. If a woman complains about a breast change, he should do a meticulous breast examination in the same way a woman would do it for herself. If a doctor feels a lump, he should explain to a woman whether or not it appears to be benign. A woman might be asked to monitor a lump that is not suspicious. (The latest techniques for aiding the diagnoses of abnormalities are described at the end of this chapter.)

Women of all ages should examine their breasts. A teenager as well as postmenopausal women should practice breast self-examination. Even when a woman does not have a menstrual cycle to guide her in the timing of her BSE, she should write a once-a-month reminder to herself on the calendar.

A doctor or nurse can instruct a woman in the proper method of breast self-examination.

BENIGN BREAST LUMPS

Most breast lumps found during the menstrual years are benign. Fibrocystic breast disease, which is covered in depth in this chapter, accounts for the majority of these benign lesions. Fibroadenomas—

movable, well-defined, painless masses—are also commonly diagnosed (see pages 604 to 605), and doctors sometimes see papillomas, fat lumps, hematomas, and duct ectasia (clogged milk ducts), the rarer types of noncancerous growths.

Considering that all these different kinds of benign conditions exist, a woman should not become immediately alarmed when she finds a lump in her breast. If she is under fifty, the lump is most likely free from cancer, but it must never be dismissed. Every breast abnormality should be examined by a doctor.

FIBROCYSTIC BREAST DISEASE (FBD)

Fibrocystic breast disease, also called fibrocystic change, is the most common noncancerous breast condition among women. One out of five women, or 20 percent of the female population, might at some time have fibrocystic breast disease.

For most women, the latter part of the menstrual cycle brings swelling and tenderness of the breast, starting at the time of ovulation and becoming more severe as menstruation approaches. At the onset of the menstrual flow, the normal breast usually returns to its relaxed, less sensitive state. If a breast continues to feel sore and tender after menstruation, a woman might have fibrocystic breast disease. A hormonal imbalance, a disturbance in the estrogen/progesterone ratio, can cause the acini and the milk ducts in the breast to expand and form cysts (fluid-filled sacs).

Generally, a cyst, since it is fast-forming, pulls on the nerves that encircle the breast tissue and causes pain. Although fibrocystic breast disease can be painless if a lump is slow to enlarge, the cysts are always tender to the touch. (On the other hand, breast cancer is slow-growing and generally consists of hard, painless lumps.)

A cyst can be almost any size, from a fraction of an inch in diameter to the size of a golf ball or a plum. Cysts do not appear before menarche but afterward, when a young woman begins to secrete hormones. Most often these growths are found in women between

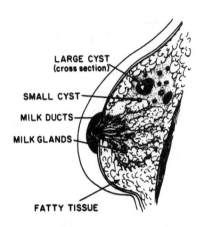

LARGE CYST
(cross section)

SMALL CYST

MILK DUCTS

MILK GLANDS

FATTY TISSUE

16-2 **Fibrocystic Breast Disease (FBD).** One out of five women will suffer from FBD, the most common breast condition in females. A single cyst, or several cysts, might develop at various locations in a woman's breasts. Most often, the cysts are found in the upper outer portions of the breast and are surrounded by the milk glands, milk ducts, and fatty tissue that are the breast's normal components. A cyst, which can be as small as a pea or as large as a plum, is a fluid-filled sac, as shown in the illustrated cross-section. If the fluid within a cyst increases in amount, the liquid can be aspirated with a needle. FBD cysts are influenced by a woman's hormonal fluctuations, and just before the onset of the menstrual period cysts enlarge and become more painful than they are at other times during the monthly cycle.

the ages of sixteen and fifty. They might appear with greater frequency as a woman enters her late thirties and forties, when there are more hormonal imbalances due to the approach of menopause. Cysts often disappear with menopause and are rarely detected after change-of-life.

Women who have had children early in life do not seem to be as susceptible to fibrocystic breast disease as women who have never been pregnant or women who have given birth when they were older. Also, women who have breast-fed their children seem to have added protection against FBD. However, there is some evidence that fibrocystic breast disease might be hereditary.

Since fibrocystic breast disease is linked to a hormone imbalance, teenagers who have not yet achieved regular menstrual cycles might suffer from cystic breasts. The disease might be seen in any woman at any time, of course, but as a woman enters her late thirties and forties her hormones become irregular again and the disease might appear for the first time or recur. Also, situations that shift the hormonal balance can bring on fibrocystic breast disease.

A woman who is on estrogen treatment or a woman who has gained weight will have more estrogen than progesterone in her body. As estrogen becomes more potent than progesterone, it will result in enlargement of the estrogen-sensitive breast tissue. The estrogen receptors in the breast will receive greater stimulation from the surplus estrogen and an increased amount of fluid will be secreted within a cyst. If enough fluid develops, a cyst grows larger and causes more pain. Depending upon how sensitive estrogen receptors are within a woman's breasts, cysts might develop in only one breast or in both breasts. Even after it is discovered, there is no way that the disease can be contained in one breast alone. Cysts do not appear in any particular pattern; they can either stand alone, be located in one general area, or be spread throughout the breasts.

What Are the Symptoms of Fibrocystic Breast Disease?

Fibrocystic breast disease is usually discovered by a doctor who is examining his patient's breasts during a comprehensive checkup, or by a woman who feels a tender lump during a self-examination and seeks help. A painful lump or lumps might exist in one or both breasts throughout the month. As the latter part of the menstrual cycle approaches, tenderness might increase. Sometimes a breast is so filled with large, tender lumps that a woman must wear a comfortable bra at all times, and she might even take painkillers. In a moderate case of the disease, a woman might have just one or two lumps in which the soreness intensifies before her menstrual period.

In a mild form of fibrocystic breast disease, the cysts might diminish and disappear after menstruation. As mentioned in the previous section, the cysts emerge due to a hormonal imbalance caused by an increase in estrogen and a weakening of progesterone.

This imbalance might have been brought on by stress or weight gain, among other factors. When a woman's circumstances change, her hormones might stabilize again and the cysts might vanish. With severe fibrocystic breast disease, the breasts are very painful and tender. Although the sore, tender lumps might become less painful after menstruation, with severe FBD they continue to hurt throughout the month and they do not disappear.

Most often, fibrocystic breast lumps are benign and a woman should not be so afraid when she discovers one that she hesitates to call her doctor. He will be able to treat the disease appropriately and give her peace of mind at the same time. A hard, painless lump that does not move with the tissue and persists, unchanged, throughout the menstrual cycles is far more suspicious than the tender, malleable, cystic lump.

Caffeine and Fibrocystic Breast Disease

Dr. John Minton, professor of clinical oncology at Ohio State University College of Medicine, was the first physician to make a connection between chemicals called methylxanthines and fibrocystic breast disease. Methylxanthines are consumed in three ways: in the *caffeine* of coffee, tea, cocoa, chocolate, certain soft drinks, and various drugs; in the *theobromine* of chocolate and tea; and in the *theophylline* of tea and certain bronchial and asthma remedies.

Dr. Minton studied forty-seven women with fibrocystic breast disease who drank four cups of coffee a day. He asked all forty-seven women to abstain from coffee for the duration of the study. Only twenty women complied, and of those twenty, thirteen or (65 percent) were free of breast lumps in one to six months. Since the Minton study in 1979, other researchers have also found improved breast symptoms and reduction in breast lumps when methylxanthines have been restricted.

The exact reason why methylxanthines influence fibrocystic breast disease is not known. It has been speculated that benign lumps might result from a buildup of cyclic AMP (cAMP) and cyclic GMP (cGMP), two biochemicals. Normally, cAMP and cGMP are held in check by an enzyme called phosphodiesterase, but methylxanthines prevent the enzyme from functioning adequately. The biochemicals overproduce and breast lumps appear. It follows, then, that these biochemicals probably work via the estrogen/progesterone receptors in the breast tissue. There are other theories about how methylxanthines operate within the body, but the main message from all the studies is that a reduction in these chemicals, which are especially prevalent in caffeine, would be beneficial.

Women with fibrocystic breast disease have a two to five times greater chance of developing breast cancer than women who do not have the disease. It is imperative for women with cystic breasts to do everything they can to eliminate the condition, and something so simple as a change in diet should not be ignored. For example, in every 12 ounces of Pepsi there are 35 mg of caffeine; Coke has 42 mg, Tab is slightly higher with 45 mg, Mountain Dew contains 49 mg, Mr. Pibb has 57 mg, and Dr Pepper has a high 61 mg. The caffeine content in the last two soft drinks approaches the 66 mg of caffeine in a cup of instant coffee, which is still much less than the 150 mg of caffeine in a cup of drip coffee. (See chart: "Methylxanthine Content of Foods and Drugs.")

If a woman is suffering from fibrocystic breast disease, she should try to cut down on her caffeine, but I do not believe that she must initiate an austerity program. A woman might have her morning cup of coffee and not feel guilty about it, and a teenager may enjoy a cola drink now and then. Automatic mass consumption of caffeine, however, is a habit that should be changed, and then there might be some improvement in the occurrence of fibrocystic breast disease.

But a woman should not expect miracles. Although the findings about methylxanthines are exciting, they are only one possible factor in the appearance of benign breast problems. These chemicals still are under investigation.

METHYLXANTHINE CONTENT
OF FOODS AND DRUGS

	Caffeine (mgs)	Theobromine (mgs)	Theophylline (mgs)
COFFEE (5 oz.)			
Regular Brewed			
—percolated	110	3	tr
—drip	150	3.5	1
Instant	66	1.5	tr
Decaf Brewed	4.5	tr	tr
Instant Decaf	2	tr	tr
SOFT DRINKS (12 oz.)			
Dr Pepper	61	tr	tr
Mr. Pibb	57	tr	tr
Mountain Dew	49	tr	tr
Tab	45	tr	tr
Coca-Cola	42	tr	tr
RC Cola	36	tr	tr
Pepsi-Cola	35	tr	tr
Diet Pepsi	34	tr	tr
Pepsi Light	34	tr	tr
BREWED DRINKS			
Tea (5 min. brew)	45	9	6
Cocoa (5 oz.)	13	73	tr
Milk Chocolate (1 oz.)	6	42	tr
DRUGS			
Vivarin Tablets	200	—	—
Nodoz	100	—	—
Excedrin	65	—	—
Vanquish	33	—	—
Empirin Compound	32	—	—
Anacin	32	—	—
Dristan	16.2	—	—

tr = less than 1 mg per serving

How Is Fibrocystic Breast Disease Treated?

In the past, fibrocystic breast disease did not receive much attention. There was no recognized form of treatment, little awareness about the condition, and an assumption on the part of doctors that if left alone the lumps would disappear. Physicians did not realize that while a woman was living with fibrocystic breast disease, she was often in severe pain. If any treatment was suggested, it was surgical removal of the lumps, which did not cure the disease.

Today, doctors have much more knowledge about FBD. A physician might attempt to help a woman overcome the condition by suggesting a change in diet and giving her newly approved medication. However, if a woman has a questionable lump, surgical intervention might still be needed to rule out malignancy.

Needle Aspiration for Evaluation of the Cyst. Sometimes, even when a doctor feels that a breast lump is in all probability benign fibrocystic breast disease, he might want to conduct a needle aspiration to verify his suspicions.

While a woman is on the examining table in the doctor's office, he might advise her of his intentions. Then the doctor will hold the breast firmly in his hand, steady the cyst, insert a fine, thin needle into the cyst, and attempt to withdraw fluid. If clear fluid is extracted, the abnormality is most likely benign. All breast fluid should be sent for cytological analysis, but many breast specialists in major medical centers do not bother. They trust the clear fluid to be a firm indication of a benign condition. If fluid is bloody it is more suspicious and definitely requires a cytological lab analysis.

A lump that does not release fluid might be a solid fibroadenoma, a benign breast condition that is seen much less frequently than fibrocystic breast disease. A cancerous mass is also solid, but it often has a rigid configuration since it might contain calcium. A skillful physician who examines the breasts of all his patients can usually sense an abnormality when he touches a lump. Further examination of a suspicious mass might be conducted through mammography, ultrasound, or other technical methods described at the end of this chapter. These screenings of the breast will show whether an enlargement has no shadow, meaning that it is benign, or whether a shadow and a possibility of abnormality exist. If the latter is true, a doctor most likely will suggest that a woman undergo a biopsy of the lump. In the past, doctors were much more indiscriminate, and they would often biopsy all breast lumps they discovered.

Danocrine (danazol). Danocrine (danazol) is the first and only drug that has been FDA-approved and designated for the treatment of fibrocystic breast disease. This medication has provided the physician with an option in the fight against FBD. Surgery is no longer the only way to treat this condition. Already, since the release of Danocrine for the treatment of fibrocystic breast disease, and with the increased knowledge research has brought, the number of surgical excisions of fibrocystic breast lumps has declined.

The effectiveness of Danocrine as a cure for this condition was discovered coincidentally when studies of Danocrine as treatment for endometriosis were conducted (see chapter 7). It was found that women with endometriosis who were also suffering from fibrocysitic breast disease were relieved of their breast pain, tenderness, and cystic lumps while they were taking Danocrine. Remember, as explained in the "How Hormones Influence the Breast" section of this chapter, certain cell tissues of the breast are estrogen receptors; in metaphorical terms, they are like keyholes waiting to be fitted with their estrogen "keys." Estrogen activates these cell receptors, stimulating them to grow and form cysts. Danocrine, an antigonadotropic agent, blocks the production of estrogen so that this hormone no longer affects the breast. Without estrogen stimulation to the cell tissue, cysticness disappears.

Danocrine also inhibits the release of the brain hormones FSH and LH, which, therefore, are not present to stimulate ovulation. Without ovulation, a woman will not experience a menstrual flow and her estrogen and progesterone will no longer fluctuate. Pain and tenderness of fibrocystic breasts, which normally increase with the hormonal fluctuation of the menstrual cycle, will, with the absence of this hormonal fluctuation, not occur.

Thus, Danocrine works in the following ways: (1) it directly blocks the estrogen that might stimulate the cell tissue receptors in the breast; (2) it arrests the menstrual cycle; and (3) it maintains a steady estrogen/progesterone level too low to generate fibrocystic breast disease.

In all studies, Danocrine has been found to be 85 to 90 percent effective in eliminating the symptoms of fibrocystic breast disease. Pain and tenderness are usually the first to subside after the initiation of Danocrine treatment. Slowly, the cysticness—the benign breast lumps—disappears. Every woman with fibrocystic breast disease might undergo a three-to-six-month or longer Danocrine treatment. Women with moderate cases might be helped by two 100-mg tablets daily, or even two 50-mg tablets daily, if the condition is especially mild. Women who are suffering severely usually need two 200-mg tablets daily, one in the morning and one in the evening.

The side effects of Danocrine used in the treatment of fibrocystic breast disease are similar to the side effects encountered when the drug is used for pelvic endometriosis. However, since the dosage is only half or less than half that recommended for endometriosis, the side effects are much diminished. The main complaint about Danocrine is that a woman experiences an initial five-to-seven-pound weight gain. After three or four months, though, as a woman's body adapts to the drug, her weight levels off and pounds begin to drop. A decrease in salt intake might help to counterbalance the weight gain. Vitamin B-complex with at least 50 mg of vitamin B_6 daily, might also aid in countering some of the side effects of Danocrine.

Other side effects include a slight oiliness of the skin, a mild case of acne, and possibly vaginitis. Since Danocrine is a derivative of the male hormone testosterone, it has sometimes caused an appearance of facial hair on women who have taken the medication for endometriosis. In the doses prescribed for fibrocystic breast disease, however, the hair growth side effect is usually not a factor.

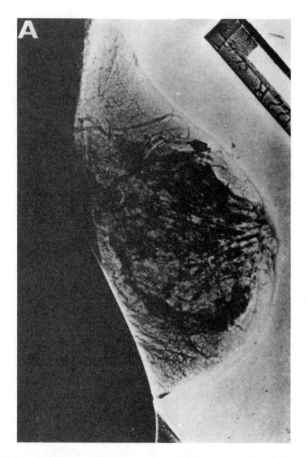

16-3 **Mammography of the Breast.** This special X ray of the breast shows a woman with fibrocystic breast disease before and after Danocrine treatment. In the left-hand X ray (A), a cyst is indicated by four arrows. The right-hand X ray (B), shows a mammogram of the same breast after Danocrine treatment. Note how the cyst in B, after six months of medication, has completely disappeared. There is also a slight reduction in breast size in response to the treatment; however, the breast will return to its normal size a few weeks after the course of medication has ended. *Reproduced by permission of Robert B. Greenblatt, M.D., Professor Emeritus, Medical College of Georgia, Augusta, Georgia.*

The cost of the drug does not change from treatment to treatment, unfortunately. Danocrine is a high-priced medication, but most women find that their health insurance policies cover at least 80 percent of the cost.

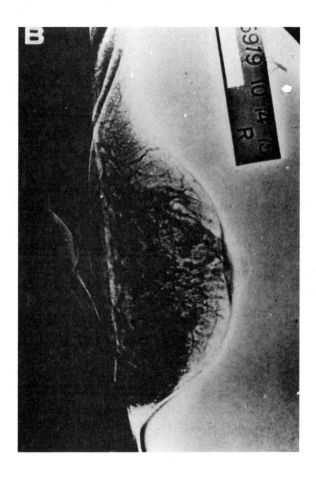

The Birth Control Pill. When a woman begins taking an oral contraceptive, even the low-dose pills with 35 micrograms of estrogen, she experiences an increase in breast size during the first few months. Afterward, her breasts will not enlarge because the pill will stabilize her estrogen/progesterone fluctuation. By eliminating the hormonal fluctuations of a normal menstrual cycle, the pill reduces the possibility of fibrocystic breast disease, which is why young women in their teens and twenties might be advised to take the pill for this condition. The pill, however, has serious side effects, which are discussed in chapter 12 (see pages 369 to 373).

Danocrine does not exhibit the side effects of oral contraceptives; most specifically, Danocrine does not cause blood clotting or the possibility of thrombophlebitis. No matter what their ages, women who have circulatory problems should be placed on Danocrine rather than on birth control pills. Women in their thirties and forties, the women who are usually faced with the most severe forms of fibrocystic breast disease, should never be on the pill anyway. For older women, Danocrine is the treatment of choice.

Vitamin E. There is some discrepancy in scientific opinion about whether vitamin E helps to eliminate fibrocystic breast disease. A Boston-based study concluded that women who took 400 mg or more of vitamin E daily for two to three months showed improvement in their fibrocystic breast conditions. Other studies have not revealed vitamin E to aid in the healing of fibrocystic breast disease, and in some instances, nodularity has even increased. What might be the definitive studies on vitamin E and its relation to fibrocystic breast disease are only now under way.

In the meantime, perimenopausal women seem to find relief from change-of-life symptoms with vitamin E. It might follow, then, that if a woman in her forties has fibrocystic breast disease, she might be making her "change" easier and her disease less severe if she takes vitamin E. Such a woman might take 400 to 800 mg of vitamin E every day for two or three months. If she sees no improvement in her condition, she need not continue the vitamin, but there is a chance that she might feel better in general.

Progesterone. At least three studies in France have shown that when 10 mg of a progesterone cream are applied to the outside of the breast, 5 mg penetrate to the breast tissue below the skin. The progesterone treatment, administered for about nine days a month for three months, gave 70 percent of the women in the studies relief from breast pain. The effectiveness of the progesterone treatment seems to come from the fact that it counteracts the excess estrogen. Practically speaking, the local application of progesterone cream, available at health food stores and specialty pharmacies, is easier and more convenient than intramuscular injections.

NOTE: It is important to mention that minor pain or tenderness in the breast can often be relieved by a comfortable support bra and aspirin, or aspirin-related compounds such as Midol. By restricting her fluid and salt intake about a week before her period, a woman can also reduce water retention and ease breast pain. However, she should use diuretics for this purpose only under a doctor's supervision.

Does Fibrocystic Breast Disease Lead to Cancer?

It has been reported that patients with fibrocystic breast disease have a 2.5 to 4 times greater chance of developing breast cancer than women who have never had fibrocystic breast conditions. There is considerable research being conducted into the true relationship between fibrocystic breast disease and cancer, but so far nothing definite has been established. It is difficult to find a single answer to the question "Does fibrocystic breast disease lead to cancer?" because there are so many histological types of FBD, meaning that various cell-and-tissue structures make up different forms of the disease. Were there only one kind of fibrocystic breast disease the answer would be easier to give.

Generally, if a woman's fibrocystic breast condition appears benign on physical examination and clear fluid can be aspirated, it is most likely benign. If a sonogram or mammogram (breast screenings that are explained at the end of this chapter) is obtained and either one indicates that the condition is benign, a woman need not worry about malignancy. A problem arises only if there is a suspicious mass on physical examination, if the mass cannot be aspirated, and if the mass is confirmed as being suspicious or abnormal on ultrasound or mammography. Then a biopsy should be performed.

If the pathological findings show a benign breast biopsy, a woman might have a slightly higher risk of developing breast cancer than a woman who has never had a fibrocystic breast disease. On one hand, the well-known breast specialist Dr. Susan Love and associates made a strong case that cystic breasts were not a prelude to breast cancer in their work done in the early 1980s. However, researchers have shown that the presence of breast cysts might increase the risk for breast cancer mostly when a woman has a family history of breast cancer and/or she has been diagnosed with atypia (precancerous breast cells).

The best conclusion that can be made about fibrocystic breast disease and cancer is that although women who have FBD seem subject to a slightly higher incidence of breast cancer, rarely does fibrocystic breast disease lead to cancer.

QUESTIONS ABOUT FIBROCYSTIC BREAST DISEASE AND OTHER BREAST PROBLEMS

How Can I Help My Daughter?

My daughter is twenty years old. Her breasts are not large, but she has to wear a bra day and night because her breasts are tender all of the time. She is taking a minimum amount of vitamins C and E, but they don't seem to be doing anything. As a mother I want to help her get well. Her doctor says her condition is due to a hormone imbalance and she has to live with it. Is there anything I can tell her that might give her more comfort than his advice that she "live with it"?

—N.V., Portland, Oregon

Breast size has nothing to do with the pain that can be associated with fibrocystic breast disease. As a cyst enlarges it pulls on the nerves and the breast begins to feel sore. The condition is probably due to a hormone imbalance, but Ms. V.'s daughter does not have to be resigned to a future of pain. There are steps she could take toward relief.

First, Ms. V.'s daughter should cut down her caffeine consumption. As explained in the "Caffeine and Fibrocystic Breast Disease" section of this chapter, a reduction of the methylxanthine chemicals, which are especially prevalent in caffeine, seems to help eliminate the disease. After cutting back on caffeine but continuing her vitamins, if Ms. V.'s daughter is still suffering, she might be placed on low-estrogen-containing birth control pills. The first few months on the pill her breasts will become large and tender, but a few months after that, she should definitely feel better on the medication.

If she cannot or does not want to take birth control pills, this young woman might be a perfect candidate for treatment with Danocrine (danazol). By taking 200 to 400 mg of Danocrine every day for three to six months, Ms. V.'s daughter might show definite signs of improvement.

After treatment, studies have shown, fibrocystic breast disease might recur. Not all women will experience a recurrence, but the ones who do will have cases less severe than their original conditions.

Can I Breast-Feed with Fibrocystic Breast Disease?

I am seven months pregnant and I'm worried. I want to do what's best for my baby by breast-feeding at least for the first six months after he or she is born. The problem is that I had cystic breasts before I got pregnant and I'm afraid that I might have trouble breast-feeding after childbirth. I keep imagining the cysts stopping the milk from coming out. Will I have to forgo breast-feeding my baby?

—H.C., Auke Bay, Alaska

Women who have fibrocystic changes can definitely breast-feed. They will have the same amount of milk as any other nursing mother. Indeed, it is expressly recommended that women with fibrocystic breast disease nurse their babies because they will then be using their breast tissues for their natural purposes. And by breast-feeding, a woman might possibly be gaining added protection against FBD.

Breast-feeding, however, might not affect the incidence of breast cancer. What research has shown is that timing of childbearing—having a child early in life, or at least before the age of thirty—might be important in decreasing the probability of breast cancer. Once a woman is over thirty, the arrival of subsequent children has statistically no importance in inhibiting breast cancer.

As for Ms. C., she need not be concerned that breast cysts will block her milk flow. She will have no trouble providing her baby with all the nourishment he or she requires.

What Is the Difference Between a Fibrocystic Mass and a Fibroadenoma?

For the last ten years I have been having operations to remove breast tumors. I had three removed from my right breast and four from my left breast. One time a surgeon told me that I had fibrocystic breast disease, but my own doctor has said that I have fibroadenomas. I have not been able to learn much about the difference between fibrocystic lumps and fibroadenomas and I would like to because I'm scheduled for another surgery. I really want to stop going into the hospital for these operations. Are there any alternate treatments for these diseases?
                                                    —E.B., Modesto, California

Ms. B. should get a definite diagnosis of her condition from a doctor she trusts. If she has fibrocystic breast disease, her lumps will be fluid-filled sacs that seem to appear overnight. They will hurt right away, and as they enlarge, the cystic lumps will become more painful. A doctor might aspirate her cysts, and if clear fluid is extracted he will know, without a doubt, that she has fibrocystic breast disease. If fluid is not aspirated, she might still have FBD, however. There are many occasions when a doctor cannot extract a clear liquid from an FBD cyst and he manually re-examines the density of the lumps. If no fluid is released and the lumps are very firm Ms. B. might have fibroadenomas.

With a fibroadenoma, a benign mass or lump of fibrous tissue forms. It might be as small as a pea or as large as an orange. Fibrous tissue is found throughout the body connecting muscle tissues. In fact, tendons are made of fibrous tissue. Fibrous tissue in the breast holds the breast in place. The formation of a fibroadenoma, a benign tumor of fibrous tissue, can occur from an unknown reason or possibly due to a hormone imbalance or from a blow to the breast. Fibroadenomas are firm, well-defined, painless lumps that are easy to move during self-examination. They grow very slowly. A doctor can often tell by the feel that a lump is a fibroadenoma. He might confirm his suspicions by asking a woman to undergo ultrasound or mammography.

Once diagnosed, fibrocystic breast disease might be treated with Danocrine medication as described earlier. But a fibroadenoma will not respond to this treatment. The only way a fibroadenoma can be eliminated is through surgery, which depends upon its size, location, and a woman's age.

Are There Any Vitamins I Could Take for Fibrocystic Breast Disease?

My doctor found a lump as big as an egg in my breast. When he aspirated it clear fluid came out and he told me I had a benign cyst. That was a few months ago. Since then he has found more cysts. He says he doesn't think they're anything to worry about, but he would like to do a biopsy. The last cyst he aspirated had no fluid in it. I am in my forties and just beginning to go through the change. I wonder if menopause could be a reason for my condition. Also, are there any vitamins I could take for cystic breasts? I would like to avoid surgery if I could.

—D.P., Cheyenne, Wyoming

This woman is in her forties, a time when fibrocystic breast disease increases due to the strong hormonal fluctuations that come from approaching menopause. After menopause, cystic lumps often disappear because a woman's estrogen level drops.

During this perimenopausal time, Ms. P., since she has been diagnosed as having fibrocystic breast disease, might be helped by vitamin E, 400 to 800 units daily. Vitamin B_6, 50 to 100 mg daily, might also help to ease the effects of her hormonal shifts. Her cysticness might also be reduced if she cuts down on caffeine (see chart, "Methylxanthine Content of Food and Drugs," on page 594).

If Ms. P. tries these approaches and still finds no relief, then she might agree to the biopsy. Given a normal biopsy result, she might be placed on Danocrine medication to lessen her cysticness and make her lumps easier to monitor. In many patients in whom there is no suspicion of cancer, Danocrine is recommended to make their conditions more manageable.

I've Tried Everything and My Cysts Still Don't Go Away

I am thirty-one years old and the mother of two children. Both my aunt and my mother had breast cancer, and I'm worried. I went to a breast surgeon about a year ago because I had a painful lump in my breast. He sent me for a mammogram and then scheduled me for surgery. After he removed the lump and had it analyzed, he told me that I had fibrocystic breasts. He gave me Demerol and Tylenol with codeine and a couple of painkillers. He said there was nothing else he could do for me. I went to another doctor, who aspirated my breast and told me to come back every six months for a checkup. I have pain in my breasts all the time. I've tried vitamin E, and I've cut out caffeine entirely. I only drink decaffeinated tea. I don't want to live on painkillers, but I don't know what else to do. The cysts don't go away and I'm afraid they might lead to cancer due to my family history. I feel like I've exhausted all possible cures, unless you can tell me something new.

—D.A., Sacramento, California

Until recently the medical establishment fairly ignored fibrocystic breast disease because there was no sanctioned treatment for the condition. Doctors would prescribe tranquilizers or painkillers and women would continue to suffer. Finally, now it is realized that women with fibrocystic change might be at slightly higher risk of breast cancer than other women. Doctors and women are beginning to pay attention to FBD.

Ms. A. is a young woman who has already given birth to two children. By bearing offspring when she was under thirty, Ms. A. has already reduced her risk of breast cancer. Studies have shown that women who have no children, or who postpone childbearing, have a higher-than-average incidence of breast cancer. If Ms. A. also keeps her weight down, she will be lowering her risk even further. An overweight woman produces excess estrogen in her fatty tissue, and an estrogen increase raises the possibility of breast lumps. The slimmer woman has less estrogen-producing tissue and less likelihood of promoting breast disorders.

Since it has clearly been established that Ms. A. has a benign breast condition, she is a good candidate for Danocrine, probably 400 mg every day for six months, maybe twelve months in her case. She should also cut down her salt intake and take extra vitamin B-complex during the treatment. Her cysts should melt away and make her breasts easier and less painful to examine.

With her family history, Ms. S. might also be a candidate for *tamoxifen* or *raloxifene,* two of a new class of drugs called SERMs (selective estrogen receptor modulators), which have been shown to lower the risk of breast cancer in healthy women who are in high-risk groups. Raloxifene's 76 percent protection has lately outdistanced tamoxifen's 50 percent.

How Can Danocrine Help If My Breast Lumps Are Really Cancer?

I had a biopsy for a lump in my breast and the doctor told me it was benign. I've heard that a new medication called Danocrine can make breast lumps disappear, but how can you be sure that the lumps aren't cancerous while you're taking the medicine? I only know about my lump because I had a biopsy.

—F.Q., Clifton, New Jersey

Breast cancer is a contraindication to Danocrine (danazol). Before prescribing Danocrine treatment a doctor should first exclude the possibility of breast cancer. If a doctor cannot aspirate a cyst and his sense of touch tells him that the lump is suspicious, he should recommend that a woman undergo either a mammography or thermography breast screening. If on these tests the lump still appears to be suspicious, he will probably need to perform a surgical biopsy during which he will remove the mass. Pathological lab analysis of the excised tissue will tell him whether or not the biopsy tissue is cancerous. If a condition is benign, Danocrine might be recommended.

There have been cases in which women who have had breast cancer have been placed on Danocrine. The medication lowered their estrogen levels and the disease did not spread during the time of treatment. Danocrine certainly did not cure the cancer, but because it blocked the estrogen receptors in the breast, it effectively halted the proliferation of cancerous cells. So if it is given before a doctor can accurately diagnose a lump, Danocrine might even be beneficial.

Is a Mastectomy the Cure for Fibrocystic Breast Disease?

I am thirty-two years old. I have fibrocystic breast disease for which I've had two mammograms that show no signs of cancer. There was one suspicious lump and the doctor did a biopsy, which proved completely benign. My breasts are full of cysts, though, and the doctor did not stop there. He kept saying that the masses were very large and just because one biopsy was negative, that didn't mean that every biopsy would be. I asked about the negative mammograms. Didn't they mean I didn't have cancer? He seemed doubtful and then said that doing a biopsy on one lump was like having a bunch of marbles. "Just because you pick up one white marble that doesn't mean that there isn't a black marble in there," he told me. When I questioned him about Danocrine treatment he said, "No way do we fool around with hormones. You need a mastectomy on both breasts." Remove both my breasts with no sign of malignancy? I was horrified. I talked to all my friends and they

convinced me to go to other doctors. Finally I found a physician
who treated me with Danocrine and the cysts have started to go
away. But I can't stop thinking about how I could have lost my
breasts. And how many women are getting mastectomies because
they think that surgery is the only way to cure fibrocystic breast
disease?

—B.H., Louisville, Kentucky

I have received numerous letters and phone calls from women
who have been told by surgeons that no treatment short of mastectomy could be recommended for fibrocystic breast disease. However,
several patients who were told they needed surgery were instead
placed on Danocrine by other physicians. These women improved so
dramatically that the thought of surgery would have been absurd.

If a biopsy shows a case of borderline malignancy, then Danocrine
might not have the desired effect on breast lumps. In such a case, a
woman might be advised to have a lumpectomy, but generally,
women should not be allowed to be frightened by knife-happy surgeons who want to remove their breasts. Danocrine is the FDA-
approved medication for the treatment of diagnosed fibrocystic
breast disease. Drug therapy should certainly come before surgery.

When Is a Breast Biopsy Necessary?

I've had two operations to have breast lumps removed and each
time, the lumps were benign. Now my doctor has found another
lump he wants to biopsy. I don't know why I have to go back into
the hospital again when the lumps are always benign. The
mammogram I had indicates that the lump is probably not cancer
but fibrocystic breast disease. How many times can a doctor make
you go for a biopsy?

—D.S., Saginaw, Michigan

A few years ago, when doctors were afraid that fibrocystic breast
disease might be cancerous, they performed biopsy after biopsy.

Sometimes a surgeon would only remove a small portion of the entire mass and after the operation a woman would still be suffering.

Now scientists have learned that fibrocystic breast disease does not necessarily lead to cancer, although the incidence of cancer is slightly higher for women who have this benign condition. Ms. S. has been diagnosed as having fibrocystic breast disease and she does not need additional biopsies. Naturally, if a new suspicious lump did develop, Ms. S. might be advised to have a mammogram. If her mammogram showed an abnormality, a breast biopsy would then be indicated.

With her present condition Ms. S. might benefit from treatment with Danocrine. Some patients stay on the medication for a year or longer, if a doctor is carefully supervising the treatment. Even if she has a recurrence of FBD after her treatment ends, the disease will return in a much milder form.

Considering the constancy of her condition, Ms. S. might also be monitored through ultrasound or one of the other noninvasive breast-screening methods described at the end of this chapter.

When Is a Mammogram Necessary?

I am sixty-four years old. Last year I had a mammogram and then a biopsy of a breast lump. The doctor told me that I have fibrocystic breast disease. He wants to do a mammogram at least once, maybe twice, a year. I do not want to subject myself to radiation, which I will if I have mammograms. Is it really necessary for me to have them?

—W.N., Omaha, Nebraska

The American Cancer Society recommends that a woman have an annual mammogram starting at age forty to establish the normal pattern of her breast. The permitted outer limit of radiation exposure during mammography is 300 millirads per film screen view, and four views are required. This seems high when you realize that a chest X ray exposes the lungs to only 7 millirads. Any risk of exposure to radiation, however, is greater among younger women whose more rapidly dividing cells are more sensitive than among women over forty. In Ms. N.'s age group, about age sixty-five, the lifetime risk of breast cancer mortality from annual mammogrraphy is 0.04, hardly a risk at all. Considering the number of breast cancers detected early, experts feel the benefits outweigh any risk.

When a woman goes for a yearly mammogram, she should ask the attending X-ray technician whether the lowest amount of radiation is being used (see pages 623 to 624). Modern types of mammography require only small amounts of radiation to be effective. A woman should only submit to a low-dose X ray.

My Breasts Are Leaking; Is There a Cure?

I'm twenty-seven years old and I've never been pregnant. I took the pill for four years, but I stopped three years ago. Since then I've lost weight and in the last year I've lost my period. Now I notice that both my breasts have started to leak. Fluid is coming out of them. Did the pill do this to me? Is there a cure?

—R.B., Key West, Florida

This woman has amenorrhea, an absence of menstrual flow, in combination with galactorrhea, leakage of milk from the breast. This dual problem is caused by an increased prolactin level. Prolactin is one of the pituitary hormones produced most heavily during pregnancy. Prolactin stimulates the milk glands so that they are ready to produce milk at the time of childbirth. When a baby sucks on a nipple the hormone activates the release of the breast milk.

Ms. B. is not pregnant, but somehow a signal from the hypothalamus in her brain has triggered the rise of prolactin. The reason for the brain signal and the sudden hormonal increase is unknown. The surge of prolactin is not caused by the birth control pill, but it might be the result of a formation of microadenomas in the pituitary. Whatever the cause, as prolactin overproduces it leads to milk secretion from the breast and it blocks the flow of FSH and LH hormones from the brain. With the brain hormones blocked, the menstrual cycle comes to a standstill. Women who suffer from amenorrhea/ galactorrhea will often be infertile, since they are not ovulating.

Parlodel (bromocriptine mesylate), a prolactin-inhibitor approved by the FDA, treats this condition. When taken in the amount of two to three tablets daily, Parlodel blocks prolactin production, stops the secretion of breast fluid, and restores fertility by reinstating ovulation. Ms. H. can most likely benefit from treatment with Parlodel. Also, new mothers who do not want to breast-feed their babies can be given Parlodel to block prolactin production and, in turn, the formation of breast milk. While taking Parlodel, new mothers who do not want to breast-feed will not suffer from breast engorgement.

Is Breast Augmentation Safe?

I am a thirty-two-year-old mother of two daughters. I am a healthy woman, but I think I would be much happier about my body if my breasts were just a little bigger. I have seen the pictures of breast implants that appear with magazine articles about breast augmentation. I think I would like to have the operation, but I want to find out if it's safe. Are there risks attached to breast augmentation? Can anything happen with the implants? I'd like to look more attractive, but I don't want to endanger my health.
—S.B., Shaker Heights, Ohio

Every woman and man should feel good about her or his own body. When kept in good physical condition, a woman's body can be a source of pride for her. I always feel that it is not a question of "what you have" but how you use what you have that is important. However, if a woman is extremely unhappy with a part of her anatomy that medical science has made it possible for her to change, then it is her choice to elect to do so.

With today's improved silicone implants and advanced surgical techniques, plastic surgeons are performing very successful, natural-looking breast augmentations. Modern silicone breast implants are soft and pliable. Since 1992 silicone breast implants have been under scrutiny. That's when reports began linking the implants with connective tissue disorders such as rheumatoid arthritis, scleroderma, skin rashes, and lupus. In 1999, after years of investigation, a large government study was unable to prove a link between the implants and the disorders.

On occasion, an area of breast tissue might be damaged during implantation. It is theorized that as this irritated breast tissue heals, it forms scars that feel like hard capsules around the implant. Doctors are not quite sure why this *encapsulation* of an implant occurs. Capsules might form on one breast implantation, but not another, when both breasts have received implants. Encapsulation might become evident on both breasts after implantation or capsules might never appear at all. The incidence of encapsulation is not known, but this possible aftereffect of implantation, although infrequent, probably happens more than plastic surgeons would like to discuss.

When capsules form, they constrict the implant, making it firm and unnatural. A plastic surgeon can often break the capsules manually in a "popping" procedure. He "pops" the scar tissue with his fingers. A woman can follow up this treatment by massaging her breasts to prevent a recurrence. Sometimes women undergo the popping procedure several times for emerging capsules.

When popping does not bring relief to a woman, a plastic surgeon will surgically remove her implant and perform a *capsulectomy,* removal of the scar tissue. If a new implant is to be inserted, it is important that there be no bleeding or irritation of the breast tissue so that capsules do not form again.

Many women who want breast augmentation are willing to risk the possibility of capsule formation since most of the time it does not happen. In several cases I know personally, breast augmentation has been a very positive move.

Recently, a patient of mine felt depressed about her femininity and decided to undergo breast augmentation after trying unsuccessfully for years to conceive a child. After her surgery she became very cheerful and she also became pregnant. Since the silicone implant had been placed underneath her own healthy breast tissue, she was even able to breast-feed.

A woman should not assume that breast augmentation will change her mental status, but if she is deeply disturbed about her physique, then she should be permitted to choose her own course of action.

I Have an Inverted Nipple; Do I Have Cancer?

I am a twenty-eight-year-old woman with an imperfect body. I have always had an inverted nipple on my right breast but my nipple on my left breast sticks out. When I am sexually aroused both nipples are erect, so I seem to be in working order. I never liked the fact that I don't have a matching pair of nipples under normal circumstances, but now I'm more concerned about my health than my appearance. I recently read that an inverted nipple could be a sign of breast cancer. Does that mean that I either have cancer now or am in danger of getting cancer soon?

—R.F., Mt. Kisco, New York

A woman might be born with an inverted nipple because the tissue inside her breast has not completely developed and shortened ligaments pull the nipple inward. When discovered at birth, inverted nipples do not mean cancer. However, if a woman suddenly realizes that her protruding nipple has begun to turn inward, she might be seeing a warning sign that something is wrong. A growth within her breast might be pulling in the nipple, and that growth might possibly be a cancerous tumor. When performing a breast self-examination a woman should always observe her breasts and nipples in a mirror to see whether there are any changes such as nipple position.

Ms. F. mentions that her nipples become erect when she is sexually aroused. She might try to stimulate her breast herself, particularly if she intends to become pregnant and to breast-feed after childbirth. By self-stimulating the nipple, she will be stretching the breast tissue and making her nipple more supple and extruded.

I Have a Family History of Breast Cancer; Does That Mean I'll Get It?

I am thirty-five years old. My sixty-five-year-old mother just had a mastectomy. Her two sisters, my aunts, also had mastectomies over the last five or six years, and now I'm beginning to worry about myself. With so many women in my family having had breast cancer, am I likely to get it when I get a little older?
—A.Y., South Bend, Indiana

Dr. Patricia Kelly, a research geneticist in the department of epidemiology and international health at the University of California, recently published her analysis of the genetic risk of breast cancer. According to Dr. Kelly's findings, the risk of breast cancer to a first-degree relative—a mother, sister, or daughter—of a woman who has breast cancer hinges on the age of the woman when she is diagnosed. The chance of a woman's getting breast cancer depends on whether her relative's breast cancer is diagnosed before or after menopause, whether the disease involves one or both breasts, and whether breast cancer has struck one or two generations in the family.

Dr. Kelly has reported that the risk of breast cancer to the first-degree relative of a woman who has been found to have cancer in *both breasts before menopause* increases to almost nine times the risk of a woman who has no family history of breast cancer. However, the first-degree relative of a woman who has discovered cancer in *one breast after menopause* is at only 1.2 times greater risk than a woman whose family is cancer-free.

So before a woman becomes too worried about getting breast cancer because someone in the family has had it, she should find out at what age the cancer was diagnosed. If the breast cancer was found after change-of-life, the chance of a relative's getting breast cancer is statistically not that great. However, variables are wide-ranging.

Even when breast cancer strikes two generations of the same family, the risk to relatives might fall anywhere from 15 to 50 percent, depending upon the age of the patients and the spread of their diseases. The women in families with genetically linked breast cancers often develop the disease in their twenties and thirties. These women often have mutations in genes that normally prevent the onset of breast cancer. A number of these genes have been identified. It is thought that the BRCA 1 gene might be responsible for 50 percent of hereditary breast cancers, or about 5 percent of all breast cancers. If Ms. Y. wants to have a blood test to find out whether she is carrying a mutated breast cancer gene, she should meet with a qualified genetic risk assessment counselor about the ramifications of the test beforehand. She might also learn that she might be helped by the drug tamoxifen for breast cancer prevention.

Dr. Kelly has also pointed out that the presence of other types of cancers in a family should be considered when the risk of developing breast cancer is being calculated. Breast cancer is associated with the presence of ovarian cancer, brain tumors, sarcoma, leukemia, and gastrointestinal cancer. When a woman is a first-degree relative in a family where someone has breast cancer and others have associated cancers, her lifetime risk of developing tumors is perhaps as high as 50 percent.

Considering all the variables to risk that Dr. Kelly delineates, it is impossible to tell Ms. Y. exactly what her chance of getting breast cancer might be. She does not state the ages of her aunts and whether their cancers were in one breast or both breasts. Ms. Y. can certainly improve her odds, no matter what they are, by keeping her weight down, reducing her stress, and taking vitamins B, C, and A and zinc daily. Vitamin A is especially good since it stimulates the effectiveness of the immune system, which can become depleted during stressful situations.

It has been found that during their divorces, women have higher incidences of breast cancer. Stress produces steroids, which inhibit the functioning of the immune system, and once the immune system weakens, cancerous cells increase. While a woman is taking vitamin A to bolster her immune responses, she should also eat a balanced diet and alleviate her stress through exercise or other relaxing activities.

Since stress might be a controllable factor in the fight against breast cancer, Ms. Y.—and every concerned woman—might try to recognize a tension-producing situation and use the force of will-power to maintain a good emotional balance. If willpower does not work, she might use stress-relieving techniques such as exercise, yoga, or meditation.

Does DES Cause Breast Cancer?

I took DES when I was pregnant with my daughter, who is now thirty-two. She has had no problems so far, but we are not taking any chances. She goes for regular checkups with a very fine gynecologist. At first I was worried that she would develop cervical cancer, but lately I hear that she might be at high risk for breast cancer. Is this true?

—D.R., San Bernardino, California

Synthetic estrogen drugs called DES, for diethylstilbestrol, were taken by millions of pregnant women between 1938 and 1971 to prevent miscarriage. When a number of DES daughters developed a rare vaginal cancer called clear cell carcinoma, DES drew the attention of researchers. Today we know that the frequency of this cancer is low, about 1 in 1,000 DES daughters. As for breast cancer, DES daughters have not been shown to be at higher risk. Studies in the mid-1980s suggested that the women who took DES during pregnancy might have increased their risk at that time, but not since then.

The main problem facing Ms. R.'s daughter, as well as other DES daughters, is a risk of developing vaginal/cervical adenosis, a condition in which the outer portion of the cervix is not completely covered with its normal skin layer and appears denuded. A cervical or vaginal sore associated with adenosis might erupt on the abnormal skin surface and cause staining or bleeding during sex or with the use of the diaphragm.

DES daughters should be examined by a gynecologist twice a year and have a Pap smear taken each time. If during an internal examination a doctor finds any lumps or hard masses on the cervix, a colposcopy, an examination with a colposcope, a viewing instrument like a short telescope that magnifies the upper portion of the vagina and the cervix, must be performed and the suspected area biopsied. An increased risk of cervical cancer from exposure to DES has not been firmly established, however.

Most recent data indicate that there are DES-related reproductive problems. A DES daughter might have trouble conceiving, and when she becomes pregnant, she might have difficulty carrying to term. Also, these problems might be with her during all her fertile years. It might take as long as one year for a DES daughter to conceive. Once pregnant, she will be at high risk for miscarriage. Still, these facts should not discourage her. Most DES daughters do eventually conceive and become the mothers of healthy children. With this problem of fertility, though, a DES daughter who wants children might be well-advised to attempt conception earlier than a woman who has not been exposed to the drug.

Breast Cancer Can Hurt

I had a lump in my breast and pain. My doctor sent me for a mammogram and I was told I had fibrocystic breasts. I was only twenty-eight years old and not at high risk for breast cancer. A few months later I went for my yearly physical and the doctor sent me to a breast surgeon. I went into the hospital for a biopsy and to make a long story short, I had a modified radical mastectomy. Most of the health books and articles I have read have said that breast cancer doesn't hurt. Well, maybe most breast cancers don't hurt, but mine did. Doctors should not automatically think a woman has a non-cancerous condition if the lump in her breast is painful. Other women in my mastectomy support group say that their cancers hurt too.
—V.E., Tulsa, Oklahoma

Fibrocystic changes are characterized by lumpy, tender, and painful breasts. If the cysticness is dense, a doctor might recommend that a woman have a mammogram or other type of breast screening for cancer. It is unfortunate that Ms. E.'s mammogram did not detect the presence of her breast cancer. Perhaps her doctor was thrown off the track by the fact that she was experiencing pain. Generally, since cancer is slow-growing, it does not pull on nerves and is not painful. That is why cancer is such an insidious disease.

Ms. E.'s experience is extremely important for other women to consider. She might have had both fibrocystic breasts and cancer at the same time. Perhaps she had a rare cancerous lump that hurt. At any rate, her letter is a reminder that no lump, painful or painless, should be ignored. Every breast abnormality deserves a doctor's scrutiny.

Is a Mastectomy Always Necessary?

I have a fear of examining my breasts because I'm afraid if I find a lump I'll have to have my breast removed. How often is mastectomy necessary? Why can't all women have lumpectomies?
                                            —M.S., Sully, Iowa

The most profound recent discovery about surgery for breast cancer is that lumpectomy plus radiation—removal of a malignant tumor and some surrounding tissue, followed by radiation therapy to kill any remaining cancerous cells—is as good as mastectomy for treatment of early (stages 1 and 2) breast cancer. (Detailed descriptions of all the latest surgeries for breast cancer can be found in *The Complete Book of Breast Care*, by Niels H. Lauersen, M.D., Ph.D., and Eileen Stukane, published by Fawcett Columbine/Ballantine, 1998.) It is my hope that this good news about the effectiveness of lumpectomy will encourage more breast self-examination and early detection, because now, the sooner a breast cancer is discovered, the more likely it can be treated by lumpectomy.

A study of nearly 18,000 women treated for early stage breast cancer in 1994, however, found that more than half of those eligible for lumpectomy underwent mastectomy; it has become apparent that many doctors are not following national guidelines for treatment of breast cancer. National guidelines state that doctors should not use age, prognosis, or tumor type as criteria in choosing mastectomy over breast-conserving lumpectomy. If a doctor advises Ms. S. or any woman who has discovered a lump in her breast that she needs a mastectomy, she must ask "Why?" and seek a second opinion.

Could I Have Breast Reconstruction After My Mastectomy?

I had a modified radical mastectomy a year ago. My lymph modes were negative and my doctor gives me a 95 percent cure rate. He has suggested a breast reconstruction, but I feel dubious about more surgery. I guess I'd like you to give me a second opinion.
—A.L., Larchmont, New York

More than half of the women who are diagnosed with breast cancer undergo mastectomies, and statistics show that most of them have their breasts reconstructed afterward. About 38 percent of reconstructive surgeons are even offering the option of immediate reconstruction, at the time of mastectomy. (See *The Complete Book of Breast Care* by Niels H. Lauersen, M.D., Ph.D., and Eileen Stukane, for explanations of all the breast reconstruction techniques.) A breast can be reconstructed with either a saline (or the more controversial silicone gel) implant or with the body's own tissue, a portion called a "flap," from the back, abdomen, or buttocks.

Ms. L. appears to be in good physical shape for the reconstructive surgery. If she feels that a reconstruction would help her psychologically, would aid in her postmastectomy adjustment, and would benefit her relationship with her sexual partner, then she ought to start interviewing reconstructive surgeons. Breast reconstruction is more complicated than cosmetic surgery, and I would advise that Ms. L.

meet with at least three reconstructive surgeons to learn what experience each has with implants, natural tissue reconstruction, and microsurgery, for example, before choosing the surgeon who is right for her. For state-of-the-art technique, a woman's best bet is a university or teaching hospital.

A breast reconstruction can leave a woman with or without a nipple. The nipple/areola reconstruction is a second procedure that takes place months after the initial reconstructive surgery to allow the breast's swelling to subside. A skin flap for a reconstructed nipple is generally taken from the center of the breast. The areola might be a tattoo or a skin graft taken from the inner thigh crease.

I Wish I Had Been More Assertive

I have heard you tell women to ask their doctors to examine their breasts during checkups. I am a thirty-five-year-old woman who didn't do what you said. My doctor did not examine my breasts, but I was too timid to say anything. I also never examined my own breasts because, frankly, I was afraid I'd find something. Finally, on his own, my doctor examined my breasts when I went for a Pap smear. He found a large tumor and I had to have a mastectomy. I wish I had been more assertive in previous years. Maybe he could have found the tumor when it was still a tiny lump. Maybe I wouldn't have lost my breast. I just want to encourage other women to be demanding when it comes to their bodies, to be sure they always receive thorough checkups.

—M.J., Detroit, Michigan

It is essential that every woman participate in her own health care. A gynecologist should examine his patient's breasts while she is lying down on the examining table and when she is sitting upright. A woman should ask her doctor to examine her in this fashion if she notices that he might be skipping that part of the checkup. Also, a woman should be taught how to do a self-examination by the doctor or his nurse.

If Ms. J. had discovered her cancer at an earlier stage she might have been a candidate for treatment other than mastectomy. As it is, *her story is a* message *to all women to involve themselves in preventive medicine.*

Thank You for Caring

Thank you for caring enough to send me a letter regarding Danocrine treatment for fibrocystic breasts. I did change physicians. My new doctor has altered my diet as you suggested and he is hoping this change might have an effect on my breasts before he starts prescribing Danocrine. At least I've found a doctor who seems to be knowledgeable about diseases of the breast. Thank you again for your guidance.

—E.F., Marblehead, Massachusetts

It is gratifying to help women educate themselves to the options they have in relation to their health care. With combined efforts of doctors and their patients, with a shared understanding about the serious problems of the breast, we might, together, be able to treat fibrocystic changes and reduce breast cancer the way we, together, have lowered the rate of cervical cancer.

MODERN BREAST-SCREENING METHODS

Mammography

A woman has a mammogram (an X ray of her breasts) to diagnose a symptom, such as a newly discovered lump in her breast, to screen her breasts because she has a family history of breast cancer, or because she is age forty or over and is having a routine checkup. The American Cancer Society recommends that women begin having annual mammograms at age forty. Mammography screenings could begin before age forty if a woman has a first-degree relative, a mother or a sister, who had breast cancer before menopause. In that case, the rule of thumb is to take the age your mother was when she was diagnosed, subtract ten years, and the end result would be the age at which you should start having mammograms. Radiologists usually do not begin screening women younger than twenty-five years old, however.

Studies show that for women in their forties, having regular mammograms reduces their chance of dying from breast cancer by about 17 percent. Women age fifty or older who undergo mammographic screenings are 30 percent less likely to die of breast cancer. The average-size breast lump detected by a woman doing breast self-examination is one to two centimeters. A mammogram can detect a lump that is tiny, about half a centimeter, and finding a small breast lump improves a woman's chance of having breast-sparing surgery if the lump is malignant.

The best mammogram uses the high-resolution, low-dose film screen technique. (It must be remembered, however, that even with the most up-to-date technology and the most skilled technicians and radiologists, experts estimate that 10 to 15 percent of cancers are missed.) The permitted outer limit of radiation exposure during mammography is 300 millirads per film screen view—and an accurate mammography screening requires four views, two of each breast. Before undergoing a mammogram, a woman should always ask the hospital, X-ray, or mammography center whether it is using dedicated mammographic equipment with radiation exposure limited to 300 millirads. To be sure you are getting a high-quality mammogram, select a mammography facility accredited by the American College of Radiology (ACR) and the U.S. Food and Drug Administration, which began a joint program of accreditation in October 1994. At a top-notch facility, you should have no trouble finding an ACR certificate of accreditation and an FDA placard.

Mammography and Exposure to Radiation. Although 300 millirads per view is the outer limit of radiation exposure to the breast during mammography, FDA research shows that the average dose to the average female breast is more likely to be 150 millirads (a woman with large, dense breasts might require a higher level of radiation for an accurate image). By way of comparison, a chest X ray exposes the lungs to an average dose of 7 millirads of radiation. Still, most experts are not troubled by mammographic radiation; one frequently used example is that the risk of getting breast cancer from having a mammogram is about equal to the risk of getting lung cancer from smoking three cigarettes. It is felt that the benefits of 160 in 10,000 women between ages forty and fifty having their breast cancers detected early outweigh the risk that a breast cancer will arise from radiation exposure. Research presented in our book *The Complete Book of Breast Care* (Fawcett Columbine/Ballantine) shows that when a woman begins annual mammography screening at age forty and lives to age seventy-five, the estimated risk is that 13.8 out of 100,000 women might increase their risk of breast cancer mortality.

Tips for Getting the Best Mammogram. A complete breast checkup includes a breast examination by a doctor along with a mammogram. To obtain the best possible mammographic image, a woman should:

- Keep her breasts and underarm areas free from flecks of talc or antiperspirant, which can cause a misreading of a mammography image.
- Avoid breast tattoos that can shade a mammogram.
- Advise the radiologist about a breast implant or any other surgical procedure on her breast.
- Schedule her mammography screening during the first ten days of her menstrual cycle, when she is least likely to be pregnant and her breasts are less full and less tender. This timing is especially important for women in their forties, who have denser breast tissue than older women. For these younger women, studies have shown greater accuracy in mammographic readings if a screening is done in the first half of the menstrual month.

- Hold her breath and remain perfectly still; any motion can blur the image.

Thermography, Mammography's Potential Helper

Thermography's biggest asset is that it does not require radiation. The thermography technique for detecting breast cancer is based upon the visualization of heat patterns in the breast. By capturing infrared rays, different kinds of thermographic apparatus provide either black-and-white or color heat surface pictures.

In 1956, it was discovered that the skin temperature over a breast cancer was higher than over the rest of the breast. Normally the breasts are quite cool. A typical thermogram will show a pair of breasts with similar, although not identical, vascular markings. In a comparison of both breasts, the configuration caused by heat patterns will not be drastically different. However, when a thermogram is abnormal, the heat patterns of the breasts are asymmetrical. An area of excess heat causes divergent patterns to appear on two breasts that should be an almost matching pair.

The excess heat that shows up on a thermogram could be caused by a breast cancer that brings blood and, therefore, heat to the afflicted area. However, other conditions such as infection or cysticness also draw more blood and heat to an area. Research over the years has not shown thermography to have a high rate of accuracy. At times cancers do not release sufficient heat, or they are buried in breast tissue where their temperatures cannot be detected. Thermography is sometimes used in Europe as an aid in determining the aggressiveness of breast cancer; perhaps it will find a place in the United States as an aid to mammography. It is no longer in use as a sole breast-screening method, although French researchers once created a classification system for thermography readings.

In fact, Dr. Michel Gautherie, director of research at the French National Institute for Health and Medical Research in Paris, headed a French study in which approximately 58,000 women, most of whom had breast complaints, were examined. Of those 58,000, a group of 1,245 women were diagnosed as being normal or having benign disease by several methods—clinical examination, mammography, ultrasonography, fine-needle aspiration, or—when indicated—biopsy. In spite of the findings of their initial examinations, these

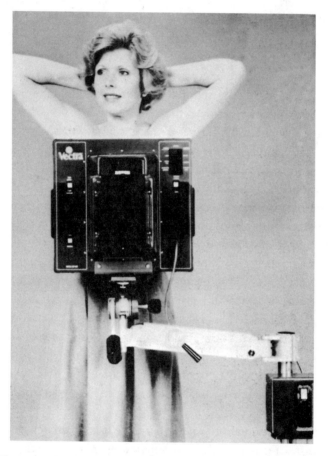

16-4 **Thermography.** Breast screening by thermography utilizes temperature changes in the breast to reveal breast conditions. In the photo, a woman demonstrating the Vectra technique stands behind thermographic apparatus. As explained in the text, configurations that indicate vascular patterns appear in color on the screen. No radiation is used in thermography and the breast is not sandwiched between metal plates as it is during mammography. *Reproduced by permission of Vectra Corporation, Miamisburg, Ohio.*

women were also screened by thermography and labeled as Th III by the French researchers, which meant that the women fell into the stage-three classification of thermogram readings.

The thermogram readings were divided into five classifications from Th I to Th V, according to the increased likelihood of cancer. Following the way the Pap smear readings are rated, thermogram readings in the first stage would be normal whereas the fifth stage would indicate abnormality. Th III would be questionable. The thermal signs might be suspicious but inconclusive. Of the 1,245 women in this TH III group, more than one third had confirmed cancers within five years. Thanks to their thermograms they could be carefully observed for the onset of the disease.

Diaphanography (DPG) or Transillumination, Another Aid to Mammography

Diaphanography, or transillumination of the breast, is another breast-screening aid that can detect abnormalities without exposing a woman to X-ray radiation. Basically, light transmitted through the breast tissue illuminates various pathological conditions, much in the way the beam of a flashlight seems to shine through one's hand in the dark.

Transillumination was first described in 1929 by Dr. M. Cutler, who found that there was a definite difference in the way normal breast tissue and pathological breast tissue could be illuminated. Dr. Cutler cautioned that overilluminating small solid tumors might make them undetectable. He warned doctors to reduce the intensity of the light they used for diaphanography.

After Dr. Cutler's findings became known, research was undertaken to find out more about the method of transillumination. Somehow, the research died in the forties and fifties, but in the sixties Dr. Charles Gros built a diaphana machine to test the transillumination method. Overillumination, the problem Dr. Cutler described, was only one of the difficulties Dr. Gros encountered. The diaphana did not succeed in promoting transillumination. Finally, the method became improved in 1976 in Sweden, where it succeeded under weak light conditions in a totally darkened room.

Ordinary low-intensity light visualizes the contents of the breast and the transilluminated organ is photographically captured on infrared film or is analyzed by a sensitive video-electronic system (closed-circuit TV with a precision color camera). One of the most evident features of breast cancer is that protein increases relative to the other breast components, fat and connective tissue. Concentrated protein absorbs the weak light and reveals breast changes. At the end of a screening, whether or not abnormalities have been viewed, a permanent picture of the transilluminated breast is always obtained.

Since 1976, when diaphanography began being used clinically, several cases of cancer that went undiscovered during other breast-screening procedures were detected through transillumination. In one study, fourteen out of sixty-two cases that were negative on

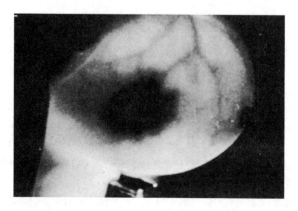

16-5 **Diaphanography or Transillumination.** Diaphanography or transillumination is another breast-screening method that does not require radiation. This promising type of screening is actually a way of scanning the breast with light waves. The transmission of light through breast tissue clearly reveals any abnormal breast mass. The mass in the photo was not found during clinical examination but it was easily detected with the transillumination technique. There are now several centers that routinely screen women's breasts by transillumination. *Reproduced by permission of E. N. Carlsen, M.D., San Bernardino, California.*

mammography were positive on diaphanography. Thus, this technique seemed very promising as a method of picking up early abnormalities, but these promises were unfulfilled.

In 1992, after studies from the National Institutes of Health (NIH) and Swedish researchers showed that transillumination was no more effective than manual breast examinations in detecting breast cancer, the FDA notified manufacturers that transillumination devices could not be marketed for primary breast screenings; however, some doctors still use transillumination as a helpful aid to other breast screenings of dense breasts and breasts that have implants.

Ultrasonographic Breast Examinations

Ultrasonography uses high-pitched sound waves to produce a picture of the internal structure of a woman's breasts. The image is much like a picture from an X ray. So far, there are no known harmful effects from ultrasonography, which is also used as a diagnostic tool during pregnancy.

A sonographer places gel on the skin of a woman's breast and uses a transducer, a device much like a microphone, to touch the skin. As the sonographer moves the transducer over a woman's breast, sound wave patterns, or echoes, are transmitted. These sound waves display the internal image of the breast on a screen. Today's ultrasound technology allows a woman to be evaluated by high-definition imaging (HDI), which has a sound beam that penetrates the breast more deeply. This increased depth gives a much more complete picture of a breast.

Most often ultrasound is used to determine whether a suspicious area on a mammogram is a solid tumor or a fluid-filled cyst. The ultrasound image helps a doctor guide a needle into the area for a biopsy or for the draining of a cyst. With improved ultrasound, however, some doctors are now recommending its use for women with very dense breasts that are difficult to screen with mammography and for young women (under age thirty-five) with a family

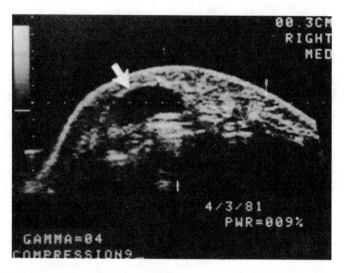

16-6 **Ultrasonsgraphy of the Breast.** This photo was obtained through a computerized ultrasonographic breast screening. During ultrasonography, high-pitched sound waves reproduce the internal structure of the breast. No radiation is required. In the photo, a fluid-filled benign cyst is indicated by the arrow. An X ray would have revealed a mass, but unlike ultrasonography, the X ray method would not have been able to differentiate between a solid mass and a cyst. *Reproduced by permission of S. N. Friedman, M.D., and J. L. Baldassare, M.D., New York, New York.*

history of breast cancer. Research among 16,000 women showed that for those women with the densest breasts, mammography detected 55 percent of breast cancers, but when mammography was combined with ultrasound, the detection rate reached 93 percent.

Mammography still remains the gold standard for detection of breast cancer, but ultrasound should be a recommended accompaniment when a woman's mammogram or manual breast examination is suspicious or unclear. At the same time, if an ultrasound screening is the only one performed when a mass is found, a woman should have a mammogram. Ultrasound readings rely on the interpretive skill of the sonographer using the equipment, however, and many sonographers are still absorbing the changes that have come with rapid advancements in technology. A woman should ask her doctor for his referral to a competent sonographer.

COMING SOON: A SHARPER IMAGE

Digital Mammography

Computer-assisted mammography, called digital mammography, is slowly becoming an option for breast screenings. A digital mammogram has no film screen or developed picture. A woman still undergoes a mammogram with a traditional X-ray detector, but her breast image travels to a computer and is enhanced on a video display terminal, which means that the radiologist can adjust the image electronically, zero in on a special area of the breast, heighten contrast, magnify, reduce the image, and locate the tiniest lesions. Digital mammography is especially helpful for picturing and evaluating dense breasts, and since the image is in a computer, it can be transmitted to doctors who are miles away for consultation. The FDA has recently approved a computer system M1000 Image Checker, made by R2 Technology Inc., Los Altos, California, which increased cancer detection from about 80 out of 100 cancers to about 88 out of 100. A drawback to digital mammography is that the computerized systems are four times more expensive than traditional mammography units.

MRI (Magnetic Resonance Imaging)

In addition to ultrasound, another way for a woman to get an inside look at her breasts without exposing herself to radiation is with MRI (magnetic resonance imaging). Hydrogen is naturally present in the water within our bodies. An MRI machine contains a magnet that stirs up the hydrogen molecules. A technologist transmits a sequence of radio waves into the magnet, which is outfitted with a special receiver coil that relays information on agitated tissues to a computer. A calculation of the time it takes molecules to return to normal distinguishes cancerous from healthy tissue. Sometimes a dye is injected into a woman's body to enhance a reading of tumor tissue. Because both the dye and the fatty tissue in the breast are bright, however, it takes a skilled MRI expert to spot trouble.

MRIs have been most helpful in screening women with silicone breast implants for signs of breast cancer or silicone leakage. The high density of the silicone obscures an estimated 22 to 83 percent of breast tissue from mammogram—but not from an MRI.

Recently, Dr. Steven E. Harms, director of magnetic resonance imaging at Baylor University Medical Center, devised a technique called three-dimensional RODEO (rotating delivery of excitation off-resonance) MRI, which he reports has twenty times better resolution of images than standard MRI. Ductal carcinoma in situ (DCIS) and lobular carcinoma in situ (LCIS), two types of breast cancer that are difficult to diagnose, had much higher rates of detection with Dr. Harms's technique. For example, with this new approach, the extent of DCIS was accurately predicted 95 percent of the time as compared with mammography's 65 percent.

PET (Positron Emission Tomography)

Research continues into PET scan tomograms, also known as nuclear breast screening. A woman is injected with a radioisotope that releases a nuclear substance called a positron. Concentrations of this isotope are taken up by cells of the breast and form "hot spots." A rapid sequence of film creates image "slices" or tomograms, which, when put together, produce a complete picture of a breast. By looking at the hot spots of a PET scan, a radiologist can find minute cancer growth and the spread of cancer in the lymph nodes, as well as get a good view of dense breasts. Sometimes false-positive results occur with a PET scan, because it can be difficult to distinguish between infections and cancer. The PET scan involves exposure to radiation, but its precision makes it worthy of continued research.

ASK ABOUT THE LATEST TESTS

Mammography remains the gold standard of breast-screening methods, the only accepted screening method in medicine. Other techniques such as ultrasound and MRI are currently used in conjunction with mammography, not alone. Still, researchers are refining breast tests all the time, and a woman should ask her doctor about whether any new, effective, safe test is available to her. Right now, screening for breast cancer involves a team: a woman who performs monthly breast self-examination, a competent mammographer, and a responsible health care practitioner—gynecologist, nurse practitioner, internist, or family practitioner—who examines a woman's breasts every year as part of her routine medical checkup.

17.

Unnecessary Surgery—
When to Get a Second Opinion

HOW A CAUSE OF CONCERN WAS BORN

A certain uneasiness about the readiness of doctors to operate began to be felt among Americans during the early seventies. The federal government stepped in and a congressional subcommittee reported that 2.4 million unnecessary operations were performed in 1974. These surgeries cost $4 billion and approximately 12,000 lives; or, more precisely, 5 percent of the quarter of a million deaths following or during surgery in 1974 could be attributed to unnecessary operations.

These figures were alarming, and the American Medical Association fought back. Unnecessary surgery was practically nonexistent, declared the powerful medical organization. The congressional subcommittee heeded this opposition and reinvestigated the issue. But three years after its 1974 report the subcommittee found that time had hardly changed its original estimates. Rather than 2.4 million unnecessary operations, the subcommittee calculated 2 million, a reduction so slight it was barely significant. The AMA notwithstanding, Americans were "going under the knife" more than they should for tonsillectomies, appendectomies, hysterectomies, gallbladder operations, coronary bypass surgeries, prostate removals, and even hernia repairs. Today, thanks to health care reforms enacted over the years, second opinions are routine, patients are skeptical, and operations such as appendectomies and tonsillectomies, which were once considered commonplace, are not. *What has not changed dramatically, however, are invasions of the uterus. Hysterectomy is running second to cesarean section as the most common surgical procedure in the United States.* What is going on? . . .

Approximately 80 percent of all surgery performed in the United States is considered "elective," not a life-or-death matter. A woman or a man elects to have an operation after learning that a particular surgery will improve her or his health, but the operation might not be needed to correct a life-threatening situation. Of course, this decision to have an operation is based upon what a doctor advises, and sometimes something besides his patient's health might be influencing a physician. He might have the chance to do surgery that adds to his prestige or that provides him with an opportunity to teach medical students. Personal motives might lead him into performing an *elective but unnecessary* operation. And do not forget, surgery also puts money into a doctor's pocket.

"Unnecessary surgery" might mean that a man has a coronary bypass when he could have been treated with medication or a woman allows her ovaries to be removed because a doctor convinces her that she will be preventing ovarian cancer. Physicians tend to recommend the operations that are currently "in fashion." Years ago, tonsils and adenoids, as soon as they became slightly enlarged, were removed. The appendix was considered a useless organ that could be casually cut out. For example, a doctor who was removing an ovarian cyst could often excise a woman's appendix at the same time because the appendix was "just there," next to his knife. Today, the tonsils, adenoids, and appendix are known to produce immune antibodies that fend off disease, and they are far from readily removed. Since the realization of the importance of these organs, the number of tonsillectomies and appendectomies has markedly dropped; these operations are no longer "stylish."

It was the federal government's 1974 report on unnecessary surgery that placed tonsillectomies, appendectomies, and so many other types of common operations under scrutiny. People became so much more aware of the rise in surgical procedures that they questioned their doctors. Today, even the circumcision of a baby boy—another operation that used to be considered routine—is the subject of controversy. But where is the concern about gynecological procedures?

Hysterectomies, D & Cs, laparoscopies, uterine suspensions, cone biopsies, and cesarean sections abound. The proliferation of these gynecological operations must be curtailed. Before agreeing to any of these procedures, in order to protect herself from unnecessary surgery, a woman should *always* seek a second opinion—even, if possible, in the case of a C-section.

HOW TO STOP UNNECESSARY SURGERY—
THE VALUABLE SECOND OPINION

Recently a woman arrived at my office for a second opinion. She was suffering from severe cramps and heavy bleeding. Her doctor had diagnosed her condition as "nerves" and had prescribed tranquilizers. When her symptoms worsened, he told her that obviously the only way to relieve the pain would be through hysterectomy. The woman was only thirty-four years old and she did not want to lose her uterus. She and her husband had just reached the stage in their marriage where they were ready to start a family. After I examined her, I realized that her condition could be controlled with hormone therapy. Today she is in good health with all her organs and is the proud mother of a baby girl.

If this patient had not been informed enough to realize that a second opinion was necessary, if she had not thought that her doctor's recommendation was a strange way to cure her condition, she might easily have become another surgical statistic. Many women have told me similar stories of how they have been saved from the knife by a second opinion.

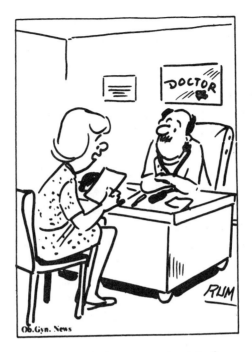

"You call this a second opinion?
Why, it's no better than the first."

17-1 Reproduced by permission of the artist, Francis H. Brummer (RUM), and Ob. Gyn. News,
Rockville, Maryland.

One of the most significant studies to back up the practice of second opinions was conducted years ago by Dr. Eugene G. McCarthy of Cornell University Medical College in New York. He found that 34 percent of 3,171 patients who were told they needed surgery voluntarily sought a second opinion and learned that they did not need operations. Dr. McCarthy also studied a second group in which 17 percent of the patients who went for mandatory second opinions were advised against surgery. For the next three years, Dr. McCarthy followed the study patients who did not have surgery on the advice of second-opinion doctors. Only a small percentage of these patients subsequently needed operations.

When the findings of the McCarthy study and other investigations became known, many insurance companies started second-opinion programs to spare their policyholders from unnecessary trauma and unnecessary death, and also to save company money. In another study of 6,000 New York, New Jersey, and Connecticut union members with mandatory second-opinion health insurance, roughly 20 percent were told they did not need surgery by their second-opinion doctors.

Second-opinion doctors are important adjuncts to initially consulted physicians. Surgeries, particularly hysterectomies, mean money to private physicians. Also, an operation provides training for interns and residents. And, of course, one must not forget that much unnecessary surgery is performed because a certain percentage of physicians are incapable of practicing medicine properly. The Federation of State Medical Boards once estimated that at least 5 percent of the country's medical practitioners were not conscientious or lack competence. A physician might be practicing while he is ill, while he is addicted to drugs or alcohol, or without the latest knowledge of modern surgical procedures.

However, there are many fine surgeons who perform surgery only when it is needed. Unfortunately, with all the publicity about the extensiveness of unnecessary surgery, good doctors are also suspected of bad performance, of undertaking unneeded operations. These competent physicians ignore any accusation, continue to consider the interests of their patients, and become examples for others to follow.

I personally see a great number of women for second opinions, and I'm amazed and confused by the fact that many of them seem more inclined to believe bad, rather than good, news. If I tell a woman that, in my opinion, she does not need the surgery that she initially was told was necessary, she is likely to look at me in disbelief, leave my office, and return to her original doctor. Many women feel that they surely must be sick if their first doctors told them that they needed operations. Why do people want to believe the worst?

Even the Massachusetts study from the *New England Journal of Medicine* points out that patients who received second opinions against surgery sought third-opinion doctors who concurred with the original physicians.

In many cases of unnecessary surgery, especially gynecological procedures, the psychological damage to patients is often more overwhelming than the physical damage. A woman must educate herself to the procedure that is being recommended to her. Hysterectomies, D & Cs, laparoscopies, uterine suspensions, cone biopsies, and cesarean sections haunt many women who have written the letters in this chapter. The ramifications of these operations, as the letters and answers reveal, are far-reaching. A woman who is facing any of these operations should, after learning all she can, seek a second opinion.

HYSTERECTOMY, PERFORMED ON ONE IN THREE WOMEN IN THE UNITED STATES

From 1980 through 1993—the most recent year for which figures are available—8.6 million U.S. women had hysterectomies. Over the years, the number of women who annually lose their uteri has not changed dramatically. In 1978 in the United States, 644,000 hysterectomies were performed; in 1993, the count was 546,683, and it is estimated that in the first year of the newest century, about 600,000 hysterectomies will be performed. In the United States, by age sixty, one in three women will be without wombs. This is one of the highest rates of hysterectomy in the world. In Italy, one in six women have had hysterectomies by age sixty, and in France, only one in eighteen.

What is even more shocking is how many young women are undergoing hysterectomy. Each year, rates are highest among women from forty to forty-four years old. Of all hysterectomies performed, more than half—55 percent—are among women thirty-five to forty-nine years old.

Several surgical options fall into the category of "hysterectomy." I am committed to giving a woman who is facing this operation, all the facts:

Technically, a *total or complete hysterectomy* entails removal of the uterus and the cervix. The word *hysterectomy* has Greek origins—*hystero* means "uterus" and *ectomy* means "excision." The cervix might be left intact in certain emergency cases; for example, when a hysterectomy is performed in association with a cesarean section or due to severe infection. But usually the cervix—the lower part of the uterus that meets the vagina and is called the "mouth of the womb"—is excised with the uterus because it could be the source of cancer later in a woman's life. Strictly defined, a hysterectomy does not include removal of the ovaries and tubes.

If a woman's uterus and both ovaries have been removed, she has had a *total hysterectomy with bilateral oophorectomy.* If her uterus and tubes are excised, she has undergone a *total hysterectomy with bilateral salpingectomy.* Consequently, if a woman has had her uterus, ovaries, and tubes removed, she has experienced a *total hysterectomy with a bilateral salpingo-oophorectomy.* The terminology is confusing, but it is important to decipher the medical jargon because a doctor might say he is going to give a woman a "total hysterectomy" and he might mean anything from removing her uterus alone to taking out all of her reproductive organs. If he says he intends to perform a "partial hysterectomy" he might mean that he is going to leave the ovaries and the Fallopian tubes, but in precise medical language "partial hysterectomy" means removing only part of the uterus and leaving the cervix.

A woman should ask her doctor to be specific when he discusses hysterectomy with her. Due to the variety of terms, he might inadvertently be misleading her. A woman should know exactly where she stands. When the ovaries and tubes are removed, a menstruating woman will immediately experience surgical menopause, as described in chapter 13.

It is interesting to note that the number of hysterectomies considerably varies from one part of the country to another. The lowest incidence of hysterectomy occurs in the Northeast, followed by the West, then the Midwest; the highest rate of hysterectomy is in the South. Hysterectomies are performed on the average of 5.5 per 1,000 women age fifteen and older.

Racial differences are not really factors in hysterectomies. Recent surveys find that across the board, three conditions prompt most hysterectomies: *fibroid tumors, endometriosis,* and *uterine prolapse.* Among women under age thirty, hysterectomy is linked to *menstrual disturbances* and *cervical dysplasia* (abnormal, probably precancerous, cells). *Endometriosis* is the most frequent diagnosis for women ages thirty to thirty-four; *fibroid tumors* lead the list of reasons for hysterectomies among women thirty-five to fifty-four years old, and *uterine prolapse* or *cancer,* for women age fifty-five and older. The high numbers for hysterectomy are baffling, since today GnRH agonist medications can successfully treat fibroid tumors and endometriosis, and many more doctors are performing myomectomy, a surgery to remove fibroids alone. With improved alternate treatments available, many experts questions why so many women continue to undergo hysterectomies.

When Is a Hysterectomy Needed?

It might be that in about one third of the hysterectomies performed, healthy uteri are removed. Second opinions more often reverse gynecological procedures than other kinds of operations advised for women and men. It is my constant recommendation that second opinions be sought in connection with hysterectomies. The slight decline in the number of wombs removed in this country is most likely due to increasing awareness among women from the spread of information about unnecessary surgery, a practice that must continue. Since most hysterectomies are elective, not life-or-death surgeries, there is usually a month from the moment the decision to proceed with the operation is made to the scheduled date of surgery. A woman has ample time to investigate her need for surgery and to seek a second opinion. It has been reported that in many

Roman Catholic hospitals, hysterectomies help doctors sidestep the church's ruling that forbids all forms of birth control, including tubal sterilization. A uterus should never be removed as a means of contraception. The fact that hysterectomies are so blithely recommended is frightening, although there are times when a hysterectomy is a lifesaving measure or a way to protect a woman's health.

A hysterectomy is the treatment of choice for:

- Cancer and precancerous lesions of the uterus, ovaries, and Fallopian tubes.
- Untreatable uterine damage caused either by severe infection or by surgical trauma produced during an abortion or during a delivery in which bleeding cannot be stopped.
- Excessive uterine bleeding that cannot be controlled by repeated D & Cs or hormone therapy.
- Uterine prolapse, when a sagging uterus descends into the vaginal canal or beyond because supporting muscles and ligaments have weakened. This condition can lead to urinary incontinence, bladder infections, back pain, and constipation.
- Cases of endometriosis that cannot be cured by GnRH medications or other therapies and do not respond to alternate avenues of treatment, as explained in chapter 7.
- Fibroid tumors that are so large that they would be dangerous or impossible to remove during a myomectomy, as described in chapter 15.

In all other instances in which hysterectomies are recommended, second opinions should be sought, and it would probably even be wise to consult a second-opinion doctor for the circumstances mentioned above. When cancer has been diagnosed, a woman should seek the opinion of an oncologist—a cancer specialist—at a reputable medical center or major cancer institute in addition to her gynecologist's. Considering the seriousness of cancer, a gynecologist should automatically refer his patient to a trustworthy oncologist when the diagnosis of cancer is confirmed. If surgery is recommended for precancerous lesions, a woman should consult an oncologist for additional testing before her operation. A condition that has been termed "precancerous" might have been misinterpreted during the original laboratory analysis.

Vaginal or Abdominal Hysterectomy?

A hysterectomy can be performed either through the vagina or through an incision in the abdomen. Although most hysterectomies are abdominal, more and more doctors are doing vaginal hysterectomies. The vaginal approach is not an option, however, if a woman has a narrow vaginal canal or a large uterus—larger than the size of a twelve-week pregnancy.

Often, a vaginal hysterectomy is performed in combination with vaginal plastic surgery to tighten up the vaginal muscles, an operation sometimes needed after the traumatic delivery of a large child. Many vaginal hysterectomies are performed for the purpose of sterilization. Today, questions are being raised about the ethics of choosing a vaginal hysterectomy as a means of sterilizing a woman. It is doubtful that such a procedure will ever gain acceptance among caring physicians, and a woman should be highly skeptical of a doctor who suggests that she be sterilized with a hysterectomy.

Abdominal hysterectomy is advised when the problem is large fibroid tumors or when scar tissue from a previous operation has resulted in pelvic adhesions. In these situations, a vaginal hysterectomy would be dangerous. Also, vaginal hysterectomies are more difficult in women who have never given birth or who have given birth to only one or two children. When a woman has delivered only once or twice her vagina has not been weakened as much as it might have been if she had borne several babies.

An abdominal hysterectomy can most often be accomplished through a Pfannenstiel or bikini incision, a cut below the upper edge of the pubic hairline. The fine, thin, Pfannenstiel scar will be hidden by pubic hairs and eventually will disappear completely. If a woman has been advised to have an abdominal hysterectomy, she might ask her doctor if he would perform such an incision. As he proceeds with the abdominal surgery a doctor will cut through the various abdominal tissue layers and enter the abdominal cavity. He can then safely perform the hysterectomy, but his speed and skill are going to be important factors in his patient's recovery.

During a vaginal hysterectomy a doctor will insert a speculumlike instrument into a woman's vagina and shine a light into the vaginal operative field. The operation can also be performed as a laparoscopically assisted vaginal hysterectomy (LAVH), as long as a woman's uterus is small and free from pelvic adhesions or obstructions. A surgeon makes three or four tiny incisions in a woman's abdomen, and through the openings inserts the narrow laparoscope (see page 679) and other instruments he needs to cut or move uterine tissue. The entire operation is performed through the vagina and no abdominal incision is needed. The doctor holds the cervix with a surgical tool and opens the top of the vagina. Subsequently, he ties and severs all ligaments and blood vessels to the uterus, and finally, he removes the uterus by drawing it through the vagina.

Whenever possible, a vaginal hysterectomy would be the procedure of choice since a woman usually recovers faster after having undergone the vaginal surgery. Indications for a vaginal hysterectomy, however, are much rarer than for an abdominal hysterectomy.

WARNING: *Usually it is not necessary to remove the ovaries of a menstruating woman during a hysterectomy.* A doctor might say that he wants to remove the ovaries to prevent ovarian cancer, an insidious disease that does not have obvious symptoms. However, studies have indicated that it would take 7,500 oophorectomies in order to prevent one death from ovarian cancer! Ovarian cancer, which accounts for only 4 percent of all cancers in women, is more frequently discovered after menopause in women between fifty-five and sixty-four years old. Therefore, a woman over fifty-five who is undergoing a hysterectomy should also have an oophorectomy because she is at high risk for ovarian cancer. There is no reason, however, to remove the ovaries of a younger woman who has not reached menopause simply because she is having a hysterectomy. A woman who never undergoes a hysterectomy is not going to have her ovaries excised for prophylactic purposes, so why should a woman who needs a hysterectomy suddenly be told she must have her ovaries removed?

Routine oophorectomy does not make sense in a younger woman because she will be thrown into abrupt surgical menopause. Without her ovaries, a woman will suffer a drop in estrogen and progesterone and she might begin to experience change-of-life symptoms along with metabolic changes, osteoporosis, and possible weight gain. A healthy woman under fifty should impress upon her doctor her need to retain her ovaries after hysterectomy. If he is not willing to listen, it is her right to seek a second opinion. However, if a woman has had breast, bowel, or uterine cancer, her risk of ovarian cancer is increased and all doctors might advise her to have her ovaries removed at an earlier age if she is undergoing a hysterectomy.

The Latest Alternatives to Hysterectomy

Endometrial Ablation. This technique is sometimes used to treat women for heavy menstrual bleeding. A woman's uterine lining, her endometrium, is destroyed, usually by laser or electrocautery, often during a hysteroscopy. This destruction of the uterine lining allows a woman to retain her reproductive organs. (Endometrial ablation does not prevent conception, so unless a woman uses birth control, she can conceive. However, the conception will usually be unable to implant itself in her destroyed uterine lining and can often lead to ectopic pregnancy.) Medical experts thought endometrial ablation would cut the rate of hysterectomies, but the procedure is not widely used. We have learned that after endometrial ablation, women might sill suffer cramping, pain, and discomfort.

Uterine Balloon Therapy. For this procedure a physician guides a narrow catheter with a small balloon through a woman's vagina and cervix, and into her uterus. He then inflates the balloon with a saline solution pumped through the catheter. The balloon expands to the size of her uterus. The fluid is heated to 188 degrees Fahrenheit for eight minutes, and the heat destroys her uterine lining, the endometrium. The doctor then drains the fluid and removes the deflated balloon. This is another technique that is not widely used. Gynecare, the makers of Thermachoice, the balloon device used for the procedure, have reported 80 percent effectiveness but I, like many other doctors, feel it is too early to tell. We are waiting for further follow-up studies.

Physical Complications After Hysterectomy

My stand against unnecessary hysterectomies is, in part, based upon the physical complications that I know can occur. At the extreme, there are one or two deaths for every 1,000 hysterectomies. These deaths are caused by anesthesia complications, bleeding, or infection. A great percentage of women experience "successful" hysterectomies and are still faced with immediate complications such as adverse reactions to anesthesia or internal bleeding that requires blood transfusions, not to mention the fact that potentially fatal embolisms—blood clots—can travel to the heart and the brain.

In a Canadian study, women who had hysterectomies were followed to see whether any of them would need hospitalization as a result of their operations. Within two years, 30 out of 1,000 women who underwent abdominal hysterectomies and 43 out of 1,000 women who had vaginal procedures were back in the hospital.

The women with abdominal hysterectomies mostly suffered from infections, hernias developing in poorly healed wounds, and fistulas. (A fistula is an abnormal passage for an organ to another organ or to the body surface. There is a fistula, for example, when the bowel leaks into an opening into the vagina.) Vaginal enterocele, a protrusion of the bowel into the vagina, afflicted the women with vaginal procedures. Women from both groups were treated for hemorrhaging and pelvic adhesions that in some cases blocked their bowels.

These serious complications do not even take into account posthysterectomy problems that women endure on their own. Urinary incontinence and pelvic pain become almost daily fare for many women who have had hysterectomies. Under the circumstances, it is not surprising that newer studies have indicated that women should be placed on antibiotics after their hysterectomies to lessen their difficulties. After a vaginal hysterectomy, in particular, a woman is susceptible to an increased possibility of infection. If a woman feels any sign of infection such as increased pain and fever after her surgery, she should ask her doctor whether he thinks she might have an infection. Before surgery, a woman might be able to reduce her postoperative problems by planning to have her hysterectomy at a hospital that is recognized for its quality care.

The hospitals with reputations for providing the best care from the most thorough doctors usually have the lowest rates of complications. Most surgery-related death comes from improper administration of anesthesia. At well-known teaching hospitals and major medical centers, informed anesthesiologists and the most up-to-date equipment exist to provide a commendable level of safety for surgical procedures. A woman should select a highly accredited hospital in her area when she finds that a hysterectomy is unavoidable.

Feelings After Hysterectomy

Every woman feels differently about the loss of her uterus. Certainly a woman who has had uterine cancer, severe bleeding, or any other painful problem that has incapacitated her, might feel better after her hysterectomy because a troublesome abnormality has been removed. The Nurses Association of the American College of Obstetricians and Gynecologists surveyed forty women with a median age of thirty-eight a few weeks after their hysterectomies. These either married or divorced women with an average of two children were in the lowest socioeconomic group. One third of the women had undergone hysterectomies for cancer, 41 percent had fibroids, and the rest of the women had hysterectomies as a result of endometriosis, pelvic inflammatory disease (PID), or cystocele-rectrocele, also called a vaginal prolapse or dropped bladder.

When questioned, 75 percent of these women felt positive about the surgery, but their good feelings were because their fears about cancer had been removed with their wombs. The women also felt freed from other problems such as heavy bleeding, abdominal pressures, backaches, and headaches. Seven out of eleven women who said they had new self-images expressed deeper feelings of femininity, and as far as sexuality was concerned, 62 percent reported no change in the way they regarded their sexual partners and 87 percent had no worries that their hysterectomies would affect their sexual activities.

This small study among a select group of women on a low socioeconomic level shows just how difficult it is to generalize about women's feelings after hysterectomy. These women who were already mothers might have been relieved that they no longer had to worry about menstruation or contraception. Also, their problems of survival might have been so great that the loss of a uterus might have seemed minor in comparison. However, the significant psychological impact of a hysterectomy often does not show up until three months to three years after surgery, and most women do not reveal themselves to be as positive as the women in the Nurses Association's study.

Even in cases where women have been told that they might have lost their lives if they had not had hysterectomies, a certain ambivalence begins to present itself. Unless women have had cancer, they often wrestle with the question of whether or not their hysterectomy was really necessary. If a woman begins to conclude that her operation was superfluous, then she might experience rage, depression, or both. For emotional as well as physical reasons, a woman should be very cautious about agreeing to a hysterectomy.

When a woman's menstruation is stopped before her change-of-life is due, she might be faced with conflicts and questions about her own femininity. If a woman has not had children, she might feel that she is less of a person, or she might mourn her inability to become a mother. Unless it is absolutely necessary, a woman should never undergo a hysterectomy.

Psychiatrists report that women even dream and fantasize about their lost uteri. A uterus marred by fibroid tumors might be perfectly smooth in a dream. When they go to bed, perimenopausal women might hear babies crying at night or dream of becoming pregnant. Thinking they have become unattractive, women might dream of accidents that disfigure their faces.

The reaction of a woman's husband or a significant loved one is important to her psychological recovery. Once a hysterectomy has been accomplished, it is important that family and friends support a woman in the fact that the surgery was needed. Recovery and emotional conflict will be eased if a woman feels that her value and desirability have remained unchanged by her hysterectomy.

Sexual Response After Hysterectomy

Decades ago, in 1947, Dr. E. W. Munnell wrote in a paper titled "Total Hysterectomy": "Not only does this study deny the idea that the cervix is a necessary organ to be stimulated in order to achieve orgasm, but it also shows that neither uterus nor ovaries are necessary for its attainment. . . . Where there are changes in libido or sexual satisfaction following hysterectomy, the cause of these changes is undoubtedly phychogenic." In other words, any sexual differences a woman might experience after hysterectomy are "all in her head."

Since the time of Dr. Munnell's statement, doctors have felt that science has given them the right to tell women that they would feel no sexual changes after their hysterectomies. Doctors have even suggested that women might enjoy sex more because they will not have to worry about menstruation and possible conception, and a 1999 study conducted at the University of Maryland medical school supports this theory.

However, it is important to remember that organs involved in the sexual response are removed during hysterectomy. There might be almost half a million oophorectomies—ovarian removals—performed in conjunction with hysterectomies every year. When a fertile woman's ovaries are removed, her hormone production stops and she is, in effect, castrated. Many women feel a reduced sex drive without their hormones, and their sexual despondency is physically, not psychologically, rooted. Also, during the excitement phase of sexual arousal the uterus becomes engorged with blood much in the way the man's penis does when he is sexually stimulated. Without her uterus, a woman might feel as if her body is not as sexually responsive.

Recent studies conducted in the United Kingdom show that 33 to 46 percent of women who have had hysterectomies with or without oophorectomies report a drop in sexual response. The theory that diminished sexual desire after hysterectomy is "all in the head" can no longer be accepted. These new revelations by women were investigated by conscientious researchers who concluded that hormonal shifts—specifically, a reduction in the hormone androgen—after ovaries were removed definitely had an impact on sexuality. Also, Dr. Munnell notwithstanding, anatomical changes had to be considered. The cervix became identified as a site of sexual stimulation that was needed for some women to achieve orgasms. Women who had lost their cervixes and uteri through hysterectomies knew what they were missing and they told investigators that they were responding differently.

Of course, women who have suffered severe bleeding, pain, and pressure in their abdomens before their hysterectomies often feel relieved after their operations and they might even enjoy better sexual responses within themselves. In the University of Maryland study, over 1,100 women were surveyed, and the number of women who reported having orgasms rose from 62.8 percent before surgery to 72.4 percent one year after surgery. Even in the U.K. studies, more than half the women surveyed reported the same or increased sexual response after their hysterectomies. Sexual drive might be altered less after an essential-to-life hysterectomy than after a hysterectomy performed unnecessarily. Overall, sexual response after hysterectomy is definitely an area that requires more research, but at least now there is no doubt that there are physical causes for a woman's altered feeling.

QUESTIONS ABOUT HYSTERECTOMY

Many women have had surgery without information, without knowing that they would experience emotional, physical, and sexual changes after hysterectomy. By the time the women who wrote the following letters learned about the many adjustments they would face after hysterectomy, it was too late for them to change their minds. By reading their stories and understanding their frustrations and difficulties, more women—and men also—can realize the horror and trauma unnecessary hysterectomy can create. Problems we all might share surface. These letters can help more people become better informed, and with information, every woman can know how to ask the right questions and when to look for a second, or maybe even a third, opinion.

My Hysterectomy Has Practically Turned Me into an Invalid

I was thirty-four when I had a hysterectomy. Today I feel like I'm thirty-six going on a hundred. When the doctor operated, he left my ovaries to make my recovery easier, but nothing has been easy. After the surgery I developed an abscessed hematoma, which put me back in the hospital for almost three weeks. While I was being cured with intravenous antibiotics I had back pains, hot sweats, and cold chills. When I went home I had pain and swelling in one leg, which the doctor later diagnosed as sciatica. The pain in my leg was rivaled by constant headaches. I didn't know what part of my body would fail me next, but I didn't have long to wait before I found out. I developed vaginitis, which lasted almost a year. No matter what I did, my vaginal infection continued. Then an ovary that was supposed to make my life easier developed a cyst and both my ovaries started to hurt. With all this I have become extremely stressed. I never used to feel depressed, but now I'm depressed all the time. I'm surprised my husband doesn't divorce me, but I guess he sees that I'm trying to hold on. I'm seeing a therapist and going to group therapy to try to keep my moods under control. I didn't have

cancer and now I'm wondering if I really needed that hysterectomy.
My body was ruined and I'm afraid my life is going down the
drain too.

—C.W., Gates Mills, Ohio

This letter clearly indicates that complications after hysterectomy can be horrendous. Ms. W. did not receive the proper care during her surgery. Since she developed a hematoma, it appears that her doctor did not thoroughly tie off her blood vessels. Also, he does not seem to have operated under sterile conditions since she abscessed and became infected. The backache and sciatica she mentioned are signs that a surgical instrument damaged the nerves in her back and leg. All things considered, it appears that her doctor was not a competent gynecological surgeon.

Another aftereffect of the surgery—vaginal infection—frequently occurs; in fact, vaginitis is expected. Hysterectomies cause hormonal changes that alter the vaginal environment and make it a breeding ground for germs. Ms. W.'s headaches could also be caused by a hormonal imbalance brought on by the surgery.

Naturally, Ms. W. has become stressed. The prolonged infections and discomforts she has endured would make anyone stressed, depressed, and tense. It is difficult for me to know whether she really needed a hysterectomy, but I do believe that when a woman is faced with the possibility of losing her reproductive organs, she must seek a second opinion. One would hope that a different, competent surgeon would have been more exacting and would have worked to diminish the internal bleeding. A capable physician would also have administered the proper antibiotics to ward off internal infection. Now Ms. W. is left to heal herself, but she is certainly doing her best to restore her health. She is wise to continue her group therapy for stress management. She might also take daily doses of stress-reducing vitamins such as vitamin B_6 (50 mg or more) and vitamin E (800 units or more). In addition, proper nutrition and exercise might help her body to become strong and resistant to disorder.

Since My Hysterectomy, Sex Feels Like Knives Cutting into Me

I'm sixty-two years old, the mother of three children, and I have had two hysterectomies. My first hysterectomy was eight or nine yours ago and many D & Cs followed it. Finally the doctor said he wanted to do a second hysterectomy. I agreed to the surgery and ever since I have been in tremendous pain during intercourse. Sex feels like knives cutting into me. I cry while my husband and I are making love. Afterward, I hurt when I urinate. I have had estrogen injections. I have used creams, and I even took garlic pills for a while. Nothing has helped and my marriage is being destroyed. What has happened to me?

—M.H., Deaumont, Texas

Ms. H.'s complaint is added proof that a woman can experience a variety of problems after hysterectomy. Since Ms. H. had two hysterectomies, she probably retained her cervix after the first operation, and during the second surgery her doctor removed the cervix and possibly some adhesions. After a hysterectomy, the organs left behind can become bound together by dense bands called adhesions, which often hurt during bowel movements and can lead to incapacitation.

Skillful surgery can prevent adhesions, but when less-efficient techniques are used, infection and internal bleeding—conditions that promote the formation of adhesions—might result. It is not clear why Ms. H. needed several D & Cs, but obviously they were not helping her condition.

If Ms. H. had adhesions after her first hysterectomy, her second surgery would only have created more adhesions. During sexual intercourse, her husband might be thrusting against her adhesions and causing her pain. Also, she might possibly have a vaginal obstruction or a vaginal stricture—a narrowing of the vagina—resulting from her second hysterectomy.

Ms. H. should seek a second opinion from a competent gynecologist at a teaching hospital or major medical center to find out what the source of her dyspareunia—pain during intercourse—might be. She might need surgery to remove a vaginal obstruction or to correct a vaginal stricture.

It is also possible that exercise, vitamins B and E, and regular application of hormone creams or K-Y jelly to her vagina might make sexual intercourse a less painful, more enjoyable experience. Even so, Ms. H. might never completely return to her normal self. Problems were inflicted upon her during her two hysterectomies, and these conditions cannot be totally corrected.

I Have Fibroid Tumors; Is There Any Alternative to a Hysterectomy?

My doctor told me I was pregnant after he examined me internally. He said he was positive and I didn't need a blood or urine test. I went for a second opinion and sure enough, I wasn't pregnant at all. The second doctor said that I had large fibroid tumors which have swollen my uterus to the size of an eighteen-week pregnancy. He wants me to come back in a month and if the tumors are still large or growing, he says he would like to do a hysterectomy. I am thirty-five years old and I want to have at least one child before I stop menstruating. I don't want to lose my uterus. Is there any alternative to hysterectomy?

—E. P., Brushton, New York

Ms. P. should try to find a doctor who will perform a myomectomy, an operation to remove her fibroids while leaving her uterus intact. As explained in chapter 15, a myomectomy performed with the tourniquet technique and an injection of pitressin into the uterine wall will decrease the chance of complications arising after surgery. There is no need for Ms. P. to undergo a hysterectomy. Even if she were in her forties, she should not agree to a hysterectomy because she has fibroid tumors if a myomectomy is possible.

Doctors have often advised women over fifty to have hysterectomies with oophorectomies as methods of treating their fibroid tumors. Many patients in my office are women over fifty who have large fibroids, and I merely monitor the tumors, which seem to shrink after change-of-life. There is no reason for a woman of any age to submit to a hysterectomy when her problem is fibroid tumors, and the ovaries, which might continue to produce hormones until a woman is fifty-five or sixty, should certainly not be removed. As mentioned earlier in this chapter, although a doctor might say that he wants to remove a woman's ovaries to save her from ovarian cancer, studies have shown that it would take 7,500 oophorectomies to prevent one death from cancer of the ovaries. A woman should undergo an oophorectomy during a hysterectomy only if she is over fifty-five, a time of life when she is at high risk for ovarian cancer.

Ms. P. is still young enough to conceive a child, and she should seek out a skilled surgeon to perform her myomectomy. She might investigate doctors at teaching hospitals, which are today's centers for training physicians in the latest myomectomy techniques.

How Can I Restore My Childbearing Ability?

I gave birth to a son, fathered by my first husband, when I was twenty-three. After childbirth, I had heavy bleeding for months. The doctor put me in the hospital, where he did a hysterectomy. After the surgery he told me that I had had three fibroids. I feel that this surgery was unnecessary since fibroid tumors can be removed without hysterectomy. Now I am twenty-seven and I have remarried. My second husband has never had any children and I wonder if it is possible to get an artificial uterus through surgery. I read somewhere that an artificial womb was created in Australia and I wonder if I could have this operation. Perhaps, since I still have my ovaries, I could be an egg donor for my own baby?
—A.S., Las Vegas, Nevada

Since Ms. S. had only three fibroid tumors, she certainly could have had a myomectomy. This surgery would have controlled her bleeding but still allowed her to remain fertile.

Today, many women like Ms. S. remarry and want children with their current husbands, but their wombs have been removed. This is why I advise caution and consultation with a second-opinion doctor before a hysterectomy becomes a fait accompli. *There is no way to reverse a hysterectomy.* It is impossible to create an artificial womb. Uterine transplants have been performed among animals, but a human uterus has never been, and might never be, transplanted. Science has not been able to overcome the problem of the body's rejection of the foreign, transplanted organ.

Ms. S. still has the ability to become a mother through the process of egg retrieval (see pages 275 to 276), which is usually performed in conjunction with in vitro fertilization (IVF). Ms. S. would take fertility drugs to induce superovulation, have her egg development monitored through ultrasound, and have her eggs retrieved during a minor procedure using a vaginal ultrasound probe. Then her eggs would be fertilized in a laboratory dish with her husband's sperm. Three or four days later, a woman who had agreed to carry the fertilized egg, or embryo, through its nine-month development and to give birth to Ms. S.'s baby, would become the recipient of the fertilized egg through IVF. Perhaps Ms. S. has a close relative who would consider such an arrangement. This reproductive technology has already created a grandmother who gave birth to her own grandchildren.

Ms. S.'s plight should be a lesson to all women to hesitate when they hear their doctors advise hysterectomies. Seek a second opinion, and do not agree to surgery unless it is absolutely necessary.

My Doctor Lied to Me and I Nearly Died

I am a forty-nine-year-old mother of three teenagers. When my children became old enough to take care of themselves, I started working as a hospital volunteer. I got to know the doctors pretty well. When I had a problem I asked one of the surgeons what I should do. I was bleeding all the time, had backaches, headaches, and no energy. The doctor examined me and said I had a tumor the size of a grapefruit and I had to have my uterus removed. I wasn't sure if I liked that idea so I went to the head of the department and asked him for a second opinion. The head surgeon confirmed the first doctor's opinion, but I told him I didn't want the operation unless he would assure me that he would only remove my uterus if the tumor was cancerous. He said he would not cut unless he found cancer and he would even show me his report after the operation. I went into the operating room feeling that I would not lose my womb unless I had a disease that could kill me. Well, the operation almost killed me. During the surgery I was given two transfusions because I bled so much. I was rushed to intensive care after the operation because the doctors were worried that they would lose me. After I recovered, I learned that my uterus, tubes, and ovaries were gone. The doctor said I didn't have cancer but he gave me a total hysterectomy anyway. "I always do a total hysterectomy on women over forty-five," he said. Now I am constantly suffering. I have hot flashes all the time because I stopped taking estrogen pills. I'm afraid the estrogen medication will give me breast cancer. I have no desire for sex and my husband will probably start having an affair soon. I am sinking into a depression that grows deeper every day. Why did my doctor lie to me?

—P.D., Orlando, Florida

This is a very sad story. This woman thought she could trust the head surgeon and she could not. She did seek a second opinion, but her experience shows that it is often important for a woman to bring someone with her when she goes for a second-opinion consultation. If Ms. D.'s husband or a close friend had heard the doctor's promise to perform a hysterectomy only if cancer was confirmed, Ms. D. could have sued. Obviously, her surgeon had no intention of keeping his promise, but without a witness, Ms. D. would have a difficult time suing for malpractice.

Now she is left without organs and with a mistrust of the medical profession. Her depression is a sign of her anger. She might find that a compassionate therapist can help her to face her rage and release it. Ms. D. should also remember that, no, she does not have her reproductive organs, but the rest of her body is still in good health. Ms. D. should try to keep her resistance high by eating a proper diet and exercising. If menopausal symptoms incapacitate her, under the careful supervision of a doctor she could take low-dose estrogen replacement therapy (see chapter 13). The lowest possible dose of estrogen brings minimal increased risk of breast cancer.

I Went for a D & C and the Doctor Did a Hysterectomy

I become pregnant with my first child when I was thirty years old. Everything looked fine until the third month. I went for my regular checkup and the doctor couldn't hear the baby's heartbeat, which is usually apparent after eleven or twelve weeks. The doctor ordered an ultrasound test and then told me I would have to go into the hospital for a D & C. I had some spotting but nothing heavy. I was admitted for the D & C, but I left the hospital having had a hysterectomy. The doctor said that my placenta was low and when he started scraping I began to bleed. He scraped harder and faster and punctured the uterus and an artery. Finally he had to make an incision and remove everything. I had two transfusions in the process. Now I am supposed to accept the fact that I can never have a child. Everything happened so suddenly. In a way, I feel like my life is over.

—K.O., Windber, Pennsylvania

There is a condition called *placenta accreta* in which the placenta firmly attaches itself to the uterine wall and can be removed only through a D & C. Placenta accreta is a relatively rare occurrence, but it is seen in women who have had a number of D & Cs or abortions. Also, if the placenta does not expel itself immediately after childbirth, placenta accreta is probably the reason. Ms. O. might have had a case of placenta accreta that necessitated a D & C. Before surgery, her doctor should have explained her condition to her and informed her that she faced a chance of losing her uterus if uncontrollable bleeding occurred during the operation.

Prior to surgery, the doctor should have administered uterine-contracting medication such as oxytocin or ergotrate to control the bleeding and make the D & C easier to perform. If medication had not controlled the bleeding, the doctor could have packed her uterus with gauze to create hemostasis—a stoppage of the blood flow—and possibly avoid hysterectomy. Also, he might have tried to give her vitamin K to help the blood coagulate more easily. The puncture Ms. O.'s doctor made in her uterus seems to indicate that he was not particularly skillful in conducting the surgery.

Unfortunately, stories like Ms. O.'s are commonplace. The fury and despair that arise after surgery could be avoided if doctors would communicate with their patients and be honest about the seriousness of their patients' conditions. Any time a hysterectomy might be a possibility, a woman should be told.

I Wish I Hadn't Had a Hysterectomy; My Vagina Is Bulging

A doctor removed by uterus when I was seventy-five years old and I wish I had never agreed to the hysterectomy. I felt fine. Now I am eighty and I have a huge bulge coming down into my vagina. This condition is uncomfortable but is it dangerous? What should I do? I'm not anxious to go back to my doctor because he gave me the hysterectomy in the first place.

—N.L., Baltimore, Maryland

Ms. L. is experiencing a prolapse of the vagina. After a hysterectomy, the ligaments that hold the vagina often weaken. The vagina sags, which is another way of saying that a prolapse occurs. Sometimes vaginal plastic surgery is performed to tighten the vaginal muscles and correct the prolapse, but considering Ms. L.'s age, surgery would be dangerous. The thin vaginal tissue of an eighty-year-old woman, even if it withstood the procedure, would be slow to heal.

Ms. L.'s vaginal prolapse could possibly be corrected with a pessary ring, a circular rubber device available in different sizes, which supports vaginal tissue. If the pessary does not work and the prolapse continues, Ms. L.'s doctor might consider performing vaginal surgery on her. However, surgery should be suggested only if Ms. L.'s problem becomes incapacitating, since her age makes any type of operation very risky.

I Was Told I Needed a Hysterectomy, but Now I'm Pregnant

Three months before I became pregnant my doctor told me I needed a hysterectomy. He said I had tumors that might be cancerous and I would have to lose my uterus. I couldn't bear the thought of being unable to have children. Out of my own fear and on the advice of friends, I refused to go into the hospital. Now I'm two months pregnant and my new doctor says there is nothing wrong with my uterus. I'm trying to get the records from the first doctor to see why he thought there was a problem. I think there might be a case of malpractice here, especially since the doctor refuses to talk to me. Anyway, I'm glad I didn't lose my uterus and my chance to have a child.

—G.K., Jersey City, New Jersey

This woman was right to act as she did. If a woman feels nothing is wrong with her she should certainly hesitate to agree to a hysterectomy. Ms. K. might have benefited from a consultation with a second-opinion doctor, and I would advise any woman to seek a second opinion whenever her instincts tell her a physician is rendering a questionable diagnosis. In the instance she describes, she did not look into a second opinion, but her pregnancy shows that she followed the correct course. Friends also advised her correctly and I recommend this good communication, this positive networking, among all women.

My Doctor Is Using a "Cancer Scare" as a Reason to Give Me a Hysterectomy

I am fifty-two years old and still menstruating. My periods last about ten days, with six of them heavy. I go for regular checkups and feel fine. I've had two children and never had any major operations in my life. My doctor has been telling me that it's not normal for a fifty-two-year-old woman to have a period. He says that it is just a matter of time before I get uterine cancer if I don't let him give me a hysterectomy. I think that this "cancer scare" is unnecessary. I have had uterine biopsies and they have been benign. I do not want an operation. Is there any truth in what he is saying?

—F.R., New Orleans, Louisiana

Ms. R. does not need a hysterectomy. It is true that if a woman has irregular bleeding, particularly if she is taking estrogen, she might need a uterine biopsy to make sure that she has no abnormalities. Ms. R. had more than one biopsy and her condition is benign. She feels good; thus there is no reason for her to worry because she is menstruating at age fifty-two, and there is definitely no indication for hysterectomy.

Women today, particularly women in good health, can menstruate well into their fifties. Also, if a woman is heavy, the fatty tissue in her body will produce estrogen, which encourages menstruation to continue.

Every six months, an older menstruating woman should have a checkup with a Pap test. As long as the Pap smears are trouble-free and a woman has no sign of abnormality, she need not concern herself about uterine cancer. A woman who is about to experience menopause and is being pushed to have a hysterectomy at this time should refuse to be coerced. When a hysterectomy is advised, a woman should seek a second opinion and prevent a doctor from freely using his scalpel.

I Woke Up After Surgery with a Complete Hysterectomy at Twenty-one Years Old

A few months after my wedding, my doctor found a small cyst on my ovary which he said he could cut out in a simple operation. I went into the hospital to have the cyst removed. When I came out of the anesthesia I found out that I had had a complete hysterectomy except for one ovary. The doctor never explained anything before or after the operation; he never even visited my room in the hospital. I was only twenty-one when that hysterectomy happened ten years ago. It changed my life. My husband and I adopted a baby, but I never got over the fact that I couldn't have a child of my own. I had a nervous breakdown and was institutionalized for a long time. When I came out I had developed an addiction to tranquilizers which took me years to overcome. In the middle of everything, I learned that I had endometriosis and that my only remaining ovary had to be removed. I have since found out the ovaries should only be removed if they're cancerous. Now I've lost everything. Do you think the doctor who did my first surgery discovered cancer? Will I have to take hormones forever?

—B.U., Rochelle, Illinois

Ms. U.'s story is heartbreaking. She was a newlywed when her doctor removed her uterus, at least one tube, and one ovary. She should try to retrieve her records to learn whether her ovary was cancerous, but I doubt it. The confirmation of ovarian cancer would have required the removal of both ovaries. It is possible that even at the time of her original surgery Ms. U. was suffering from endometriosis, since it was diagnosed at a later date.

Ms. U.'s endometriosis could have been treated with medication that would have melted her endometrial cysts. Every attempt should have been made to treat her condition with methods other than surgery. Today she is a thirty-one-year-old woman with no reproductive organs. Since she does not have ovaries to produce hormones, she will have to take hormone medication the rest of her life, or at least until she reaches the age of menopause. Without hormones, Ms. U. risks the onset of osteoporosis, a thinning and weakening of the bones partially due to estrogen depletion. With vitamins—particularly vitamins B_6, C, D, and E—exercise, and hormone replacement, she should be able to keep her body in good shape. She should be placed on the lowest possible dosage of any hormone replacement medication she might need. My hope is that, as far as her emotional health is concerned, the worst is behind her and she will be able to raise her adopted child as a loving, happy person.

I Have an Ovarian Cyst and the Doctor Wants to Do a Hysterectomy

I have heavy bleeding each month. I also have a small ovarian cyst. Pap smears show no sign of cancer, but my doctor wants to do a hysterectomy. I do not want to have an operation, but I don't know what my alternatives are. Can you help me?
—T.H., Goldsboro, North Carolina

As mentioned in chapter 15, an ovarian cyst often disappears spontaneously if it is allowed to remain through two or three menstrual cycles. If a cyst does not disappear by itself, surgery, which is explained in chapter 15, might be indicated.

Ms. H. might be experiencing heavy bleeding because her estrogen level, which has risen due to the presence of the ovarian cyst, is triggering an excessive flow. It is also possible that the cyst ruptured, spilled hormones into the abdomen, and heavy bleeding was provoked. Neither of these events is a reason for hysterectomy.

If the cyst disappears in a short time, Ms. H. might be advised to have a D & C to eliminate any endometrial tissue that might be present in her uterus, but most often no treatment is needed. If the ovarian cyst does not disappear within a month or two, she might need surgery to remove the cyst alone. Whether the cyst stays or goes, a hysterectomy should not be undertaken. A small ovarian cyst is never reason enough to remove a uterus.

I Have Heavy Periods; Do I Need a Hysterectomy?

Lately I have had very heavy periods. I have been bleeding in clots. I think my problem might be stress, which also makes me eat more. Right now I am thirty-five pounds overweight. My doctor said he would try to give me hormones to stop the bleeding, but if they don't work then I would probably need a hysterectomy. I am only twenty-eight years old and I do not want to lose my uterus. Do you think I could really be faced with an unavoidable hysterectomy?

—C.A., Eckert, Colorado

Naturally, a hysterectomy is not the treatment of choice when the problem is heavy bleeding. Ms. A. might have heavy periods because she is overweight. Estrogen produced by excess body fat might cause the thickening of her uterine lining. Her bleeding, therefore, increases as the built-up endometrium—the uterine lining—sheds itself.

Ms. A. might be a candidate for oral contraceptives while she tries to lose weight. The birth control pill will manage her hormone production and regulate her flow. After a few months to a year on the pill, she should experience less bleeding. After she stops the pill, she should continue to have a regular cycle, providing that she loses weight and exercises often to keep her body fit. Once again, she should certainly not have a hysterectomy.

I Had a Hysterectomy for Endometriosis and Since Then Life Has Been a Living Hell

I had a hysterectomy for endometriosis and afterward my whole system went crazy. Life has been a living hell. Suddenly I can't control my water retention and I've gained twenty pounds. My hormone pills nauseate me and I always feel like I'm on the verge of vomiting. I've developed high blood pressure, and worse, the endometriosis hasn't been cured. Last week I learned that the pain in my abdomen was from a new growth of endometriosis. Sometimes I think I should jump out the window.

—Y.T., Norristown, Pennsylvania

When a woman is faced with incurable cancer or uncontrollable bleeding that will not stop no matter how a doctor tries, then a hysterectomy is advised. But a hysterectomy should not be treated like the solution to all problems in the pelvic area. As pointed out in chapter 7 and many other times in this book, a hysterectomy is not the treatment of choice for endometriosis.

Before a woman agrees to have a hysterectomy she should find out exactly why her doctor thinks she needs it. Then she should investigate her condition, its symptoms and its treatments, before she concludes that she has no choice but to take her doctor's advice.

Ms. T. did not need a hysterectomy for her endometriosis. Endometrial tissue grows, among other places, outside the uterus in the pelvic cavity. A hysterectomy will not eliminate the condition. Ms. T. should have been given Danocrine or a GnRH agonist drug such as Lupron and Synarel, perhaps for six months to a year, before the endometrial tissue would have disappeared completely (see chapter 7). After Danocrine therapy, she might have had to undergo surgery to remove pelvic adhesions and perhaps sever the uterosacral ligament and nerves that support the uterus. Often when certain nerves are cut, pain that has accrued from years of the disease is eliminated. If endometriosis recurs, medication might be readministered.

Ms. T.'s situation is tragic, but she should do her best to keep her body fit. To help her overcome her recurring endometriosis, she should certainly be treated now.

I Have an Enlarged Ovary; Do I Need a Hysterectomy?

Ten years ago I had a mastectomy. Today I am sixty-four years old. I had considered myself pretty healthy recently, that is until the last time I went to the doctor. He said he could feel an enlarged ovary and that I might need surgery. I went for a second opinion and the second doctor recommended a hysterectomy. Do you think it's safe for someone with my health history to undergo an operation at sixty-four?

—J.C., El Paso, Texas

After menopause, an enlarged ovary could be a sign of an abnormality or malignancy. In Ms. C.'s case, it is impossible to predict what might be causing her ovarian mass, but women between fifty-five and sixty-four are at high risk for ovarian cancer. Ms. C.'s risk is also heightened by the fact that she has had breast cancer. It seems that Ms. C. should have surgery at least to remove the enlarged ovary.

If lab analysis shows any sign of malignancy in the removed ovary, Ms. C. should have a total hysterectomy with removal of the remaining ovary. If lab analysis indicates that the excised ovary is benign and the other ovary, on biopsy, is also benign, obviously she can decline to have a hysterectomy. At the moment, however, Ms. C. needs surgery to learn why one ovary is enlarged.

I Have Adenomatous Hyperplasia; Do I Need a Hysterectomy?

My doctor wants to do a hysterectomy because I have adenomatous hyperplasia. I am in so much pain that sometimes I can't even wear slacks or panty hose. Sexual intercourse hurts, too. I am forty-five years old and even though I don't want any more children, I don't want to lose my organs either. I went for a second opinion and the second doctor told me I didn't need the surgery. Still, I am in great pain. Frankly, I'm in a quandary over whom to believe.

—S.V., Newport, Arkansas

Adenomatous hyperplasia is a condition in which the lining of the uterus—the endometrium—has been overstimulated by estrogen. During adenomatous hyperplasia the uterine lining becomes very thick and a recognizable tissue pattern develops. If allowed to continue, the tissue of adenomatous hyperplasia might evolve into precancerous lesions and uterine cancer, and it is because of this deadly potential that this condition must be curtailed.

It is now suggested that a woman with this condition be treated with progesterone medication such as Provera, 10 mg twice a day for ten to fourteen days. Progesterone changes the configuration of the adenomatous hyperplasia tissue. After progesterone treatment, a woman usually will bleed because she is shedding the diseased uterine lining with its abnormal tissue. As soon as her bleeding stops, she will require a formal D & C in the hospital. The D & C should remove any adenomatous hyperplasia tissue that has not been sloughed off naturally. It is suggested that a woman repeat the complete treatment—progesterone medication followed by a D & C— one more time. After adenomatous hyperplasia has been overcome. A uterine biopsy should then be performed every year for the next few years to make sure that the adenomatous hyperplasia does not return.

If the double therapy does not change the uterine lining, a woman might consider an endometrial ablation (see page 645) to destroy the uterine lining, but hysterectomy is usually advised. There is too high a risk that adenomatous hyperplasia might bring on precancerous lesions to advise anything but hysterectomy when progesterone therapy is not successful.

A woman who has had adenomatous hyperplasia should avoid estrogen medication. If such a woman is placed on hormone replacement therapy, she must always take progesterone medication such as Provera as described in chapter 13.

Finally, in response to Ms. V.'s dilemma, adenomatous hyperplasia is a condition that is much more understood today than it used to be in the past. The disorder does not create an immediate reason to do a hysterectomy. After it is diagnosed, adenomatous hyperplasia should be properly treated with the progesterone/D & C procedure described above. If this treatment does not eliminate Ms. V.'s condition, then endometrial ablation or hysterectomy might be necessary last resorts.

I Have Severe Menstrual Cramps and the Doctor Suggested a Hysterectomy

> *I am in great pain each month just before my period arrives. My cramps are so severe that I cannot get out of bed sometimes. I just lie there with a heating pad on my stomach. My doctor has prescribed tranquilizers and painkillers, but I don't like to take them because I'm afraid I'll become addicted. Lately he has started saying something about ending my pain with a hysterectomy. I am thirty years old and I don't want a hysterectomy. Surely there must be another way for me to find relief.*
>
> —D.E., Lanoka Harbor, New Jersey

We know that menstrual cramps are caused by a rise in prostaglandins, hormonelike substances secreted by uterine tissue twenty-four hours before menstruation. Aspirin NSAIDs such as Motrin and Nuprin and aspirinlike medications like Midol block the production of prostaglandins and reduce the severity of menstrual cramps. Motrin or Midol tablets taken four times a day from twenty-four hours before the onset of a woman's menstrual flow up to a few days after menstruation begins often bring relief to a woman suffering from cramps.

As mentioned in chapter 3, when cramps are extremely painful, prescription NSAIDs such as Motrin, Anaprox, or Ponstel, one to two tablets taken four times a day, have been found to act like "wonder drugs" in the way they free women from their discomfort. Ms. E.'s doctor should prescribe an antiprostaglandin medication for her. Vitamin B-complex with vitamin B_6 might add to Ms. E.'s relief, and the cramp-relieving exercises suggested in chapter 3 might also prove helpful. A hysterectomy is definitely inappropriate, especially since Ms. E. is still of childbearing age.

Ms. E. should try an antiprostaglandin medication, because if her cramps continue to go untreated she might develop a case of endometriosis. If she does not feel better with an antiprostaglandin agent, then she might be a candidate for the birth control pill. The pill should regulate her cycle and diminish her pain. However, if the pill is not completely effective, she might be placed on GnRH agonist medication, which will halt her period and give her organs a "pelvic rest" during treatment.

How Long Can I Be on Estrogen After a Hysterectomy?

I am twenty-five years old. After three operations my doctor finally gave me a hysterectomy when I was twenty. He removed my uterus and both ovaries. For a while I took two estrogen tablets a day, but now I'm down to one a day. I've heard that estrogen can cause uterine cancer. I don't have a uterus so I'm wondering if I have to worry. Can estrogen cause breast cancer? Also, how long can I safely remain on estrogen? Can a person stay on hormone pills for a lifetime?

—M.D., Anchorage, Alaska

When a woman's ovaries remain after a hysterectomy, she does not need hormone replacement. Her ovaries should continue functioning into her fifties. If the ovaries of a young woman have been removed during a hysterectomy, she will need estrogen medication, such as Premarin, to prevent drying and thinning of her skin tissue and weakening of her bones, which might mean osteoporosis, and to ward off general change-of-life symptoms. A woman in Ms. D.'s situation should be given the lowest possible dose of estrogen, to be taken daily in a cycle of three weeks on and one week off. If estrogen is not prescribed right after a hysterectomy with oophorectomy, osteoporosis will set in. Ms. D. might help to reduce her need for hormones with vitamins B, E, and D; calcium; and exercise. Even so, Ms. D. should probably remain on estrogen until the point in her life when she would normally be going through menopause.

When a woman takes estrogen after a hysterectomy she does not have to combine it with progesterone because the estrogen/progesterone balance is only needed to prevent uterine cancer. Since no increased incidence of breast cancer in hysterectomized women taking estrogen has been reported, progesterone does not have to be included in estrogen replacement therapy for the purpose of preventing breast cancer.

I Took DES; Do I Need a Hysterectomy?

Before my daughter, who is now twenty-nine, was born, I took DES to avoid a miscarriage. I gave birth naturally and have never had a serious gynecological problem. My daughter is checked by a doctor every six months. She seems to be fine. The trouble now is that my doctor tells me that I have a small lesion on my cervix. He says he wants to do a hysterectomy, because I took DES twenty-nine years ago. I know the DES is dangerous for my daughter, but is it dangerous for me too?

—G.Q., Hastings, Minnesota

It has become known that DES daughters under twenty years old are subject to an increased incidence of vaginal/cervical cancer, but *cervical abnormalities in DES mothers have not been reported.* There has been some suggestion that DES mothers were at higher-than-average risk for breast cancer while taking DES, but DES mothers have not been shown to have higher rates of breast cancer.

Ms. Q.'s doctor seems to be confusing the facts about DES. I suggest that Ms. Q. consult a second-opinion doctor for his advice on treatment of her condition. Her present doctor is not as informed as he should be.

Pelvic Inflammatory Disease (PID) and Hysterectomy

I am thirty years old. Two years ago a pain in my lower abdomen was diagnosed as an abscessed tubal infection. My doctor removed

*one tube and one ovary. I was fine for a year, but then the pain
started again. I found out that my other tube was infected and I
had PID. I did not want further surgery. My doctor put me on
tetracycline for three months, but nothing happened. The antibiotic
seemed to have no effect on my condition. The pain and
inflammation increased and finally I was admitted to the hospital
to have a hysterectomy and removal of my other tube and ovary.
Now I am on Premarin. I'm afraid that I have lost my personality
with my organs. I hate taking hormones and I wish I had never
heard of PID.*

—A.I., Hampton, Virginia

As a result of the growing number of "silent" infections caused by
the rampant spread of sexually transmitted diseases such as chlamydia, pelvic inflammatory disease (PID) is seen with much greater
frequency today than it was a few years ago. Many women like Ms.
I. are given inadequate antibiotic treatments and their infections
become more severe. Organs abscess and women end up on operating tables losing their wombs.

Modern combinations of antibiotics can effectively fight PID, but
doctors must be informed of these combinations in order to administer them. Ms. I.'s doctor gave her tetracycline, which is not enough
to conquer PID. Tetracycline is used to treat superficial vaginal
infections, but it is powerless against deep-seated, extensive pelvic
inflammatory disease.

PID is best treated with a so-called triple therapy, a combination
of three powerful antibiotics administered intravenously. One
woman wrote to me that she overcame her PID after she was given
intravenous triple therapy comprised of ampicillin, Cleocin (clin-
domycin), and Garamycin (gentamicin sulfate). In this way she
avoided a hysterectomy and she is now the proud mother of a son.

Knowledgeable physicians who are associated with large medical
centers and teaching hospitals are currently informed about the latest antibiotic therapies for PID. Obviously, Ms. I.'s doctor did not
have the newest information, but her case is not unusual. I have

frequently seen young women in their twenties who have had complete "pelvic cleanouts" in which all their organs were removed to cure PID. Women must ask for the proper antibiotic therapy for PID if their physicians tell them that hysterectomy is the only way to find relief. If a doctor does not respond to a woman's suggestion, she should seek a second opinion.

Ms. I. is now faced with a future that must include hormone replacement therapy as part of her daily life, when most likely her surgery could have been entirely avoided. Her experience should not have to be relived by other women. A woman who is suffering with PID should seek out a doctor who knows how to treat the disease.

Before Giving Informed Consent

Many women who undergo hysterectomies for necessary reasons feel better after their surgeries, but as the preceding letters show, many times women feel robbed of their organs, frustrated, and depressed after their operations. If only they could be given second chances to make new decisions. . . .

Women who are told they need hysterectomies should always hesitate before they say yes to surgery. All patients are asked to sign an *informed consent* before surgery. A doctor might request that the form be signed either in his office or in the hospital after a woman has been admitted. Before signing, a woman should research her gynecological problem in health books and magazines and she should get a second opinion. Local women's health groups, health collectives, or the closest chapter of Planned Parenthood might be able to recommend trustworthy physicians.

A woman should read an informed consent carefully, and she should grant her permission to remove only diseased organs. She should never sign away her organs until her own instincts, her friends, her loved ones, and at least two doctors have told her that she has no other choice.

DILATATION AND CURETTAGE (D & C)

One out of seven women will have a D & C—opening of the cervix and scraping of the uterine lining—during her lifetime. Dilatation and curettage, D & C, is performed even more frequently than hysterectomy. In the past, D & C has been referred to as the "bread and butter" of the gynecologist because the procedure used to be performed on practically every woman who had a little irregular bleeding.

Women who have signs of abnormal bleeding usually visit their doctors to find out whether they need D & Cs. A D & C might be indicated if a woman experiences irregular menstrual bleeding or spotting after intercourse or between periods. This abnormal bleeding might be occurring because there is an excessive amount of tissue built up in the uterine cavity; in other words, the endometrium—the uterine lining—has become unusually thick. At the extreme, an overgrown uterine lining, a condition called *endometrial hyperplasia*, might develop and possibly might change into *adenomatous hyperplasia*, a potentially precancerous condition described in a preceding section on hysterectomy (pages 666 to 668).

Bleeding might also be the result of irregularities in the uterine cavity due to submucous fibroids or endometrial polyps. Polyps, which are usually benign, can become irritated and bleed during exercise or intercourse. (Endometriosis might cause irregular bleeding, but as discussed below, this condition cannot be cured by a D & C.)

A D & C might also be used as a routine diagnostic procedure to monitor the uterine linings of women who are taking hormone medication or to screen women who are bleeding during or after menopause. Bleeding after change-of-life could be an early sign of cancer. In addition, a D & C might be necessary to remove any tissue left behind after a miscarriage or to dislodge an IUD that has become imbedded within the uterine wall.

All the above situations offer legitimate reasons to perform D & Cs, but researchers are finding that a young or perimenopausal woman who bleeds irregularly is usually experiencing dysfunctional bleeding due to a hormonal imbalance, a condition that can only be treated medically, not with a D & C.

If a woman is bleeding profusely, it is fairly certain that she is suffering from a physical problem such as fibroid tumors, endometrial polyps, or uterine hyperplasia; a D & C might help her. On the other hand, prolonged scanty bleeding is more likely due to a hormonal imbalance than to a buildup of uterine tissue. Today, doctors have a greater understanding of the endocrine system and they are able to measure hormonal levels in the body. A woman can be tested for a hormonal imbalance through a Pap smear or a blood test, and if such a condition exists, she might be treated with birth control pills or progesterone tablets. It is useless to perform a D & C on a woman with dysfunctional bleeding due to a hormonal imbalance, because she has no excess tissue to remove during a scraping.

If a woman's doctor tells her that she needs a D & C, she should not be reluctant to ask him why. As mentioned, there are very real reasons for doing D & Cs. Some women cannot become pregnant before they have D & Cs because their uterine linings are so thick that childbearing is prevented. A woman who spots between periods or has very heavy periods might be harboring an excessive amount of uterine lining and she might need a D & C. However, a woman who notices minimal bleeding, light spotting on and off, probably has a hormonal imbalance that can be corrected with medication and she does not need a D & C. A woman should always ask questions, and if a doctor does not give satisfactory answers, she should seek a second opinion. Often it helps to have a friend or a relative present during consultation with the doctor. Sometimes another person has a different perspective on what the doctor is saying and is able to ask objective questions.

When a woman learns that her condition definitely requires a D & C, she might inquire about whether her doctor could perform a suction curettage or a mini D & C, also called a Vabra aspiration, in his office. With an office procedure she will save money and eliminate the ordeal of hospitalization. A woman who has suffered an incomplete miscarriage or a woman who is experiencing bleeding after an abortion can especially benefit from suction curettage in a doctor's office that is equipped for such a procedure.

Usually only local anesthesia is needed during a suction curettage. The doctor inserts a suction curette—a small, hollow catheter—through the cervix into the uterus. Vacuum pressure applied to the curette creates suction and the excess uterine tissue is removed as the physician gently rotates the instrument inside the uterus.

In contrast, a D & C performed in the hospital usually is conducted under general anesthesia and costs about $1,000. Although health insurance often covers the bill, general anesthesia adds more than cost; it increases the risk of surgery. General anesthesia can cause complications that make a hospital D & C a potentially dangerous procedure. My observation is that anesthesia deaths often occur during common procedures like D & Cs, rather than during intricate major surgeries. The reason for the higher fatality rates during the simpler operations, I think, is that anesthesiologists are less attentive when minor procedures are being performed on healthy people.

When a woman must have a hospital D & C, after she is anesthetized the doctor enlarges her cervical opening by inserting a series of smooth metal rods called dilators, each one larger in diameter than the one preceding it. When the cervix is sufficiently opened, the physician introduces a curette, a metal rod with a spoonlike scraping edge that is especially molded to remove the uterine lining (see figure 5-5, page 133). A D & C can be a one-day hospital procedure, and if all goes smoothly, a woman does not have to stay overnight; in fact, many hospitals now have outpatient facilities for minor surgeries such as D & Cs.

As mentioned before, a D & C is not always without complication. A doctor can, for example, perforate the uterus or lacerate the cervix, two injuries that could result in internal bleeding. If the doctor, during such complications, judges that no organs have been damaged, he might just observe his patient to make sure that her vital signs remain stable and that no abnormalities surface. A hysterectomy should not be a doctor's first thought after a uterine perforation or a cervical laceration. In fact, one question a woman might ask her doctor before she agrees to a D & C is how he would handle a perforated uterus or other complications.

QUESTIONS ABOUT D & C

I Have Irregular Spotting Throughout the Month; Do I Need a D & C?

I do not bleed heavily, but I have had spotting throughout the month for the last five months. The bleeding comes at different times, not just the middle of the month when it would be from my ovulation. I have been under a lot of stress with a new job in a new state and my doctor—my former doctor from my previous residence—tells me that I will be fine once I have adjusted. The bleeding has become so annoying, though. I always wear tampons because I'm never sure when I'll be spotting. I'd like to do something to stop the flow. Do you think a D & C would help?
—K.N., Fort Worth, Texas

Since Ms. N. has spotting in between her periods, she is experiencing dysfunctional bleeding due to a hormonal imbalance. Estrogen and progesterone should increase in the last two weeks of her menstrual cycle, causing the uterus to relax and the uterine lining to thicken. When estrogen and progesterone diminish sooner than expected in the menstrual cycle, the uterine lining stops developing and begins to shed itself. The lining, however, has not had sufficient hormonal stimulation to build itself up, so the sloughed-off endometrium creates a light, spotty flow. This hormonally induced abnormal bleeding cannot be cured with a D & C.

Treatment with progesterone medication such as Provera, 10 mg twice a day for five to ten days, might bring her relief. Progesterone will alter her uterine environment, settle any uterine contractions, and halt the bleeding. After she ends her course of medication she will begin to bleed again. Such a treatment might also reset her hormonal fluctuation and make her periods regular again.

I Had a Few D & Cs and Now I'm Told I Need a Hysterectomy

I am thirty-eight years old. Two years ago I had an ectopic pregnancy and one tube and an ovary were removed. I've been bleeding heavily ever since. My doctor performed a D & C, but the bleeding didn't stop. Then he gave me two different kinds of hormones and another D & C, but the bleeding still continued. Finally, I had a third D & C and my blood pressure rose so high the doctor sent me to an internist. My blood pressure has been lowered, but I still bleed almost every day. Now my doctor thinks that my remaining ovary is just dysfunctional and I need a hysterectomy to remove my uterus, tube, and ovary. I am in great discomfort, but I don't want a hysterectomy. Do I need yet another D & C?

—I.C., Loveland, Colorado

Ms. C.'s period might be managed with hormone medication. Since she is only thirty-eight, she could take birth control pills for a few months to try to regulate her cycle, or she might be given a cyclic estrogen/progesterone combination. Ms. C does not mention her weight, but if she is overweight, the estrogen produced by her body's excess fatty tissue could be contributing to her heavy flow. If extra pounds are a problem she should try to eat a proper diet and slim down. Also, daily vitamins, especially vitamin B_6, might aid her attempt to change her condition.

Most likely, Ms. C. has dysfunctional bleeding and a D & C would not be helpful. However, if none of the aforementioned suggestions change her condition and her bleeding cannot be controlled, she might be advised to have a hysterectomy. Should a hysterectomy be the only way to cure her condition, she should not allow her remaining ovary to be removed during the surgery. At thirty-eight years old, Ms. C. is too young to have to experience the menopausal symptoms that would be likely to arise once her ovary has been excised.

I've Had Heavy Bleeding Since My Tubes Were Tied; Do I Need a D & C?

Before my tubal ligation, my period was eight days long and heavy for four of those days. Since I had my tubes tied three years ago, I've had a fifteen-day period with seven heavy days. I'm nervous and depressed even after my period is over, I think maybe I need a D & C, but my doctor doesn't listen to me.
—Y.E., Yardley, Pennsylvania

As explained in chapter 12, after tubal sterilization women sometimes experience irregular bleeding. Sometimes too large an area of a tube is severed or burned during sterilization and the blood supply to the ovary is impaired. An irregular blood supply causes a hormonal imbalance that brings on abnormal bleeding. Ms. E. now has heavy bleeding and symptoms of premenstrual syndrome, but her early menstrual history shows her to have had heavy bleeding as a younger woman. She might have had a hormonal imbalance before her surgery and now her imbalance might be all the more aggravated. A D & C will probably not help her.

I have seen many women undergo D & C after D & C for heavy bleeding after tubal sterilizations. These women sometimes end up with hysterectomies that could have been avoided if they had not had their tubes tied.

If Ms. E. is under thirty-five, birth control pills for a few months might help to regulate her cycle. After she stops the pills, her problem might be gone. If abnormal bleeding continues after the pill, then she might be helped by Danocrine (danazol), Lupron, or Synarel. Taken for a few months, one of these medications might shrink her uterine lining and reduce the size of her ovaries. Her organs will receive a "pelvic rest," and after the treatment her bleeding might be diminished and her cycle should be regulated.

Should all medical treatments appear ineffective, a D & C might have to be advised, but Ms. E. should seek a second opinion on the procedure. A D & C can cause great frustration when it is performed unnecessarily.

LAPAROSCOPY, THE BAND-AID PROCEDURE

A laparoscopy, a surgical procedure used for both diagnostic and therapeutic purposes, sometimes helps to avert major surgery. During a laparoscopy, an electrically lighted tubular instrument, a laparoscope, is inserted into a woman's abdomen through a small incision in her navel. This procedure is usually conducted under general anesthesia, but it can be done using local anesthesia combined with an analgesic. The local anesthetic is given before the doctor makes the tiny incision, which is later covered by a Band-Aid.

By looking through a laparoscope, which is really a medical periscope, a doctor can view a woman's internal organs and attempt to diagnose a pelvic problem she might have. Pelvic pain, the presence of ovarian cysts, or infertility can provide good reason for a doctor to perform a laparoscopy. If during the procedure a doctor notices any abnormalities of the ovaries or the tubes, he can insert a needle through the hollow laparoscope and aspirate or remove biopsy sample cells from these organs. (It is interesting to note that aspiration during laparoscopy is also the technique used to extract an egg from an ovary for in vitro fertilization.)

A laparoscopy is often used to identify endometriosis, which is sometimes difficult to diagnose. Endometrial growth can be located behind the uterus on the ligaments, or it can be hidden inside tissue. A physician has to be dexterous and skillful to find it. He must position the scope underneath the uterus to view the buried endometriosis. However, many physicians are not adept at using a laparoscope. A woman might undergo a laparoscopy and wake up after the surgery without a diagnosis of endometriosis when she, indeed, has the disease. It is also possible that instead of solving a pelvic problem

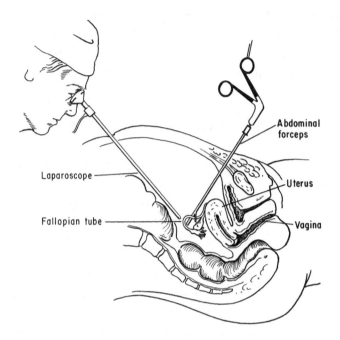

17-2 **Laparoscopy.** A laparoscopy, also referred to as a Band-Aid procedure, is an operation in which a surgeon inserts a laparoscope (an electrically lighted surgical periscope) through a tiny incision in a woman's abdomen after her abdominal cavity has been distended (expanded with the aid of carbon dioxide). The doctor can view a woman's internal organs through the laparoscope to determine whether there are any abnormalities such as pelvic adhesions or endometriosis. Through an accompanying small incision, a doctor can insert tubal forceps or other helpful surgical instruments. Minor operations for removal of adhesions, biopsies, and tubal sterilizations can be performed with the use of these surgical tools. In the drawing, tubal forceps are being used to grasp a Fallopian tube.

a doctor might create one by jabbing the instrument into the bowel or by damaging or burning the intestines or other internal organs during cauterization. When executed correctly, however, a laparoscopy is an important technique for helping a gynecologist evaluate pelvic disorders and sparing a woman a longer, more involved operation.

When used as a therapeutic measure, laparoscopy has refined the art of tubal sterilization. Gaining a direct view through a laparoscope, a doctor can lift a Fallopian tube and either graft, cauterize, or place a ring on the tube to prevent conception from occurring.

Infertility surgeons are using laparoscopy in conjunction with very fine instruments that make sterilization a much less scarring procedure. Older doctors who are less skilled in the current method of tubal sterilization through laparoscopy might awkwardly perform the procedure. It is not unusual to see a woman who has had a laparoscope inserted into an unsightly incision made between the pubic hair and the navel. Since a medical instrument is being guided into and out of the incision, sometimes the opening becomes irregular and heals into an unattractive scar.

This unnecessary scarring is unfortunate because a woman will carry a mark that shows she has been "fixed" forever.

When a woman has been advised to undergo a laparoscopy, she should ask her doctor if he intends to make the incision deep inside her navel to avoid scarring. I perform many laparoscopies, and I usually make the horizontal incision about a quarter of an inch across the deepest inner recess of the navel. When the incision heals, there is no visible scar. If a woman's doctor tells her that he plans to operate through an obvious abdominal incision, she should consult a physician who is more skillful.

The laparoscopy has been very important in advancing women's health care, but even so, the procedure can be performed unnecessarily. Sometimes a woman who is suffering with pelvic pain could be diagnosed as having a pelvic infection or pelvic endometriosis from her symptoms without the need of a laparoscopy. Before agreeing to a laparoscopy, a woman who has the slightest doubt about whether she really needs the procedure should get a second opinion.

QUESTIONS ABOUT LAPAROSCOPY

Do I Need a Second-Look Laparoscopy?

Six months ago I underwent a laparoscopy to see if I had endometriosis and to what extent it existed. The doctor determined that I had endometriosis on the bowel, ovaries, and behind my uterus,

but he said that I did not have a bad case. He put me on Danocrine
for six months and told me that he might "take another look" when
I finish with the medicine. Do I need this second-look laparoscopy?
I don't want to submit to another dose of anesthesia if I don't
absolutely have to. Is there any other way he can tell if the
endometriosis is gone?

—B.F., Somerville, Massachusetts

Ms. F. seems to have received proper treatment. Her physician performed a laparoscopy to diagnose her endometriosis and now she is on Danocrine. She should stay on the medication for six to nine months, after which her doctor should perform a pelvic examination to determine the state of her endometriosis. He should be able to tell on examination whether the disease has diminished and her organs are healthy without the aid of a laparoscopy.

If Ms. F. wants to conceive, she might be advised to have a hysterosalpingogram—an X ray of her uterus—after Danocrine treatment. If the hysterosalpingogram shows that her tubes are open, she should try to conceive. After six months, if she is still not pregnant, her doctor might recommend another laparoscopy followed by microsurgery to free pelvic adhesion, should any be diagnosed during the laparoscopy. After surgery she might be placed on Danocrine for a few months to increase her fertility when she stops the medication.

If Ms. F. does not want to become pregnant, she might be placed on the birth control pill as a deterrent to the return of endometriosis.

I Have an Ovarian Cyst; Is a Laparoscopy Necessary?

I am twenty-seven years old. Recently my doctor discovered an
ovarian cyst that he said could be dangerous. He wants to do a
laparoscopy, but I'm leery of the procedure. I've read that cysts
might disappear by themselves and I'm wondering if I should wait
and avoid surgery. Do you think a second opinion would help?

—E.S., Sunnyvale, California

It is very possible that this young woman has a functional ovarian cyst that might disappear in a month or two. Her doctor should wait until she has completed at least two menstrual cycles, and if the cyst does not go away he should then evaluate it through ultrasonography. Depending on what he sees on a sonogram, a doctor might elect to put Ms. S. on birth control pills for a few months to reduce her cyst.

If Ms. S.'s cyst persists in spite of this treatment, a laparoscopy could be called for to allow the doctor to view the growth directly. He can then decide whether it is a dermoid, endometrial, or solid cyst. During a laparoscopy he can even aspirate cells from the cyst for lab analysis.

Thus, a thorough laparoscopy is not immediately necessary to the treatment of an ovarian cyst, but it certainly is a valuable diagnostic procedure to be used when an ovarian cyst lingers. Ms. S. might ask her doctor to see if her cyst will respond to alternate treatments before he attempts a laparoscopy. If he insists that a laparoscopy must be done right away, then she would be wise to consult with a second-opinion doctor.

UTERINE SUSPENSION AND THE TILTED UTERUS

A tilted, also called retroverted, uterus is a normal biological occurrence, a genetic trait like an inverted nipple. In the past when a doctor discovered that a woman had a tilted uterus he tended to make an issue of his finding. Patients with tilted uteri were routinely convinced that they needed surgery—*uterine suspensions*—to have their uteri turned forward to enable them to bear children.

However, a uterine suspension is a major surgical procedure. During an exploratory laparotomy, the surgeon lifts the uterus into its correct position by shortening the ligaments that hold the uterus in place. A uterine suspension usually requires seven days in the hospital and four to eight weeks for recovery.

Today we know that if a woman has a tilted uterus her mother probably has one too, and the mother did conceive the daughter. If no abnormality is diagnosed in connection with a tilted uterus, a woman has no cause for concern. A *tilted uterus will not result in infertility unless it has been moved backward by endometriosis or pelvic infections.* A uterine suspension might be advised if such underlying problems are pulling a uterus out of position and harming the tubes. If a doctor blames a woman's infertility on a tilted uterus alone, she should seek a second opinion. A uterine suspension to move the womb forward will not change a woman's ability to bear a child if a tilted uterus is her only problem. Only when a pelvic disorder such as endometriosis is tilting the uterus should a uterine suspension be indicated.

The Doctor Moved My Uterus and I Miscarried

I had delivered two children by natural childbirth. During my third pregnancy I went to a new doctor, a physician at a clinic. The doctor said my uterus was retroverted, which I already knew, but he said it was too far back and would have to be moved forward. I didn't want him to move my uterus, but he did it anyway. The pain was unbearable. I could hardly walk from the car when I got home and that night I bled and bled. When I went back to the doctor he turned my uterus some more and I bled more heavily. Finally I had to be put into the hospital for a D & C after a miscarriage at fifteen weeks of pregnancy. I have not been the same since.

—W.W., Lake Forest, Illinois

This woman was mistreated. She had no problem with a tilted uterus. She had previously given birth to two children with apparently no problem, and obviously, since she was already pregnant, she had no difficulties conceiving. There are too many misconceptions about the tilted uterus. A woman who is born with a tilted uterus like her mother's must believe that she has no abnormality or need for surgery. Anyone who tells her that it will be difficult for her to become pregnant and deliver her baby is wrong.

Mismanagement of Ms. W.'s case was probably the cause of her miscarriage. It seems that the doctor pushed her uterus too hard with his fingers and thus probably stimulated the miscarriage. A tilted uterus requires medical attention only when it has been pulled backward by endometriosis or other pelvic disorders. If a woman is advised to have surgery for a tilted uterus, she should certainly seek a second opinion.

THE CONE BIOPSY AND CERVICAL CANCER

During a cone biopsy, a surgical procedure performed through the vagina, an outer cone-shaped portion of the cervix is removed. If a woman's Pap test (described on pages 687 to 691) has indicated a Number 5, it could mean *carcinoma in situ,* an early, localized stage of precancer that is found on the surface of the cervix but not deep within the tissue. A colposcopy, as described below, is indicated to carefully view the cervix. If any abnormal tissue is seen, multiple cervical biopsies should be obtained to determine whether the lesion is benign or malignant. If the biopsies are negative and the Pap smear remains abnormal, cells might be located deep within the tissue and a cone biopsy might be recommended. Carcinoma in situ shows up before cancer starts to spread. In a situation in which a woman with carcinoma in situ has completed her family, *a hysterectomy might be advised to assure the arrest of the cancer.* A woman who wants to remain fertile and objects to a hysterectomy can be treated with a cone biopsy. She will subsequently need a Pap smear two to three times a year.

A cone biopsy is major surgery conducted with the patient under general anesthesia. There is a concentrated blood supply in the cervix that can cause extreme bleeding during the operation. A cone biopsy is more intricate than one might think. A patient usually stays in the hospital two to three days. After the surgery a woman must avoid sexual intercourse for several weeks. Approximately ten to fourteen days after the operation the sutures begin to disintegrate. Before that, sexual activity might tear the sutures and the surgical incision, which has not had time to heal, might begin to hemorrhage; this bleeding might even happen spontaneously if a woman is too physically active. Hemorrhaging causes many women to be readmitted to the hospital for resuturing of the cervix after their cone biopsies. It might take up to three or four weeks to completely recover from a cone biopsy. During this time, intermittent bleeding might be expected.

If a Pap smear has indicated *cervical dysplasia*—a collection of abnormal cells on the cervix—a doctor might emphasize that he must proceed with a cone biopsy. Whether a cone biopsy would be the treatment is this case is debatable.

A cone biopsy is not always called for in the case of cervical dysplasia, which can range from mild to severe. Rather than agreeing to a cone biopsy for this condition, a woman should seek a second-opinion doctor who will perform a colposcopy followed by a cervical biopsy. A colposcopy is an examination with a colposcope, a magnifying instrument that enables a doctor to pinpoint the area of abnormal cell growth. By staining the cervix with acetic acid and viewing the cervix through the colposcope, a doctor can identify any dysplastic cells and know exactly where to perform a biopsy. Cells might be either punched out or scraped for laboratory analysis.

If the pathology report indicates that the dysplasia has advanced to the point of carcinoma in situ, a woman, depending on her age and her desire to have children, might be treated with a hysterectomy or a cone biopsy. However, there are various stages of cervical dysplasia that are not nearly as severe as carcinoma in situ, truly a condition unto itself.

Cervical dysplasia is not cancer; it is merely a sign that all cells are not perfectly normal. The dysplastic cells, after they are clearly classified through pathological testing, might be treated by either laser surgery, cryosurgery, or electrocautery, techniques described at the end of this section.

Considering the range of diagnoses that can result from colposcopy and cervical biopsy, a woman should not allow herself to be pushed into having a cone biopsy. She might seek a second opinion from a gynecological oncologist, a doctor who specializes in the treatment of gynecological cancers. A dysplasia is not cancer, but a gynecological oncologist knows how to treat this condition and it is most likely that he will recommend colposcopy and cervical biopsy to start.

To find a good gynecological oncologist a woman might contact her local chapter of the American Cancer Society or she might ask for referrals from the physician referral services of a well-known cancer center such as Sloan-Kettering Memorial Hospital in New York or M. D. Anderson Hospital in Dallas, Texas. A woman who learns that she has a Class 2 Pap test indicating cervical dysplasia should resist the recommendation of a doctor who automatically tells her she must have a cone biopsy. Before she submits to any surgery she must know the degree of her problem.

HOW A PAP TEST SIGNALS TROUBLE

A Pap test can identify cervical cancer that is perhaps ten years away. But when Dr. George N. Papanicolaou, father of the Pap test, first began to lecture on his method of cancer detection he was laughed at. It was the 1920s and no one believed that any sort of test could discover a cancer before it occurred. Yet Dr. Papanicolaou determinedly continued his cell studies in his laboratory at New York Hospital–Cornell Medical Center. By taking a small swab or scraping from the cervix—the mouth of the womb-staining the cell sample with his special solution, and viewing it under a microscope, he was able to differentiate normal and abnormal cells. After examining cervical cells from many, many women, Dr. Papanicolaou realized that he saw cell patterns that could indicate inflammation and vaginal infections, but he also noticed cell changes that warranted observation. After following the women with the cell changes for several years, he watched the cells develop into cervical cancer.

PAP TEST

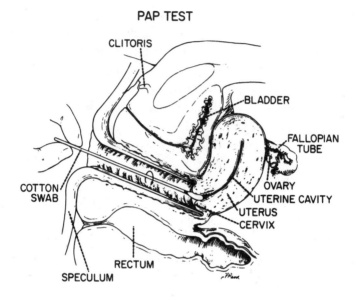

17-3 **The Pap Test.** The drawing depicts a cross-section of a woman's reproductive organs. To obtain a smear from the cervical canal during a Pap test, a doctor opens the vagina with a speculum, visualizes the cervix, inserts a cotton swab into the cervical canal, and rotates the swab, as illustrated in the drawing. A few cells from inside the cervix will adhere to the swab. These endocervical cells are transferred to a glass plate that is sent to a lab for analysis.

The Pap test started to become a routine part of a woman's gynecological checkup in the fifties, and since then the number of female deaths from cervical cancer has dropped by 70 percent. Dr. Papanicolaou has tremendously improved the health of all women, and I would always feel proud of my profession when I saw his name on old charts in the laboratory where I was trained in New York Hospital.

An estimated 16,000 cases of cervical cancer are discovered every year in the United States. Still, 5,000 deaths occur annually, and really, with the Pap test it is tragic that any woman would die from cervical cancer. When detected early through a Pap test, cervical cancer can be cured almost 100 percent of the time. Women must continue to have regular Pap smears.

PAP TEST

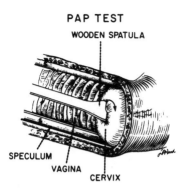

WOODEN SPATULA

SPECULUM

VAGINA

CERVIX

17-4 **The Pap Test.** During a Pap test a doctor will obtain a swabbed sample from inside the cervix, as illustrated in figure 17-3. A physician will also obtain a scraping from outside the cervix, as illustrated in the above drawing. During this stage of the Pap test, a wooden spatula is inserted into the vagina and gently pressed against the cervix. As the spatula is rotated, a few cervical cells will adhere. The spatula is then removed from the vagina. The extracted cells are smeared onto a glass slide that is sent to a lab for analysis.

The cause of cervical cancer is still not known, but a number of factors have been linked to development of the disease. There seems to be a high incidence of cervical cancer among women who became sexually active at young ages, at least before they were twenty, among women who have had multiple sex partners, and among women who have given birth when they were in their teens or early twenties. Infection with certain strains of the human papillomavirus (HPV), which leads to genital warts, is strongly linked to cervical cancer. Every so often a new cervical cancer association arises. At one time it was thought that women who had sexual intercourse with uncircumcised men were at higher-than-average risk of developing cervical cancer, but this theory is no longer held. However, it seems that the bottom line is that every sexually active woman has a chance of developing cervical cancer.

The drastic reduction in cervical cancer since the fifties gives me reason to support the annual Pap smear. I would suggest that women continue to have yearly Pap tests, and in fact, I believe that women

who are sexually active with more than one partner, or women who
have had an abnormal Pap test, should have Pap smears every six
months.

Classification of Pap Test

Besides detecting abnormal cells, a Pap test also spots inflammation and infections. The result of a Pap smear analysis is classified
according to degree of cell abnormality:

The five-point Bethesda System of grading Pap smears starts at
Number 1 for normal and goes to *Number 5* for carcinoma in situ, a
cervical cancer that has not spread.

The confusing *Number 2,* atypical squamous cells of uncertain
significance (ASCUS), or low-grade squamous intraepithelial lesions
(LSIL), might be from inflammation due to an infection such as
yeast or chlamydia, or might indicate a mild dysplasia (the presence
of abnormal cells that might be precancerous). Most of the time
these mild abnormalites disappear on their own. A physician might
want to perform an colposcopy examination of a woman's cervix
through a special well-lit magnifying instrument called a colposcope
and/or perform a cervical biopsy; on the other hand, he might simply suggest a repeat Pap smear in six months.

When a woman has a *Number 3 or 4* result that shows high-grade
squamous intraepithelial lesions (HSIL) or cervical dysplasia (abnormal cells that are likely to be precancerous), a colposcopy and
cervical biopsy are musts.

Number 5 indicates carcinoma in situ (CIS), cancerous cells on
the surface of the cervix, or the presence of a more serious invasive
cancer. A woman should undergo an immediate cervical biopsy. If
carcinoma in situ is found, a cone biopsy or a hysterectomy would be
indicated. If invasive carcinoma is diagnosed under cervical biopsy, a
woman should be referred for treatment to a gynecological oncologist, a doctor who specializes in gynecological cancer. Knowing the
latest cancer therapies, a gynecological oncologist, after learning the
results of her biopsy, will be able to wisely advise a woman.

A woman should understand Pap test classifications and not become so alarmed when she learns that she has something other than Number 1 that she agrees to major surgery without consulting a specialist. Only unquestionable cancer requires radical treatment.

New Technology to Sharpen the Pap Test's Accuracy

Technological advances have led researchers to develop ways of improving the accuracy of the classic Pap test. These techniques are still new, more costly, and might not be covered by health insurance.

The *ThinPrep* Pap test is a new method of collecting and preparing cervical cells to make microscopic readings easier for technicians. ThinPrep readings are somewhat more accurate than traditional readings, but a woman's health insurance might not cover the ThinPrep. Collected cells from a Pap smear are not spread directly onto a slide; instead, the swab with the cells is rinsed in a vial of preservative solution. This solution suspends the cells and separates them from blood, mucus, and other materials. Then a thin, even, layer is prepared on a slide from the clean cells in suspension.

PAPNET and *AutoPap* are computerized rescreening methods for Pap tests. Although each depends on a different technology, they both are designed to help give a second, more accurate reading of abnormal cells. The value of these methods over manual rescreening, which has always been done, is still being debated. Automated microscopes scan the cell slides in conjunction with computer programs that help identify abnormal cells.

QUESTIONS ABOUT THE CONE BIOPSY

Did I Really Need a Cone Biopsy?

I went to my doctor for a pain I have in my lower right side ten days to two weeks before my period. The doctor did a smear and put me on intravenous antibiotics for several days in the hospital. After

I got home I still had the pain so I went to a health care clinic for a second opinion. The gynecologist at the clinic did another Pap smear and gave me cream for a vaginal infection. The smear showed that I had bad cells in my cervix, but the doctor said not to worry and he put me on antibiotics for more than a month. Then another letter from the clinic said that my smear really showed the start of cancer. I showed this letter to a third gynecologist, who put me in the hospital to perform tests, he said. Later he told me he had done a cone biopsy and he would let me know if I needed a hysterectomy. Thank God I didn't have to have a hysterectomy, because I am only twenty and someday I want to have children. Right now my Pap smears are always normal, but the pain that originally sent me to a doctor has never gone away. I feel that since two letters said two different things, maybe I didn't have cancer. I still have my pain and I would like your opinion as to whether I really needed that cone biopsy.

—J.A., Waterbury, Connecticut

Rarely does a twenty-year-old woman need a cone biopsy. This woman went for second and third opinions and still ended up with what was probably unnecessary surgery. Her experience reinforces my belief that women must research and understand their individual health problems while they are consulting with doctors. Also, Ms. A.'s additional physician consultation should have been with a gynecological oncologist after she was given word that her Pap test might have detected cancerous cells.

Sometimes laboratory tests are interpreted differently by different labs. Ms. A.'s letter leads me to believe that two different pathologists examined her smear and classified their results, which did not match, at separate times. Then she received two letters. The discrepancy that might arise in determining the results of a Pap test offers yet another reason for women to have annual Pap smears. What is normal one year might be abnormal the next.

As for Ms. A., she should have been treated with a colposcopy examination and a cervical biopsy to determine the extent of her problem. Once her condition was known, the next appropriate treatment could have been advised. Now she has lost part of her cervix, which could make her more vulnerable to miscarriage or premature birth.

Her pain was never cured, but her symptoms compare to symptoms of endometriosis. Since antibiotics were ineffective against the pain, endometriosis, which does not respond to these drugs, might very well be her problem. A skillful physician could perform a laparoscopy to look for endometriosis, and if he is able to diagnose the disease, he could administer Danocrine, Lupron, or Synarel to dissolve the endometrial growths (see chapter 7).

In sharing her experience, Ms. A. has done all women a service. She has shown that a woman must add her own researched knowledge of her health problem to her doctor's advice in order to receive optimum care.

My Doctor Saved Me from a Cone Biopsy

I was told I had a Number 3 Pap smear. My doctor examined me with a colposcope and said my cervix was clean. The lesion, he said, was probably inside my cervix and the only way to get it out would be with a cone biopsy. I got scared and went to another doctor. He looked at me during a colposcopy and said my cervix showed nothing. Then he told me that high on the inside of the cervix there was an area of tissue that could be the problem. He did something called an endocervical curettage in his office. I had local anesthesia and he scraped away all the tissue. My Pap smears have been normal since, and I want this doctor to be my physician for life. He saved me from a cone biopsy and I have great faith that he will always take good care of me.

—G.C., Linwood, New Jersey

Cervical cancer frequently develops in the squamous columnar junction, an area where the other cells meet the inner cells high on the inside of the cervical canal, the opening that leads from the vagina to the uterus. This passage is also called the *endocervix*. When Ms. C. had an *endocervical curettage*, she underwent a procedure in which the cells inside the endocervical canal were removed by gently scraping them as would be done during a D & C.

Ms. C.'s first doctor apparently did not consider the possibility of a lesion in the squamous columnar junction, but her second doctor did. Ms. C. could have had a cone biopsy without reason. From now on, she knows that if her Pap smear indicates an abnormality, she can undergo another endocervical curettage. A second opinion saved her from major surgery. She was able to walk out of her doctor's office instead of having to spend days in the hospital and weeks of recovery.

Modern Treatment of Cervical Dysplasia

If a Pap test shows that a woman has the cell changes associated with cervical dysplasia, and a coloposcopy and cervical biopsy reveal *severe* dysplasia verging on early malignancy, a cone biopsy might be called for to remove the outer abnormal portion of the cervix. However, if a doctor performs a colposcopy, sees an area of abnormal cells, undertakes a cervical biopsy, and learns that a woman has *mild to moderate* dysplasia, he has a choice of treatment.

Laser Surgery. There are no long-term studies available yet on laser surgery because it is so new, but it looks promising and some-day might become the treatment of choice for cervical dysplasia. The laser is a concentrated beam of light that replaces the scalpel as a surgical tool. After a doctor has positioned a speculum in a woman's vagina, he focuses the laser beam on the abnormal cells on the surface of the cervix. The water in the body's cells actually absorbs the high-intensity beam. Cells vaporize when they are the target of a laser. The laser also cauterizes and seals off blood vessels to prevent bleeding during a surgical procedure. The laser technique for removing dysplastic cells on the cervix takes four to fifteen minutes in a doctor's office, and patients who have undergone the treatment report little or no pain. Healthy normal cells seem to regenerate faster with laser surgery than with cryosurgery or electrocautery. There seem to be no noticeable complications and women have healed in three weeks.

Since it is new, laser surgery is controversial. Some physicians claim it is no better than the standard treatments, cryosurgery and electrocautery, while other doctors boast of great success. If a woman's doctor suggests laser surgery as a treatment for her cervical dysplasia, he is offering her one of the most modern techniques in medicine. However, laser beams are extremely powerful and penetrating and could cause more damage than good in the hands of an unskilled laser surgeon.

Cryosurgery. Cryosurgery is a surgical procedure in which the outer cervical cells are destroyed through a freezing technique. During the procedure a doctor situates the speculum in a woman's vagina in order to view the cervix. He then places a cryosurgical probe against the cervix and freezes the area. The frozen tissue eventually dies, sheds itself, and is replaced by new healthy tissue when cryosurgery succeeds. Often, however, women have reported recurrences of cervical erosions and dysplasia after being treated with cryosurgery. It is thought that cervical erosion is sometimes due to abnormal pH in the vaginal environment. Therefore, cryosurgery, which is usually somewhat painful, is not always curative and should be weighed carefully against other treatments. When cryosurgery is suggested as a treatment for cervical dysplasia, a woman might want to consult a second-opinion doctor.

Loop Electrosurgical Excision Procedure (LEEP). This technique is the latest electrosurgical method. A wire loop that has an electric current running through it becomes a knifelike surgical instrument that facilitates the removal of abnormal cells.

Electrocautery. During this procedure a woman is also on the examining table with the speculum placed within her vagina. An electrocauterizer applied to the cervix burns off the abnormal cells. Since it does not hurt to be cauterized on the cervix—there might be some cramping but there is no specific pain—anesthesia is not necessary. After the dysplastic cells are burned, they shed and are replaced by new, healthy cells. As with cryosurgery, however, elctro-cautery might not be a permanent cure. (Laser surgery has not been in use long enough to know whether its effectiveness is enduring.) Cervical dysplasia might return and treatment might have to be repeated. A woman who has cervical dysplasia might want a second-opinion doctor to help her decide the best treatment for her condition. Only if laser surgery, cryosurgery, and electrocautery fail to treat a moderate dysplastic lesion should a cone biopsy be considered.

CESAREAN SECTION: THE MOST COMMON MAJOR SURGERY IN THE UNITED STATES

For years, childbirth by cesarean section accounted for only 3 or 4 percent of all deliveries, but during the late 1960s a gradual increase began. Between 1968 and 1977, cesarean childbirths tripled, and in 1978 the national cesarean rate was 15.2 percent. By now, the rate has reached 21 percent of all deliveries, making cesarean section the number-one surgery in the United States. Why? "Fewer abnormal or damaged babies are being born," the doctors claimed in their defense. But is that entirely due to cesarean births? The question women have started to ask is, "Why are there so many cesareans?"

In 1979, the National Institute of Child Health and Human Development (NICHD) set out to answer the question by organiz-ing a task force to review childbirth by cesarean section. The task force published its report in 1980 and it is still valid today. The fig-ures showed that one of the major reasons for the increased inci-dence of cesarean births was a condition called *dystocia,* or CPD (cephalo-pelvic disproportion), the disproportionate size of a baby in relation to its mother's pelvis; in other words, it was judged that babies were too large for their mothers. Yet today's babies are really no bigger than babies were years ago. The difference is that today doctors are no longer performing difficult and dangerous forceps deliveries. The less traumatic cesarean birth has become the preferred procedure for dystocia.

Another reality the task force documented is that when a woman has one cesarean, she often ends up with repeat cesareans. Thirty-one percent of all cesarean births were repeat cesareans. The task force also found that 12 percent of cesareans are done for breech births and 5 percent for fetal distress. One look at the percentages showed that the increase in cesarean births could not be blamed on fetal monitoring, as many doctors and women had thought, but on new philosophies permeating obstetrical care. Still, one of the main frustrations facing women who undergo cesareans is that they are later told that subsequent children must also be delivered abdominally. Doctors used to abide by the credo "Once a cesarean, always a cesarean." This thinking, however, is changing. It is now becoming an accepted fact that a woman can have a safe vaginal delivery after a cesarean section. As doctors become more willing to practice vaginal deliveries after C-sections, one hopes the cesarean birth rate will begin to drop.

Since many of today's new mothers are older women subject to more medical problems than younger women, doctors want to guarantee healthy babies, and the result is more first-time cesarean deliveries. These women then increase the numbers of those who are candidates for repeat cesareans. The American College of Obstetricians and Gynecologists (ACOG) is supporting the recommendation that the increasing number of women who have had cesareans be allowed to deliver vaginally. A committee for the organization reviewed twenty-five studies in which more than 28,000 women who delivered vaginally had had previous C-sections. Based on its findings, ACOG recommends that *if a woman has previously had a low uterine incision for her cesarean, she can safely be allowed a vaginal delivery, providing that the difficulties that led to the first cesarean do not exist in the second delivery and that the woman goes into spontaneous labor.* If labor does not occur spontaneously, it is not advised that a woman who has had a C-section be induced. This change in approach to cesarean sections is now encouraged by doctors and hospitals.

There is a breed of obstetricians, the perinatologists, who specialize in delivering older women and women who have problematic pregnancies. Pregnant women can seek out perinatologists who are trained to guide women through high-risk pregnancies and natural deliveries. Also, a pregnant woman and her husband could question the woman's obstetrician about his attitude toward cesarean section well before the baby is due to arrive. If a doctor believes that a cesarean is always necessary after a woman has had a previous cesarean birth, then it would seem that he is advocating unnecessary surgery, since many of his pregnant patients would be able to deliver vaginally. A woman who encounters such a doctor might want to find a different obstetrician to guide her through her pregnancy. To avoid unnecessary cesarean sections, women must interview their doctors, research physicians' records for cesarean births, and choose the doctors who value the intention of every expectant mother who hopes to have natural childbirth.

QUESTIONS ABOUT CESAREAN SECTION

Is the Statement "Once a Cesarean, Always a Cesarean" True?

I had to have an emergency cesarean section with my first child. She was in a breech position and the doctor said that if I delivered her normally I would have run the risk of having her strangle on the umbilical cord. Now I am pregnant again and the doctor says I will always have to deliver by C-section. He also tells me that I might have to deliver in the eighth month because of the way the incision was made on my abdomen. He explained that he does not want to stress my scar or rupture my uterus. Is everything he tells me true? I want to deliver my baby naturally. Is the saying "Once a cesarean, always a cesarean" some kind of unwritten law?
                                                —M.J., Woodstock, New York

The saying "Once a cesarean, always a cesarean" was coined by Dr. Edward Cragin on Might 12, 1916, when he addressed the Eastern Medical Society in New York City. Dr. Cragin was a respected physician with Columbia Presbyterian Medical Center in New York, and his pronouncement was universally accepted by the obstetrical community in the United States. Even in 1968, 80 percent of obstetricians who were surveyed said that they felt cesarean section was the best way to deliver the second child of a woman who was given a cesarean section for her first child.

Recent studies, however, have challenged this belief, and it is now found that a normal delivery can easily be performed after cesarean birth. It is imperative that before a woman undergoes a cesarean section she ask her doctor what kind of incision he intends to make in her uterus. The significant cut is not the incision made in the abdomen but the internal incision in the womb.

The lower portion of the uterus is called the lower segment (or lower flap), and if a *transverse incision* was made in the lower segment, this area is usually covered by the bladder afterward and is strengthened. Following this type of incision, the chance of rupturing the scar during natural childbirth is very slim. However, there is another type of cut, the *classical incision,* a vertical uterine incision that weakens the womb. If this type of incision is made during a cesarean section, a repeat cesarean would be indicated.

A woman who has had a transverse incision, called "low flap cesarean section," would be able to deliver vaginally if the problems of her previous delivery did not recur. As long as the newborn is not unusually large, there is no reason why natural childbirth cannot be attempted in such a woman's case. Her uterus would be strong. Many doctors would still say "We're afraid of rupture," but studies have shown that if a woman is carefully monitored and allowed to go into labor, she should be successful at delivering vaginally. If a problem arises and she needs a C-section, at least she would have been given every opportunity to fulfill her wishes. I have vaginally delivered babies born to a great number of women who have previously delivered by cesarean section. I've met women who have traveled

from far distances where they could not find doctors who would permit them to have natural childbirth.

Ms. J. experienced a breech birth baby, but if her next pregnancy
is a head-first delivery, she will probably give birth naturally with no
problem. If her second baby moves into a breech pose, she can lie on
her side with the lower half of her body elevated for the last two
months of pregnancy. This position might cause the fetus to turn
into a normal delivery position without manipulation. Also, a new
medication called Yutopar (ritodrine), a uterine relaxant, can be used
by an obstetrician to calm the uterus for a few minutes to make it
easier for him to turn the baby into a head-first position.

The rate of cesarean deliveries has increased dramatically in the
last decade chiefly because there has been a great tendency for doctors to overrate the problem if labor is difficult or prolonged.
Overreactions have also occurred if the fetus is in a breech position
or is in distress. In addition, much of the increase is due to repeated
cesarean sections. If the conventional wisdom that nurtured "Once a
cesarean, always a cesarean" continues, one fourth or more of future
U.S. births will be by cesarean section.

Women who have had cesarean sections should find out what
types of incisions were used in their procedures. Every woman who
has had a low flap cesarean section should be able to deliver vaginally, naturally, without worry. If a doctor is not willing to give her a
"trial of labor," a woman, along with her husband, should look for
another doctor well ahead of her due date.

Did I Really Need a Cesarean?

*My doctor said I was a textbook case during my pregnancy. I
had no problems. My husband and I had been trying to conceive for
a long time and we were very excited. We took every Lamaze class!
We waited for the baby to come but my contractions didn't start
until two weeks after my due date. I had been in labor for four
hours when my obstetrician told me that nothing was happening.
He said he wanted to speed the labor and he injected me with*

oxytocin. Labor became excruciating, but he said that he didn't want to give me any painkiller because I had elected to have natural birth. He didn't tell me much more until after I had had oxytocin for three hours. Then he said, "Since you're not making progress, I'm going to give you a cesarean." My husband and I asked him to wait a little longer, maybe the labor would improve, but he said waiting might be dangerous for the baby. He gave us no choice. I still don't understand how he reached his decision. Why couldn't we have more time?

—J.P., Oklahoma City, Oklahoma

It is unfortunate that Ms. P. did not receive a more thorough explanation of her condition from her doctor. From the letter, it is difficult to determine whether she definitely needed the cesarean, but since her pregnancy had continued two weeks beyond her due date, the baby might have grown too large for a natural delivery.

However, every woman should know that when labor is speeded by oxytocin, the contractions become much stronger and more painful, and often the pain prevents labor from progressing. Ms. P. should have been given an epidural anesthetic that could have completely eliminated her pain. (An epidural anesthetic involves an injection of local anesthesia into the area of the lower spine. This injection numbs the nerves in and around the uterus and provides a safe form of pain relief.) Then, if labor had been allowed to continue, she might have been able to deliver vaginally. Had a fetal monitor been used during stimulated labor in association with an epidural, and had the baby's heartbeat remained stable, there would have been no reason to believe that the baby was in danger, as the doctor had said.

An average length of labor for a firstborn is approximately ten hours. Ms. P. was laboring for only seven hours. It is possible that if she had had another doctor, he might have waited longer and permitted a vaginal delivery. Many doctors will ask other doctors for second opinions when their patients are having problematic labors. Usually, if a second opinion is obtained from a competent physician and two doctors, together, feel that there is sufficient indication for a cesarean section, then surgery is usually the right and proper choice.

Still, an obstetrician should always discuss his decision with the expectant couple and explain the need for the cesarean. If Ms. P. had been told that her cervix had only opened to a certain degree and did not look as if it would dilate further, then both she and her husband would have realized that their baby would not fit through her pelvic structure. Ms. P. would have been confident that her doctor had acted appropriately.

GENITAL COSMETIC SURGERY

Vaginal tightening, more technically called *posterior repair of the vagina,* is surgery that doctors have been performing for years, usually in connection with treating a prolapsed uterus. As a woman ages, her muscles and ligaments can weaken and her uterus can sag into her vagina. This *uterine prolapse* sometimes leads to hysterectomy and the posterior repair of the vagina, a removal of a portion of vaginal mucosa and a suturing, or tightening, of the muscles. Women who do not have uterine prolapse, but feel they are losing sexual pleasure because their vaginal muscles have been weakened by childbirth or age, sometimes have the same surgery. This is not unusual, but what is unexpected today is a reported rise in interest in cosmetic laser surgery for:

- vaginal tightening alone
- cosmetic reconstruction of the labia minora and labia majora
- a combination of both vaginal tightening and cosmetic surgery on the labia

There are legitimate reasons for altering labia. I have known some women who cannot exercise properly and, in fact, are quite uncomfortable because their labias are so large. The corrective surgery for this situation can be performed in a doctor's office or a freestanding clinic, but it is usually not covered by health insurance. Purely "cosmetic" vaginal tightening and labia reconstruction by plastic surgeons charging thousands of dollars gives me pause. I would encourage all women, unless they are in medical need of genital surgery, to appreciate the beauty of their female genitalia. Also, vaginas can be naturally tightened through Kegel exercises (see page 444), eliminating the need for this expensive ($2,000 to $4,000) and exotic cosmetic surgery.

The Bottom Line

Better Health Care—
You Can Make the Difference

MORE THAN ONE SOLUTION

When our mothers became ill they often suffered in silence because culture and religion had made their imprints on yesterday's women. They accepted pain and suffering as necessary components of womanhood. A woman went to a doctor only after she had reached the limits of her endurance and was extremely sick. Then she never doubted her physician. A doctor's skill was revered by his patients, and his advice, which was highly regarded, was strictly followed. Doctors were sacred beings!

This view of a doctor as a god was also perpetrated by medical schools, where students were taught that their professors were sacrosanct individuals whose words should never be questioned. Twenty years ago, earnest medical students were learning that many women's complaints, menstrual cramps included, were psychological, "all in their heads." Today's aspiring doctors know better.

Extensive research during the past decade has redefined many previously misunderstood women's complaints. For example, endocrine studies have shown that the pain from menstrual cramps is real and that, if not treated, problems such as endometriosis and infertility might arise. There is no reason for a woman to suffer in silence, since many gynecological disorders can be cured with newly developed remedies. And sometimes a doctor even has a choice of cures.

Still, although medical students and informed physicians know about the latest treatments, a woman might find herself the patient of a doctor who is still following "yesterday's philosophy." He might administer painkillers and tranquilizers to alleviate her symptoms and never investigate or treat the cause of her ailment.

Contemporary women realize that doctors can no longer be considered gods. A doctor's words must not be unquestioningly heeded because often there is more than one solution to a problem. Frequently a woman requires a second opinion, but more important, she needs to know how to talk to the doctor she has initially chosen. By educating herself about her bodily functions, a woman will be less hesitant about talking to her doctor. However, as the letters in this book show, for all women to become active partners in their own health care the female body needs to be demystified even further.

WOMEN'S NETWORKS

The women's movement and the sexual revolution have shaped attitudes, and now women feel freer about expressing their health concerns and sharing their experiences. A woman who keeps her medical worries a secret from the people who love her might not know whether or not she is receiving second-rate treatment. We all benefit from feedback.

Women must talk to each other and form community health groups to promote better understanding and improved health care. As mentioned before, there is often more than one solution to a medical problem. A conservative measure might be able to replace radical treatment advised by a doctor, but a patient must be informed as to what that conservative measure might be. Health groups and good communication among women who question physicians do change the way doctors treat their female patients.

It might seem that the task of altering the quality of health care is insurmountable, but think of the power that just one woman, Rose Kushner, had. In 1975, she wrote the book *Breast Cancer*[1]—now titled *Why Me?*[2]—and began her challenge of the one-step surgical treatment of breast cancer. Since Rose Kushner came forward, the two-step approach—biopsy first, followed by surgery, if needed, at a later date—has been instituted. Before her voice was heard, women who had not yet been biopsied, women who did not even know if they had breast cancer, were wheeled into operating rooms and afterward woke up with radical mastectomies. Women can change the ways of medicine for themselves and generations to follow if they will courageously discuss the ways in which they are cared for by doctors.

When communication is opened, it will soon become clearer which doctors are the most thorough, most informed, and most responsible physicians in a community. By organizing into formal health collectives or by being involved in loosely knit *women's networks*, expanding groups of like-minded women who share information with each other, women will find help in seeking out the best physicians and steering away from the greedy doctors, who might then, by discovering empty waiting rooms, change their methods of healing the sick.

MOTHERS AND DAUGHTERS

Mothers should realize that today's teenagers are more sexually active and that their daughters want sound counseling from them. A teenager needs a good understanding of her body. If a teenage daughter is suffering from severe menstrual cramps, a parent should not permit the pain to be dismissed or carelessly treated with a painkiller. A mother has a responsibility to learn about her bodily functions, not only for herself, but also for her daughter. A teenager who is afflicted with menstrual cramps might be a victim of endometriosis, and a mother should insist that her child's pain be attended to.

When a daughter becomes sexually active, a mother should help her to select a form of birth control that will not cause her problems in the future, problems that might include infertility. Sex and health education that teaches protection against STDs should be part of growing up.

Proper health education might also prevent young women from experiencing the emotional traumas associated with teen pregnancies. If they are sexually active and informed, teenagers will know how to protect themselves. Should a teenager want to bear and raise a child, she must know how to stay healthy during her pregnancy. For successful pregnancies early in life, young women could learn much from their sisters in Sweden, where the health education in schools is so extensive that small schoolchildren are taught about reproduction. By the time they are teenagers, Swedish girls have a deep comprehension of birth control, abortion for unplanned pregnancy, and the value of prenatal care. Every young woman understands that if she wants a healthy, robust baby she must nurture the developing fetus in her womb. As a country, Sweden is known to have very little problem with perinatal mortality, infant death, and it has been theorized that the reason for Swedish success in this area is the health education of its children.

TRUST YOURSELF—FOLLOW YOUR INSTINCTS

If girls begin to understand their bodies at early ages, they will grow to be astute women who not only know how to find the best physicians and the finest care, but also are wise enough to prevent health problems with balanced diets and exercise. A young woman who considers good health a priority and understands her body's responses will avoid unplanned pregnancy, sexually transmitted diseases, and many other medical worries. She will stay fit as she matures. The bottom line is: *If you listen to your body when you are young, your body will keep you healthy when you are old.*

Notes

CHAPTER 1: BECOMING A PARTNER IN YOUR OWN HEALTH CARE

1. Carl N. Degler, *At Odds: Women and the Family in America from the Revolution to the Present* (New York: Oxford University Press, 1980), p. 58.
2. By the Boston Women's Health Book Collective, Inc. (New York: Simon & Schuster, 1971).
3. Hardcover, New York: Grosset and Dunlap, 1978; paperback, New York: Playboy Press Paperbacks, 1980.

CHAPTER 3: MENSTRUAL CRAMPS ARE REAL

1. Paula Weideger, *Menstruation & Menopause* (New York: Delta Books, 1977), p. 110.
2. Nancy Friday, *My Mother/My Self* (New York: Delacorte Press, 1977), pp. 98–99.
3. Norman Cousins, *Anatomy of an Illness* (New York: W. W. Norton and Company, 1979), pp. 39–40.

CHAPTER 10: HOW YOU KNOW YOU ARE PREGNANT

1. David M. Rorvik with Landrum B. Shettles, M.D. (New York: Dodd, Mead, 1970).

1115171820

22242272829

3132353637383940

414243444648

CHAPTER 11: MISCARRIAGE, ECTOPIC PREGNANCY, AND ABORTION—DO THEY HARM YOUR BODY?

1. Hardcover, New York: Grosset and Dunlap, 1978; paperback, New York: Playboy Press Paperbacks, 1980.

CHAPTER 13: MENOPAUSE—HOW TO DEMYSTIFY THIS NATURAL PROCESS

1. See Chapter 17 for a discussion of how a hysterectomy can be performed without removal of the ovaries.

2. *Hot Flashes:* One of the vasomotor symptoms (related to the dilation and constriction of the blood vessels) of menopause. A sudden flash of heat might pass throughout the entire body. A woman will feel hot all over but the sensation is not associated with sweating or skin changes. Hot flashes occur less frequently than hot flushes.

3. *Hot Flushes:* Another vasomotor symptom of menopause. A hot flush comes from increased blood flow to the skin, brain, and vital organs as a result of sudden enlargement of the blood vessels. A woman has a sensation of heat and a red flush involving her face, neck, and upper chest. A hot flush often begins with profuse sweats frequently followed by a scarlet skin tone. Hot flushes should not be confused with hot flashes, which only produce a feeling of burning heat throughout the body. After a hot flush, body heat is usually lost and a woman might feel immediately cold.

CHAPTER 17: UNNECESSARY SURGERY—WHEN TO GET A SECOND OPINION

1. Rose Kushner, *Breast Cancer: A Personal History and an Investigative Report* (New York: Harcourt Brace Jovanovich, 1975).

2. Rose Kushner, *Why Me? What Every Woman Should Know About Breast Cancer to Save Her Life* (New York: New American Library, 1977).

Index